Managing Pain in Children

Managing Pain in Children
A Clinical Guide for Nurses and Healthcare Professionals

Second edition

Edited by

Alison Twycross
Head of Department, Children's Nursing;
Reader, Children's Pain Management,
London South Bank University, United Kingdom

Stephanie Dowden
Clinical Nurse Consultant, Paediatric Palliative Care
Princess Margaret Hospital for Children, Perth, Australia

and

Jennifer Stinson
Nurse Clinician Scientist and Nurse Practitioner, Chronic Pain
Programme, The Hospital for Sick Children;
Associate Professor of Nursing, Lawrence S. Bloomberg
Faculty of Nursing, University of Toronto, Toronto, Canada

WILEY Blackwell

This edition first published 2014 © 2014 by John Wiley & Sons, Ltd.
First edition published 2009, © Blackwell Publishing Ltd.

Registered office: John Wiley & Sons, Ltd, The Atrium, Southern Gate, Chichester, West Sussex, PO19 8SQ, UK

Editorial offices: 9600 Garsington Road, Oxford, OX4 2DQ, UK
111 River Street, Hoboken, NJ 07030-5774, USA

For details of our global editorial offices, for customer services and for information about how to apply for permission to reuse the copyright material in this book please see our website at www .wiley.com/wiley-blackwell

Library of Congress Cataloging-in-Publication Data

Managing pain in children : a clinical guide for nurses and healthcare professionals / edited by Alison Twycross, Stephanie Dowden, and Jennifer Stinson. – 2nd edition.
    p. ; cm.
  Preceded by: Managing pain in children : a clinical guide / edited by Alison Twycross, Stephanie J. Dowden, and Elizabeth Bruce. 2009.
  Includes bibliographical references and index.
  ISBN 978-0-470-67054-5 (pbk.)
  I. Twycross, Alison, editor of compilation. II. Dowden, Stephanie, editor of compilation. III. Stinson, Jennifer, 1963- editor of compilation. IV. Title.
  [DNLM: 1. Child. 2. Pain Management–nursing. 3. Evidence-Based Nursing. WL 704.6]
  RJ365
  616′.0472083–dc23
                                    2013025395

A catalogue record for this book is available from the British Library.

Wiley also publishes its books in a variety of electronic formats. Some content that appears in print may not be available in electronic books.

Cover image: Health Care & Children © Sean Warren, courtesy of iStock
Cover design by His and Hers Design (www.hisandhersdesign.co.uk)

Set in 10/11.5 pt Sabon by Toppan Best-set Premedia Limited
Printed and bound in Malaysia by Vivar Printing Sdn Bhd

1   2014

Contents

List of Contributors

Alison Twycross, Head of Department for Children's Nursing and Reader in Children's Pain Management, London South Bank University, UK

Jennifer Stinson, Nurse Clinician Scientist and Nurse Practitioner, Chronic Pain Programme, The Hospital for Sick Children; Associate Professor of Nursing, Lawrence S. Bloomberg Faculty of Nursing, University of Toronto, Toronto, Canada

Stephanie Dowden, Clinical Nurse Consultant, Paediatric Palliative Care, Princess Margaret Hospital for Children, Roberts Road, Subiaco, Perth, WA 6008, Australia

Jackie Bentley, Senior Lecturer Child Health, University of Worcester, St John's Campus, Henwick Grove, Worcester, WR2 6AJ, United Kingdom

Lindsay Jibb, Registered Nurse, Division of Haematology/Oncology, Department of Pediatrics, The Hospital for Sick Children, 555 University Avenue, Toronto, Ontario, M5G 1X8, Canada

Lori Palozzi, Nurse Practitioner, Acute Pain Service, Department of Anesthesia and Pain Medicine, The Hospital for Sick Children, 555 University Avenue, Toronto ON, M5G 1X8, Canada

Sueann Penrose, Clinical Nurse Consultant, Children's Pain Management Service, Royal Children's Hospital, Flemington Road, Parkville, Victoria 3052, Australia

Kathy Reid, Nurse Practitioner, Paediatric Chronic Pain Program, Stollery Children's Hospital, Edmonton AB, T6G 2B7, Canada

Dianne Tuterra, Child Life Specialist, Stollery Children's Hospital, Edmonton AB, T6G 2B7, Canada

Anna Williams, Faculty of Health, Social Care and Education, Kingston University and St George's University of London, Cranmer Terrace, London, SW17 0RE, United Kingdom

Foreword

I am delighted to introduce you to *Managing Pain in Children: A Clinical Guide for Nurses and Healthcare Professionals* (2nd edition). The editors, Twycross, Dowden and Stinson, are each internationally known as clinicians and scientists in pain in children. I know their work well. Together they bring a profound commitment to excellence in nursing care and their extensive experience from three continents in helping children, their nurses and their parents overcome pain.

The first edition of this book was an overwhelming success as it ensured that the best evidence was combined with a practical approach that is lacking in most textbooks. The coverage is broad and detailed and includes helpful approaches to acute, chronic and procedure pain as well as the special problems of pain in palliative care.

The integration of theory, evidence and practice is evident in the very helpful case studies that enliven the text.

Managing Pain in Children will be used by nurses, psychologists, physicians and other healthcare professionals who are committed to helping children. It is more than a book; it encompasses the distilled wisdom of the best clinicians and scientists in the field. This text will serve as a trusted colleague in guiding your clinical practice. Keep it close; you will consult it often.

Patrick J McGrath OC, PhD, FRSC, FCAHS
Integrated Vice President Research and Innovation,
Capital District Health Authority and IWK Health Centre;
Professor of Psychology, Pediatrics and Psychiatry
Canada Research Chair, Dalhousie University
Halifax, Nova Scotia, Canada

CHAPTER 1

Why Managing Pain in Children Matters

Alison Twycross

Department for Children's Nursing and Children's Pain Management,
London South Bank University, United Kingdom

Anna Williams

Faculty of Health, Social Care and Education, Kingston University and
St George's University of London, United Kingdom

Introduction

Despite the evidence to guide clinical practice being readily available, the management of pain in children is often suboptimal. This chapter will start by providing a definition of pain and pain management and will highlight the consequences of unrelieved pain. Children's views about the effectiveness of their pain management will be discussed, and commonly held misconceptions about pain in children detailed. The factors thought to influence pain management practices will be outlined. Information about pain management standards published in several countries will be discussed. How well children's pain is currently managed will be considered alongside the issue of professional accountability. Finally, the ethical imperative for managing children's pain effectively will be examined.

What is Pain?

'**Pain** is whatever the experiencing person says it is, existing wherever they say it does' (McCaffery 1972).
'**Pain** is an unpleasant sensory and emotional experience associated with actual or potential tissue damage, or described in terms of such damage. Pain is always subjective. Each individual learns the application of the word through experiences related to injury in early life' (International Association for the Study of Pain [IASP] 1979, p. 249).

Managing Pain in Children: A Clinical Guide for Nurses and Healthcare Professionals, Second Edition.
Edited by Alison Twycross, Stephanie Dowden, and Jennifer Stinson.
© 2014 John Wiley & Sons, Ltd. Published 2014 by John Wiley & Sons, Ltd.

These two definitions of pain illustrate that the experience of pain is both a subjective and an individual phenomenon. This is particularly clear in the IASP definition, which explains how the many facets of pain interrelate and affect pain perception. Although supporting the concept of pain as a subjective phenomenon, the original IASP definition fell short in relation to those unable to communicate verbally, including neonates and young children and cognitively impaired children. This was addressed in 2001 when the following amendment was made:

'The inability to communicate in no way negates the possibility that an individual is experiencing pain and is in need of appropriate pain-relieving treatment' (IASP 2001, p. 2).

Pain management means applying the stages of the nursing process – assessment, planning, implementation and evaluation – to the treatment of pain.

The cyclical basis of these stages is illustrated in Figure 1.1.

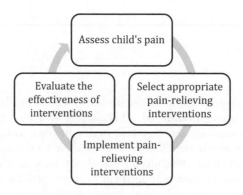

Figure 1.1   The stages of pain management.

Consequences of Unrelieved Pain

Pain has an important purpose, serving as a warning or protective mechanism, and people with congenital analgesia, who are unable to feel pain, often suffer extensive tissue damage (Melzack and Wall 1996). However, unrelieved pain has a number of undesirable physical and psychological consequences (Box 1.1). When these are considered, the need to manage children's pain effectively is clear. The results of studies demonstrating this are outlined in Box 1.2.

Children's memories of pain also influence subsequent pain experiences (Noel et al. 2012). Other consequences of unrelieved pain include:

- In a retrospective study with adults ($n = 147$), aged 17–21 years, childhood experiences of medical and dental pain were significant predictors of adults' medical pain (Pate et al. 1996).

BOX 1.1

Consequences of unrelieved pain

Physical effects

- Rapid, shallow, splinted breathing, which can lead to hypoxaemia and alkalosis
- Inadequate expansion of lungs and poor cough, which can lead to secretion retention and atelectasis
- Increased heart rate, blood pressure and myocardial oxygen requirements, which can lead to cardiac morbidity and ischaemia
- Increased stress hormones (e.g. cortiosol, adrenaline, catecholamines), which in turn increase the metabolic rate, impede healing and decrease immune function
- Slowing or stasis of gut and urinary systems, which leads to nausea, vomiting, ileus and urinary retention
- Muscle tension, spasm and fatigue, which leads to reluctance to move spontaneously and refusal to ambulate, further delaying recovery

Psychological effects

- Anxiety, fear, distress, feelings of helplessness or hopelessness
- Avoidance of activity, avoidance of future medical procedures
- Sleep disturbances
- Loss of appetite

Other effects

- Prolonged hospital stays
- Increased rates of re-admission to hospital
- Increased outpatient visits

Source: WHO (1997)

BOX 1.2

Examples of research demonstrating the effects of poor management of *acute* pain

Taddio et al. (1997)

- Data from a clinical trial studying the use of EMLA® during routine vaccinations at 4 or 6 months was used to ascertain whether having had a circumcision impacted on boys' (n = 87) pain response.
- Boys who had been circumcised without anaesthesia as neonates were observed to react significantly more intensely to vaccinations than uncircumcised boys (p < 0.001).
- Supported findings from a previous study (Taddio et al. 1995).

Grunau et al. (1998)

- Examined the pain-related attitudes in two groups of children, aged 8–10 years: extremely low birthweight children (n = 47); full birthweight children (n = 37).
- The very low birthweight group of children had been exposed to painful procedures as neonates, the other group had not.
- Children were shown the *Pediatric Pain Inventory*, which comprises 24 line drawings, each depicting a potentially painful event (Lollar et al. 1982).

BOX 1.2 Continued

- The two groups of children did not differ in their overall perceptions of pain intensity. However, the very low birthweight children rated medical pain intensity significantly higher ($p < 0.004$) than psychosocial pain, suggesting that their early experiences affected their later perceptions of pain.

Saxe et al. (2001)

- Investigated the relationship between the dose of morphine administered during a child's hospitalisation for an acute burn and the course of post-traumatic stress disorder (PTSD) symptoms over the 6-month period following discharge.
- Children ($n = 24$) admitted to the hospital for an acute burn were assessed twice with the Child PTSD Reaction Index: while in the hospital and 6 months after discharge.
- The Colored Analogue Pain Scale was also administered during the hospitalisation. All patients received morphine while in the hospital. The mean dose of morphine (mg/kg/day) was calculated for each subject.
- There was a significant association between the dose of morphine received while in the hospital and a 6-month reduction in PTSD symptoms.
- Children receiving higher doses of morphine had a greater reduction in PTSD symptoms.

Rennick et al. (2002)

- A prospective cohort study of patients ($n = 120$) in paediatric intensive care units and medical-surgical wards.
- There were no differences between wards in terms of negative outcomes; however, children in the intensive care units received more analgesics and sedation.
- 17.5% of patients expressed significant medical fears 6 weeks after discharge.
- 14% continue to express these fears 6 months later.
- Children who underwent more invasive procedures had more medical fears, felt less in control of their own health, and exhibited more signs of post-traumatic stress for 6 months after discharge.

Taddio et al. (2002)

- A prospective cohort study of babies ($n = 21$) born to mothers with diabetes and babies ($n = 21$) born to mothers with an uneventful pregnancy.
- Infants of diabetic mothers had repeated heel-sticks in the first 24–36 hours of life.
- Babies of diabetic mothers demonstrated significantly greater pain behaviours at venepuncture for newborn blood screening ($p = 0.04$).

Grunau et al. (2009)

- Infants ($n = 137$ born preterm at 32 weeks gestation; $n = 74$ full-term controls) were followed prospectively.
- Infants with significant brain injury or major sensorineural impairments were excluded.
- At 8 and 18 months, poorer cognition and motor function were associated with a higher number of painful (skin-breaking) procedures.

- Distress associated with needle-stick procedures can develop into phobic reactions (Hamilton 1995), making completion of later procedures more difficult.
- Pain affects children's anxiety, mood and general quality of life (Schanberg et al. 2003; Martin et al. 2007).
- Pain and pain-related fear and anxiety affect children's functioning and can lead to deconditioning or avoidance of activity (Martin et al. 2007; Asmundson et al. 2012).

There is increasing evidence that acute (postoperative) pain can result in chronic pain:

- The incidence of chronic postsurgical pain is between 15% and 30% of (adult) patients (Gupta et al. 2011).
- 13% of children undergoing orthopaedic surgery developed chronic postoperative pain (Fortier et al. 2011).

> Unrelieved pain has short- and long-term effects on children. It is important, therefore, to ensure that pain is managed effectively.

Children's Views about the Effectiveness of Pain Management

Pain is a biopsychosocial experience (Chapter 3) and this is why two people undergoing the same surgery or experiencing the same illness may report different pain experiences. When considering children's painful experiences it is, therefore, essential to explore children's views. Indeed the United Nations Convention on the Rights of the Child (1989) states that:

'Children's views must be taken into account in all matters affecting them, subject to children's age and maturity.'

Children's views about how well their pain has been managed have been explored in four studies in the past decade (Box 1.3). It is evident that from the child's perspective there is a need to evaluate practices. (Further discussion about undertaking research with children can be found in Chapter 11).

Although these studies highlight the fact that children continue to experience moderate to severe pain, it is worth noting that this does not necessarily impact on satisfaction with care (Twycross and Collis 2012; Vincent et al. 2012; Twycross and Finley 2013). A study by Habich et al. (2012) found no changes in patient or family satisfaction with care despite improvements in pain assessment when evaluating the effectiveness of implementing evidence-based paediatric pain guidelines. These findings suggest that children, and their families, may expect to experience pain when in hospital and may see this pain as unavoidable. Children's perceptions of good pain management emphasise a holistic approach; valuing professional competence, communication, openness, and the invitation to participate in decision-making about pain management interventions (Nilsson et al. 2011).

Additional information

Further insight into children's experiences of pain in hospital can be found in:
Kortesluoma, R.L. and Nikkonen, M. (2004) 'I had this horrible pain': The sources and causes of pain experiences in 4- to 11-year-old hospitalized children. *Journal of Child Health Care* **8**(3), 210–231.

BOX 1.3

Studies exploring children's views about pain management

Polkki et al. (2003)

- Children (n = 52), aged 8–12 years, were asked about their postoperative pain experiences and to suggest what nurses could do to improve postoperative pain management.
- Children indicated that they wished the nurses had given then more or stronger analgesic drugs, as soon as they asked for them, and that they would like nurses to ask them about their pain on an hourly basis. Children would also like nurses to provide them with *meaningful things to do* to distract them from their pain.

Kortesluoma et al. (2008)

- Children (n = 44), aged 4–11 years, were interviewed about their experiences of pain management in hospital. Children's descriptions of what helped when they were in pain included self-help strategies, the assistance of healthcare professionals and significant others, medicine, emotional support and modifying the environment.
- Children felt that healthcare professionals were not always gentle enough or did not have enough time to manage their pain adequately. They expected professionals to be competent and empathic, and to give time to help them when in pain.

Twycross and Collis (2012)

- As part of a larger study, young people (n = 17) completed a questionnaire about their pain management experience.
- Young people felt their pain management was of an acceptable level or very good. This was despite the fact that 58% of children experienced severe pain and 24% moderate pain.

Twycross and Finley (2013)

- Children (n = 8), in one Canadian tertiary hospital, were interviewed about their perceptions of pain care, and asked to rate the worst pain experienced postoperatively on a numerical scale.
- Most children (n = 10) experienced moderate to severe pain postoperatively.
- Children were, on the whole, satisfied with the care provided.
- Children reported being asked about their pain, receiving pain medication and using physical and psychological methods of pain relief.
- A lack of preoperative preparation was evident for one child.

Misconceptions about Pain

Children are still experiencing moderate to severe pain in hospital (Kozlowski et al. 2012; Stevens et al. 2012; Twycross et al. 2013). One reason for this could be the perceptions of the healthcare professionals caring for the child. A number of misconceptions about children's pain have been identified, with a comprehensive summary of these provided by Twycross (1998). The key misconceptions and a summary of the evidence demonstrating their mythological status can be seen in Table 1.1. (Other misconceptions are discussed in Chapters 2, 4 and 9.) These misconceptions have all been shown to have no scientific basis. Other reasons that may explain why pain continues to be mismanaged are discussed in Chapter 11.

Table 1.1 Key misconceptions about pain in children

Misconception	Evidence
Infants do not feel as much pain as adults	Pain pathways (although immature) are present at birth and pain impulses are able to travel to and from the pain centres in the brain (Wolf 1999; Coskun and Anand 2000; Fitzgerald 2000) Neonates exhibit behavioural, physiological and hormonal responses to pain (Franck 1986; Hogan and Choonara 1996; Carter 1997; Abu-Saad et al. 1998)
Infants cannot feel pain because of an immature nervous system	Complete myelination is not necessary for pain to be felt (Volpe 1981) Painful stimuli are transmitted by both myelinated and unmyelinated fibres (Volpe 1981; Craig and Grunau 1993) Incomplete myelination implies only a slower conduction speed in the nerves, which is offset by the shorter distances the impulse has to travel (Volpe 1981; Anand and Hickey 1987) Noxious stimuli have been shown to produce a cortical pain response in preterm babies (Bartocci et al. 2006; Slater et al. 2006)
Young children cannot indicate where pain is located	Children as young as 4 years old can demonstrate on a body chart where they hurt without knowing the names of body parts (Van Cleve and Savedra 1993) Children are able to report the intensity of pain by the age of 3–4 years (Harbeck and Peterson 1992)
Sleeping children cannot be in pain	Sleep may be the result of exhaustion because of persistent pain (Hawley 1984)

Factors Affecting Healthcare Professionals' Perceptions of Pain

Several factors have been postulated as contributing to suboptimal practices relating to healthcare professionals, patients (children and parents) and the organisation (International Association for the Study of Pain [IASP] 2010). These factors are illustrated in Figure 1.2. Research conducted in the past 10 years provides an indicator of the factors relating to children and healthcare professionals, which may affect pain management practices (Table 1.2). These factors are discussed in more detail in Chapter 11. Research relating to the factors impacting on pain management practices of other healthcare professionals has not been carried out.

> Suboptimal practices can be attributed to a number of factors. A multifactorial approach is needed to improve practice.

Pain Management Standards

Some of the pain management standards published in the last 10 years are listed in Box 1.4. These guidelines and standards provide knowledge and guidance about how pain should be managed. In the United States, the Joint Commission for the Accreditation of Healthcare Organisations (JCAHO) first published standards for pain

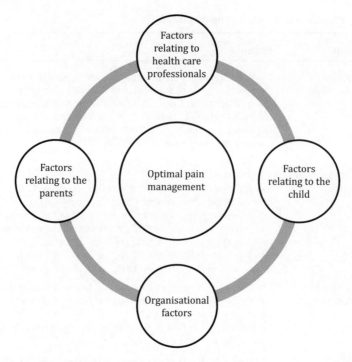

Figure 1.2   Barriers to optimal pain management practices.

management in 2001. These were updated in 2010 (Box 1.5). These standards are not specific to children, but they ensure that accreditation is dependent on each hospital being able to demonstrate that they are meeting these standards. Whether the implementation of these standards improves pain management requires evaluating.

How Effective are Current Pain Management Practices?

An increasing number of studies have focused on exactly how healthcare professionals manage children's pain. The results of key studies examining practices over the past 10 years are summarised in Box 1.6. These studies indicate that practices do not always conform to current best practice guidelines. Most of these relate to nursing practice. There is very little information regarding other healthcare professionals. It is likely that suboptimal practices would also be evident among other professional groups.

Professional Accountability and Evidence-Based Practice

Registered nurses are accountable for their actions and should practise in an evidence-based manner. In the UK, nurses' professional conduct must conform to the Nursing and Midwifery Council's (NMC) Code of Professional Conduct (2008). The clauses that relate to accountability and evidence-based practice can be seen in Box 1.7. (The Code is available from: www.nmc-uk.org/Nurses-and-midwives/The-code/.) Similar codes of conduct are in place in other countries.

Table 1.2 Factors that contribute to suboptimal pain management

Factors relating to staff	Factors relating to children	Factors relating to parents	Organisational factors
• Healthcare professionals' personal judgements, preconceived views and assumptions • Priority healthcare professionals give to pain management • Lack of knowledge about pain management (nurses and medical staff) • Nurses' belief that children exaggerate their pain scores • Nurses' belief that parents encourage their child to have pain medication when they had not asked for it • Nurses having to remind doctors to ensure analgesics are prescribed • Healthcare professionals being desensitised to pain or emotional distancing to cope with patients in pain	• Child's age • Child's culture • Child's behaviour • Child's diagnosis • Time since surgery • Non-compliance with nurses' suggestions for pain care • Child's reluctance to report their pain • Child refusing pain medications	• Reliance on behavioural cues to assess pain • Reluctance for their children to receive pain medications • Fears about the side effects of analgesic drugs • Fears about addiction • Belief that pain medications should be given as little as possible	• Ward/unit norms in relation to managing pain (patterns of pain care) • Inadequate or insufficient medication orders • Lack of time to implement physical and psychological strategies • Low staff numbers and a heavy workload • Insufficient supply of some medication • A lack of cooperation between nursing and medical staff

Source: Data from Nagy (1999); Byrne et al. (2001); Kankkunen et al. (2003); Vincent (2005); Gimbler-Berglund et al. (2008); Vincent and Gaddy (2009); Zisk-Rony et al. (2010); Czarnecki et al. (2011); Lim et al. (2012); Ljusegren et al. (2012); Sutters et al. (2012); Twycross and Collis (2012); Williams (2012); Twycross et al. (2013)

Evidence-based practice is:

'An approach to providing care to patients that involves the use of clinical research combined with clinical experience, patient characteristics, and patient preferences to make clinical decisions regarding pain treatment and management' (Joint Commission International 2010, p. 9).

BOX 1.4
Pain standards and guidelines
Australia and New Zealand

Macintyre, P.E., Schug, S.A., Scott, D.A., Visser, E.J., Walker, S.M.; APM:SE Working Group of the Australian and New Zealand College of Anaesthetists and Faculty of Pain Medicine (2010) *Acute Pain Management: Scientific Evidence*, 3rd edition. ANZCA & FPM, Melbourne. Available from: www.anzca.edu.au/resources/books-and-publications/Acute%20pain%20management %20-%20scientific%20evidence%20-%20third%20edition.pdf

Canada

Reducing the pain of childhood vaccination: An evidence-based clinical practice guideline (2010). Available from: www.cmaj.ca/content/182/18/E843.full.pdf+html

International Consensus Document

Assessment and Management of Pain in Neonates (2006). Available from: http://pediatrics.aap-publications.org/content/118/5/2231.full.pdf+html.

United Kingdom

Royal College of Nursing (2009) *The Recognition and Assessment of Acute Pain in Children*, 2nd edition, RCN Publishing, London. Available from: www.rcn.org.uk/development/ practice/clinicalguidelines/pain

Association of Paediatric Anaesthetists of Great Britain and Ireland (2012) *Good Practice in Postoperative and Procedural Pain*, 2nd edition. Available from: http://onlinelibrary.wiley .com/doi/10.1111/j.1460-9592.2012.03838.x/pdf

USA

American Society of Anesthesiologists Task Force on Acute Pain Management (2012) *Practice Guidelines for Acute Pain Management in the Perioperative Setting*. Available from: http:// journals.lww.com/anesthesiology/Fulltext/2012/02000/Practice_Guidelines_for_Acute_Pain_ Management_in.11.aspx

American Society for Pain Management Nursing (2011) *American Society for Pain Management Nursing Guidelines*. Available from: www.aspmn.org/Organization/documents/ProceduralPainMgt .PositionStatement.pdf

World Health Organization

Guidelines on the pharmacological treatment of persisting pain in children with medical illnesses. Available from: www.icpcn.org.uk/page.asp?section=0001000100330009&sectionTitle=WH O+guidelines+on+the+pharmacological+treatment+of+persisting+pain+in+children+with+ medical+illnesses

Everyone is responsible for pain management. The bedside nurse is as responsible as the analgesia prescriber, the physiotherapist or a member of the specialist pain management team; if any of these clinicians do not fulfil their role, the patient suffers. Thus all healthcare professionals have a responsibility to:

- learn and be educated about pain;
- know about pain management (pharmacological, physical and psychological strategies);
- assess and respond to patients in pain.

BOX 1.5

Topics addressed by the JCAHO Pain Management Standards

- Patients' rights regarding pain management
- Assessment and reassessment
- Managing patients' pain according to the treatment plan
- Ensuring comprehensive pain management after surgery
- Addressing pain in the hospice setting
- Educating patients about pain
- Staff and licensed independent practitioner training and competency
- Discharge communication regarding pain management

Source: Joint Commission International 2010

BOX 1.6

Studies examining pain management practices

Twycross (2007)

- Observed registered nurses (*n* = 13) on a children's surgical ward in England for a period of 5 hours per shift for two to four shifts.
- The role of the *observer as participant* was adopted, whereby the researcher could shadow the nurse and act primarily as an observer.
- Although nurses administered analgesic drugs when a child complained of pain, other practices did not conform to current recommendations and were in need of improvement.
- Nurses did not, for example, routinely assess a child's pain, nor use physical or psychological methods of pain relief on a regular basis.

Taylor et al. (2008)

- Undertook an audit of pain management practices during one 24-hour period at a Canadian children's hospital.
- A structured interview was used to collect data from 83% of the inpatients on the day of the study (*n* = 241) and a chart review was carried out.
- They found that 23% of children had moderate to severe pain at the time of the interview, and 64% had had moderate to severe pain at some point during the 24-hour period.
- Of the children in pain, 58% had received analgesic drugs but only 25% had received these on a regular basis.
- Only 27% of patients had a pain score documented.

Shrestha-Ranjit and Manias (2010)

- Carried out a retrospective audit of children (*n* = 106), aged 5–15 years, who were admitted for a surgical procedure for a fractured lower limb over a two-year period in one Australian children's hospital.
- Data were collected pertaining to the first 72 hours postoperatively.
- They found that 50% of children experienced moderate to severe pain during this period.
- Nurses were found to document pain assessments less frequently than would have been expected in the postoperative period.
- Most analgesics were prescribed on an *as-needed* basis with children receiving a lower dose than the amount prescribed.

Smyth et al. (2011)

- Explored nursing practices associated with administration of postoperative pro re nata (PRN) analgesia to children.

BOX 1.6 Continued

- A mixed methods explanatory study was carried out in one Australian hospital.
- Nurses used multiple strategies to ascertain children's need for postoperative PRN analgesia, including reference to pain assessment tools, focusing on the behavioural cues of children, involving parents and children, and drawing upon personal and professional backgrounds and experience.
- Evaluation of the effectiveness of PRN postoperative analgesia was poorly communicated.

Zhu et al. (2012)

- Reviewed medical records at one Canadian Children's Hospital on a single day in September 2007.
- Inpatient records (n = 265) were audited and data recorded on a standardised form.
- 63% of children had a documented pain assessment.
- 83% of children with documented pain received had at least one recorded pain management intervention.
- 51% of children received pharmacological therapy, and 15% received either a psychological or physical pain-relieving intervention.
- Of those assessed, 44% experienced pain in the previous 24 hours with 31.5% indicating they had experienced moderate to severe pain.
- One-third of children received opioids: 19% of these had no recorded pain assessment.
- Children (n = 131) underwent a painful procedure, 21% had a concurrent pain assessment.
- Painful procedures were accompanied by a pain-relieving intervention in 12.5% of cases; 87.5% of children had no pain-relieving interventions documented.

Twycross et al. (2013)

- Observed the postoperative pain care of children (n = 10), aged 5 years and over in one Canadian children's hospital.
- A philosophy of care on the unit was identified where pain medications were given regularly even if they were prescribed prn.
- Pain management was considered synonymous with administering analgesic drugs; physical and psychological methods seen as parents' role.
- Communication tended to focus on pain medications and there was limited documentation about pain. Pain scores were not recorded consistently.
- Actions when a pain score ≥5 was recorded varied: 30% of the time no action was taken but in 37% of cases additional action was noted.
- Recorded pain scores did not appear to guide decision-making about pain medications given.

BOX 1.7

Clauses of the NMC Code (2008) relating to accountability and evidence-based practice

- You must deliver care based on the best available evidence or best practice.
- You must ensure that any advice you give is evidence-based if you are suggesting healthcare products or services.
- You must have the knowledge and skills for safe and effective practice when working without direct supervision.
- You must recognise and work within the limits of your competence.
- You must keep your knowledge and skills up to date throughout your working life.
- You must take part in appropriate learning and practice activities that maintain and develop your competence and performance.

Pain management practices should be based on **scientific facts** or agreed best practice, not personal beliefs or opinions. The burden of proof lies with the healthcare professional, **NOT** the patient.

The aim of this book is to provide healthcare professionals with knowledge about current research and best practice guidelines in relation to managing children's pain. Each practitioner is accountable and responsible for evaluating their practices to ensure they conform to current best practice guidelines.

Managing Pain in Children is an Ethical Imperative

The United Nations, in its Declaration on the Rights of the Child, states that:

'Children should in all circumstances be among the first to receive protection and relief, and should be protected from all forms of neglect, cruelty and exploitation' (United Nations 1989).

This principle can be applied to the management of pain, particularly as evidence-based practice guidelines are available (Box 1.2). Yet there is evidence that children still experience moderate to severe unrelieved pain (Kozlowski et al. 2012; Stevens et al. 2012; Twycross et al. 2013). Failing to provide children with satisfactory pain relief can be considered a violation of their human rights. Indeed, when the consequences of unrelieved pain are taken into account, managing children's postoperative pain effectively could be considered an ethical imperative. The *Human Rights Watch report* (2009) and the *Declaration of Montreal* (2010) make it clear that failure to provide access to effective pain-relief constitutes a breach of human rights.

The Declaration of Montreal is an international initiative highlighting the ethical imperative of managing pain worldwide. It outlines three key human rights in relation to pain and its treatment, including the rights:

- of access to pain management without discrimination;
- to having one's pain acknowledged and the provision of information about pain and pain management;
- of access to pain assessment and treatment, delivered by appropriately trained healthcare professionals.

These rights imply a number of obligations for both healthcare organisations and professionals in establishing appropriate laws, policies and systems for pain management, and delivering effective pain management as part of the therapeutic relationship.

Summary

- Pain is an individual and subjective phenomenon.
- Unrelieved pain has a number of undesirable social, physical and psychological consequences.
- Children are still experiencing moderate to severe pain while in hospital. This is not necessarily reflected in the overall satisfaction with pain care.

- Children's reports of how well their pain is managed indicate areas where pain practices could be improved.
- The continuing belief in misconceptions about children's pain by some healthcare professionals may account, at least in part, for suboptimal practices.
- Other reasons for suboptimal practices include nurses emotionally distancing themselves from patients in pain; nurses managing patients' pain behaviours rather than their pain; and nurses becoming desensitised to patients' pain.
- Clinical guidelines and best practice standards have been produced in several countries to promote good pain management practices.
- Healthcare professionals' practices in some areas need evaluating to ensure that they conform to current best practice guidelines.
- Every healthcare professional is responsible for managing pain and accountable for their own practices.
- Pain management practices should be based on scientific facts not personal beliefs or opinions.
- Managing children's pain effectively is an ethical imperative. Access to adequate pain management is a human right.

Additional information

Declaration of Montreal: www.iasp-pain.org/Content/NavigationMenu/Advocacy/Declaration ofMontr233al/default.htm
Human Rights Watch: www.hrw.org/reports/2009/03/02/please-do-not-make-us-suffer-any-more-0
The IASP Special Interest Group on Pain in Childhood: http://childpain.org/
International Association for the Study of Pain (IASP): www.iasp-pain.org

---

References

Abu-Saad, H.H., Bours, G.J., Stevens, B. and Hamers, J.P. (1998) Assessment of pain in the neonate. *Seminars in Perinatology* 22(5), 402–416.

Anand, K.J.S. and Hickey, P.R. (1987) Pain and its effects in the human neonate and fetus. *New England Journal of Medicine* 317, 1321–1329.

Asmundson, G.J.C., Noel, M., Petter, M. and Parkerson, H.A. (2012) Pediatric fear-avoidance model of chronic pain: foundation, application and future directions. *Pain Research and Management* 17(6), 397–405.

Bartocci, M., Bergqvist, L.L., Lagercrantz, H. and Anand, K.J.S. (2006) Pain activates cortical areas in the preterm newborn brain. *Pain* 122, 109–117.

Byrne, A., Morton, J. and Salmon, P. (2001) Defending against patients' pain: A qualitative analysis of nurses' responses to children's postoperative pain. *Journal of Psychosomatic Research* 50, 69–76.

Carter, B. (1997) Pantomimes of pain, distress, repose and lability: The world of the preterm baby. *Journal of Child Healthcare* 1(1), 17–23.

Coskun, V. and Anand, K.J.S. (2000) Development of supraspinal pain processing. In: *Pain in Neonates* (eds K.J.S. Anand, B.J. Stevens and P.J. McGrath), 2nd edition, pp. 23–54. Elsevier, Amsterdam.

Craig, K.D. and Grunau, R.V.E. (1993) Neonatal pain perception and behavioural measurement. In: *Pain in Neonates* (eds K.J.S. Anand, B.J. Stevens and P.J. McGrath), 2nd edition, pp. 67–105. Elsevier, Amsterdam.

Czarnecki, M.L., Simon, K., Thompson, J.J. et al. (2011) Barriers to pediatric pain management: A nursing perspective. *Pain Management Nursing* 12(3), 154–162.

Fitzgerald, M. (2000) Development of the peripheral and spinal pain system. In: *Pain in Neonates* (eds K.J.S. Anand, B.J. Stevens and P.J. McGrath), 2nd edition, pp. 9–22. Elsevier, Amsterdam.

Fortier, M.A., Chou, J., Maurer, E.L. and Kain, Z.N. (2011) Acute to chronic postoperative pain in children: Preliminary findings. *Journal of Pediatric Surgery* 46, 1700–1705.

Franck, L. (1986) A new method to quantitatively describe pain behavior in infants. *Nursing Research* 35(1), 28–31.

Gimbler-Berglund, I., Ljusegren, G. and Ensker, K. (2008) Factors influencing pain management in children. *Paediatric Nursing* 20(10), 21–24.

Grunau, R.V.E., Whitfield, M.F. and Petrie, J. (1998) Children's judgements about pain at aged 8–10 years: Do extremely low birthweight children differ from their full birthweight peers? *Journal of Child Psychology and Psychiatry* 39(4), 587–594.

Grunau, R.V.E., Whitfield, M.F., Petrie, J. et al. (2009) Neonatal pain, parenting stress and interaction, in relation to cognitive and motor development at 8 and 18 months in preterm infants. *Pain* 143(1–2), 138–146.

Gupta, A., Gandhi, K. and Viscusi, E.R. (2011) Persistent postsurgical pain after abdominal surgery. *Techniques in Regional Anesthesia and Pain Management* 15,140–146.

Habich, M., Wilson, D., Thielk, D. et al. (2012) Evaluating the effectiveness of pediatric pain management guidelines. *Journal of Pediatric Nursing* 27, 336–345.

Hamilton, J.G. (1995) Needle phobia: A neglected diagnosis. *Journal of Family Practice* 41, 169–175.

Harbeck, C. and Peterson, L. (1992) Elephants dancing in my head: A developmental approach to children's concepts of specific pains. *Child Development* 63, 138–149.

Hawley, D. (1984) Postoperative pain in children: Misconceptions, descriptions and interventions. *Pediatric Nursing* 10(1), 20–23.

Hogan, M. and Choonara, I. (1996) Measuring pain in neonates: An objective score. *Paediatric Nursing* 8(10), 24–27.

International Association for the Study of Pain (1979) Pain terms: A list with definitions and notes on usage. *Pain* 6, 249–252.

International Association for the Study of Pain (2001) IASP Definition of Pain. *IASP Newsletter* 2, 2.

International Association for the Study of Pain (2010) *Why the Gaps Between Evidence and Practice*, Seattle, IASP.

Joint Commission International (2010) *Approaches to Pain Management: An Essential Guide for Clinical Leaders*, 2nd edition, Joint Commission International, Oakbrook Terrace, Illinois.

Kankkunen, P., Vehvilainen-Julkunen, K., Pietila, A-M., Kokki, H. and Halonen, P. (2003) Parents' perceptions and use of analgesics at home after children's day surgery. *Paediatric Anaesthesia* 13, 132–140.

Kortesluoma, K., Nikkonen, M. and Serlo, W. (2008) 'You just have to make the pain go away': Children's experiences of pain management. *Pain Management Nursing* 9(4), 143–149.

Kozlowski, L.J., Kost-Byerly, S., Colantuoni, E. et al. (2012) Pain prevalence, intensity, assessment and management in a hospitalized pediatric population. *Pain Management Nursing*, online early.

Lim, S.H., Mackey, S., Liam, J.L.W. and He, H.-G. (2012) An exploration of Singaporean parental experiences in managing school-aged children's post-operative pain: A descriptive qualitative approach. *Journal of Clinical Nursing* 21, 860–869.

Ljusegren, G., Johansson, I., Gimbler-Berglund, I. and Enskar, K. (2012) Nurses' experiences of caring for children in pain. *Child: Health, Care and Development* 38(4), 464–470.

Lollar, D.J., Smits, S.J. and Patterson, D.L. (1982) Assessment of pediatric pain: An empirical perspective. *Journal of Pediatric Psychology* 7, 267–277.

Macintyre, P.E., Schug, S.A., Scott, D.A., Visser, E.J., Walker, S.M.; APM:SE Working Group of the Australian and New Zealand College of Anaesthetists and Faculty of Pain Medicine (2010) *Acute Pain Management: Scientific Evidence*, 3rd edition. ANZCA & FPM, Melbourne.

Martin, A.L., McGrath, P.A., Brown, S.C., and Katz, J. (2007) Children with chronic pain: Impact of sex and age on long-term outcomes. *Pain* 128, 13–19.

McCaffery, M. (1972) *Nursing Management of the Patient in Pain*. Lippincott, Philadelphia.

Melzack, R. and Wall, P. (1996) *The Challenge of Pain, updated* 2nd edition. Penguin, London.

Nagy, S. (1999) Strategies used by burns nurses to cope with the infliction of pain on patients. *Journal of Advanced Nursing* 29, 1427–1433.

Nilsson, S., Hallqvist, C., Sidenvall, B. and Enskar, K. (2011) Children's experiences of procedural pain management in conjunction with trauma wound dressings. *Journal of Advanced Nursing* 67(7), 1449–1457.

Noel, M., Chambers, C.T., McGrath, P.J. and Klein, R.M. (2012) The influence of children's pain memories on subsequent pain experience. *Pain* 153, 1563–1572.

Nursing and Midwifery Council (2008) *The code: Standards of conduct, performance and ethics for nurses and midwives.* Nursing and Midwifery Council, London.

Pate, J.T., Blount, R.L., Cohen, L.L. and Smith, A.J. (1996) Childhood medical experience and temperament as predictors of adult functioning in medical situations. *Child Health Care* 25, 281–298.

Polkki, T., Pietila, A-M. and Vehvilamen-Julkunen, K. (2003) Hospitalized children's descriptions of their experiences with postsurgical pain relieving methods. *International Journal of Nursing Studies* 40, 33–44.

Rennick, J.E., Johnston, C.C., Dougherty, G., Platt, R. and Ritchie, J.A. (2002) Children's psychological responses after critical illness and exposure to invasive technology. *Journal of Developmental & Behavioral Pediatrics* 23(3), 133–144.

Saxe, G., Stoddard, F., Courtney, D. et al. (2001) Relationship between acute morphine and the course of PTSD in children with burns. *Journal of the American Academy of Child & Adolescent Psychiatry* 40(8), 915–921.

Schanberg, L.E., Anthony, K.K., Gil, K.M. and Maurin, E.C. (2003) Daily pain and symptoms in children with polyarticular arthritis. *Arthritis and Rheumatism*, 48, 1390–1397.

Shrestha-Ranjit, J.M. and Manias, E. (2010) Pain assessment and management practices in children following surgery of the lower limb. *Journal of Clinical Nursing* 19, 118–128.

Slater, R., Cantarella, A., Gallella, S. et al. (2006) Cortical pain response in human infants. *Journal of Neuroscience* 26(14), 3662–3666.

Smyth, W., Toombes, J. and Usher, K. (2011). Children's postoperative pro re nata (PRN) analgesia: Nurses' administration practices. *Contemporary Nurse* 37(2), 160–172.

Stevens, B.J., Harrison, D., Rashotte, J. et al. (2012) Pain assessment and intensity in hospitalized children in Canada. *Journal of Pain* 13(9), 857–865.

Sutters, K.A., Holdridge-Zeuner, D., Waite, S. et al. (2012) A descriptive feasbility study to evaluate scheduled oral analgesic dosing at home for the management of postoperative pain in preschool children following tonsillectomy. *Pain Medicine* 13, 472–483.

Taddio, A., Goldbach, M., Ipp, M., Stevens, B. and Koren, G. (1995) Effect of neonatal circumcision on pain responses during vaccination in boys. *Lancet* 345, 291–292.

Taddio, A., Katz, J., Ilersich, A.l. and Koren, G. (1997) Effect of neonatal circumcision on pain response during subsequent routine vaccination. *Lancet* 349, 599–603.

Taddio, A., Shah, V., Gilbert-MacLeod, C. and Katz J. (2002) Conditioning and hyperalgesia in newborns exposed to repeated heel lances. *Journal of the American Medical Association* 288(7), 857–861.

Taylor, E.M., Boyer, K. and Campbell, F.A. (2008). Pain in hospitalized children: A prospective cross-sectional survey of pain prevalence, intensity, assessment and management in a Canadian pediatric teaching hospital. *Pain Research and Management* 13(1), 25–32.

Twycross A. (1998) Perceptions about paediatric pain. In: *Paediatric Pain Management: A Multidisciplinary Approach* (eds A. Twycross, A. Moriarty and T. Betts), pp. 1–24, Radcliffe Medical Press, Oxford.

Twycross, A. (2007) What is the impact of theoretical knowledge on children's nurses' postoperative pain management practices? An exploratory study. *Nurse Education Today* 27(7), 697–707.

Twycross, A. and Collis, S. (2012) How well is acute pain in children managed? A snapshot in one English hospital. *Pain Management Nursing*, online early.

Twycross, A. and Finley, G.A. (2013) Parents' and children's views about pain management. *Journal of Clinical Nursing*, online May 2013.

Twycross, A., Finley, G.A. and Latimer, M. (2013) Pediatric nurses' post-operative pain management practices: An observational study. *Journal for Specialists in Pediatric Nursing* 18(3), 189–201.

United Nations (1989) *Convention on the Rights of the Child.* United Nations, New York.

Van Cleve, L.J. and Savedra, M.C. (1993) Pain location: Validity and reliability of body outline markings by 4- to 7-year-old children who are hospitalized. *Pediatric Nursing* 19(3), 217–220.

Vincent, C. (2005) Nurses' knowledge, attitudes, and practices regarding children's pain. *American Journal of Maternal and Child Nursing* 30(3), 177–183.

Vincent, C.V.H. and Gaddy, E. J. (2009) Pediatric nurses' thinking in response to vignettes on administering analgesics. *Research in Nursing and Health* 32, 530–539.

Vincent, C., Chiappetta, M., Beach, A. et al. (2012) Parents' management of children's pain at home after surgery. *Journal for Specialists in Pediatric Nursing* 17, 108–120.

Volpe, J. (1981) *Neurology of the Newborn*. Saunders, Philadelphia.

Williams, A. (2012) *Acute pain management in children: An ethnographic approach*. Unpublished PhD Thesis, St Georges, University of London.

Wolf, A.R. (1999) Pain: Nociception and the developing infant. *Paediatric Anaesthesia* **9**, 7–17.

World Health Organization (1997) How to examine the impact of unrelieved pain. *Cancer Pain Release* **10**(3). Available at: http://whocancerpain.wisc.edu/old_site/eng/10_3/impact.html (accessed January 2013).

Zhu, L.M., Stinson, J., Palozzi, L. et al. (2012) Improvements in pain outcomes in a Canadian pediatric teaching hospital following implementation of a multifaceted, knowledge translation initiative. *Pain Research and Management* **17**, 173–179.

Zisk-Rony, R.Y., Fortier, M.A., MacLaren-Chorney, J., Perrett, D. and Zain, Z.N. (2010) Parental postoperative pain management: Attitudes, assessment and management. *Pediatrics* **125**, 1372–1378.

CHAPTER 2

Anatomy and Physiology of Pain

Jackie Bentley

Institute of Health and Society, University of Worcester, United Kingdom

Introduction

The capacity to feel pain helps to protect us from harm. Knowledge of nervous system anatomy and physiology is crucial to understanding pain, its presentation and management. This chapter explores the mechanisms involved in pain perception and how this relates to the management of pain.

The Nervous System

Terminology relating to pain is defined in Table 2.1 and key nervous system structures and terms are presented in Table 2.2. The nervous system is made up of neurons (nerve cells) and can be subdivided into the *peripheral nervous system* (PNS) and *central nervous system* (CNS).

- The PNS is made up of all nervous tissues (*nerves, ganglia, enteric plexuses* and *sensory receptors*) outside the CNS. It transmits information to the CNS (via *sensory* or *afferent* neurones) and from the CNS (via motor or *efferent* neurones).
- The CNS is comprised of the brain and spinal cord. The brain integrates and interprets information from sensory neurones and determines a response.
- The dorsal area of the spinal cord acts as an information hub and is able to simultaneously direct information to the brain and down the spinal cord to the area of injury.

Misconceptions about the Physiology of Pain in Children

In the past, healthcare professionals have doubted the capacity of children and infants to feel pain and be affected by it to the same extent as adults. These assumptions were

Managing Pain in Children: A Clinical Guide for Nurses and Healthcare Professionals, Second Edition. Edited by Alison Twycross, Stephanie Dowden, and Jennifer Stinson.

Table 2.1 Key pain terminology

Term	Definition
Acute pain	Pain of short duration that can be attributed to injury or disease and is generally considered to be protective as it triggers behaviours that remove us from harm and promote recovery
Allodynia	Pain due to a stimulus that does not normally provoke pain
Causalgia	A syndrome of sustained burning pain, allodynia and hyperpathia after a traumatic nerve lesion, often combined with vasomotor and sudomotor dysfunction and later trophic changes
Central pain	Pain initiated or caused by a primary lesion or dysfunction in the central nervous system
Central sensitisation	Increased responsiveness of nociceptive neurones in the central nervous system to their normal or subthreshold afferent input
Chronic pain	Pain that persists after the initial injury and may (as in some types of neuropathic pain) occur in the absence of tissue damage. As a result it serves no protective function and becomes a health problem in itself
Dysaesthesia	An unpleasant abnormal sensation, whether spontaneous or evoked
Hyperaesthesia	Increased sensitivity to stimulation, includes both allodynia and hyperalgesia
Hyperalgesia	Increased pain from a stimulus that normally provokes pain
Hyperpathia	A painful syndrome characterised by an abnormally painful reaction to a stimulus, especially a repetitive stimulus, as well as an increased threshold
Hypoalgesia	Diminished pain in response to a normally painful stimulus
Neuralgia	Pain in the distribution of a nerve or nerves
Neuropathic pain	Pain caused by a lesion or disease of the somatosensory nervous system
Neuropathy	A disturbance of function or pathological change in a nerve: in one nerve, mononeuropathy; in several nerves, mononeuropathy multiplex; if diffuse and bilateral, polyneuropathy
Nociception	The neural process of encoding noxious stimuli
Nociceptive pain	Pain that arises from actual or threatened damage to non-neural tissue and is due to the activation of nociceptors
Nociceptor	A high-threshold sensory receptor of the peripheral somatosensory nervous system that is capable of transducing and encoding noxious stimuli
Pain	An unpleasant sensory and emotional experience associated with actual or potential tissue damage, or described in terms of such damage
Pain threshold	The least intensity of a stimulus that is perceived as painful
Pain tolerance level	The maximum intensity of a pain-producing stimulus that a subject is willing to accept in a given situation
Paraesthesia	An abnormal sensation, whether spontaneous or evoked
Placebo analgesics	'Medications' that are presented to the patient as providing pain relief, which contain no pharmacologically active ingredient
Wind-up	An increase in the excitability of spinal cord neurones provoked by repetitive stimulation of C-fibres

Source: Melzack and Wall (2008); International Association for the Study of Pain (IASP) (2011)

Table 2.2 Key nervous system terminology

Term	Definition
Action potential (nerve impulse)	Electrical signal created by changes in electrochemical energy across the membrane of the neurone
Afferent (*sensory*) neurones	Neurones that carry sensory information *to* the central nervous system
Axon	Single long process of a neurone that conducts nerve impulses towards another neurone
Cranial nerves	12 pairs of nerves emerging from the brain
Dendrite	Receiving, input portion of neurone
Descending modulation	Mechanisms that modulate nociception (may be facilitatory or inhibitory) via nerve impulses transmitted from the brain to the spinal cord. The process modulates transmission of pain signalling in the spinal cord
Dorsal horn	Found in all spinal cord levels and is comprised of sensory nuclei that receive and process somatic information. From there ascending projection emerges to transmit the sensory information to the midbrain and diencephalon
Efferent (*motor*) neurones	Neurones that carry motor information *from* the central nervous system
Excitation	Triggering of a nerve impulse. Excitation of an A-delta or C fibre will lead to transmission of pain stimuli
Ganglion	Cluster of neuronal cell bodies in the peripheral nervous system
Grey matter	Comprised of neuronal cell bodies, dendrites, unmyelinated axons, axon terminals and neuroglia
Enteric plexuses	Networks of neurones in organs and gastrointestinal tract
Inhibition	Inhibition refers to processes that impair onward transmission of nerve impulses, e.g. prevention or reduction of pain impulse transmission from primary to secondary afferent neurones in the dorsal horn of the spinal cord
Interneurones	Form connections between sensory and motor neurones in the central nervous system
Myelin sheath	Lipid and protein covering that insulates the axon enabling faster electrical transmission
Myelination	Process of forming the myelin sheath
Nerve	Bundle of axons in the peripheral nervous system
Neuroglia (glial cells)	Nerve cells that support neurone functioning (includes astrocytes, microglia, ependymal cells and oligodendrocytes)
Neurone	Excitable nerve cells (capable of transmitting an impulse and processing information) made up of cell body, dendrites and an axon
Neurotransmitters	Chemicals that influence the transmission of the impulse across the synapse by inhibition or excitation
Nociceptor	A sensory nerve ending capable of responding to noxious (painful) stimulation
Spinal nerves	31 pairs of nerves emerging from the spinal cord
Spinoreticular tract	An ascending nociceptive pathway that carries information on the emotional/affective components of pain

Table 2.2 Continued

Term	Definition
Spinothalamic tract	An ascending nociceptive pathway that carries information on the sensory-discriminative aspects of pain (i.e. the site and type of painful stimulus)
Substantia gelatinosa (SG)	An area within the dorsal horn of the spinal cord where primary afferents of the spinothalamic tract synapse
Synapse	The junction between two or more neurones
Tract	Bundle of axons in the central nervous system
White matter	Comprised of myelinated axons

Source: Melzack and Wall (1965); Almeida et al. (2004); Melzack and Wall (2008); Clancy and McVicar (2009); Macintyre et al. (2010); Tortora and Derrickson (2012)

generally based on perceptions that an immature nervous system rendered infants less able to perceive pain. However, recent advances in our understanding of pain physiology make it difficult to deny the experience of pain in infants and therefore in children. These misconceptions are presented in Table 2.3 along with the factual evidence that can be used to refute them.

Pain Mechanisms

The mechanisms involved in pain perception (nociception) can be divided into four processes: transduction, transmission, perception and modulation. The integration of these processes is illustrated in Figure 2.1.

Transduction: The conversion of stimuli to electrical impulses

Nociceptors are unmyelinated, free nerve endings. They are found in somatic tissues (i.e. skin, cornea, mucous membranes, bones, joints and blood vessels) and in smaller numbers in visceral tissues (i.e. gastrointestinal tract and organs). Their concentration is highest in areas most prone to injuries (i.e. hands and feet) or in regions of the body needing additional protection (i.e. corneal, dental and some visceral tissues) (Charlton 2005). There are two types of afferent nerve fibres that have different nociceptors:

- *C fibres* – very small-diameter unmyelinated fibres that conduct impulses slowly;
- C-fibre *nociceptors* are polymodal, responding to a range of potentially harmful stimuli, including chemical, thermal and mechanical;
- *A-delta fibres* – larger diameter, myelinated fibres that conduct impulses faster;
- A-delta *nociceptors* respond to mechanical and thermal stimuli.

(Melzack and Wall 2008; Patel 2010)

Activation of nociceptors

The activation of nociceptors is essentially a chemical process as nociceptors have receptors that respond to different mechanical, thermal or chemical stimuli. These chemicals impact the degree of response and thus pain intensity. (Details of this

Table 2.3 Misconceptions about the physiology of pain in infants and children

Misconception	Evidence
Infants cannot feel pain as their nervous system pathways are not fully developed	Evidence summarised by Beggs and Fitzgerald (2007) and Anand et al. (2007) identifies the responsiveness of nociception changes in early embryonic life and continues to be refined into adulthood. Sensory neurones extend into the epidermis in the neonate, and later retract into the dermis. This may mean the newborn infant has a lower threshold for responding to handling and skin-breaking procedures (Beggs and Fitzgerald 2007). The mechanisms involved in descending inhibition of pain appear to develop in the latter stages of gestation and the first few days of life (Anand et al. 2007) and are not fully functional until childhood. Therefore, some of the mechanisms that moderate or override incoming pain stimuli are less effective in the neonate. This suggests that infants are *more* sensitive to pain than adults.
Myelination is not complete at birth, therefore pain transmission is inefficient	Pain is transmitted on both myelinated and unmyelinated nerve fibres. Myelination progresses rapidly in the first few months of life (Neill and Bowden 2004). Impulse transmission can occur along *A-delta fibres* before they are fully myelinated but does so more slowly (Loizzo et al. 2009). Myelination is not necessary for conduction along *C fibres* (these fibres do not become myelinated).
Infants and children suffer no adverse consequences as a result of pain experiences	Experiencing pain is one factor associated with reduced growth of infants born before 32 weeks gestation (Vinall et al. 2012). Infancy is a period of rapid nervous system development and, therefore, a time when the nervous system is highly influenced by experiences such as pain (Neill and Bowden 2004). Beggs and Fitzgerald (2007), Bouza (2009) and Loizzo et al. (2009) suggest that the evolution from acute pain to persistent chronic pain in infants transpires through neuroplastic adaptation in the peripheral and central nervous systems, to the extent that they are more sensitive to pain (see *plasticity*, p. 32).
Infants and young children have no memory for pain	Taddio et al. (1995) found that male infants responded more vigorously to immunisations at 4–6 months if they had been circumcised a birth.

chemical process and the impact on inflammation are outlined in Box 2.1.) The process involves the following stages:

1. Nociceptors are not uniformly sensitive and the receptor sites will be activated by sufficient mechanical, thermal or chemical stimuli liberated to reach a *threshold*;
2. When the threshold is reached, the nerve terminal is depolarised and an impulse (*action potential*) is created;
3. In the presence of persistent stimuli (such as inflammation), nociceptors become sensitised and capable of transmitting further nerve impulses at lower thresholds;
4. Under these conditions action potentials are generated by stimulation through touch or movement at levels that would not normally be interpreted as painful.

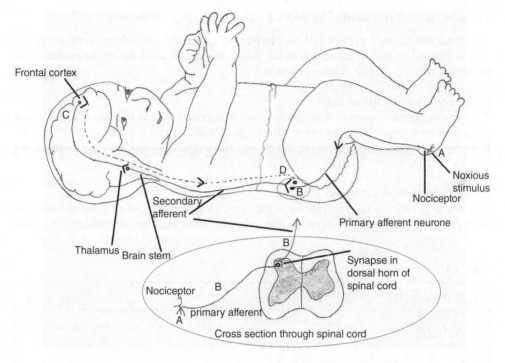

Figure 2.1   The stages of nociception: transduction (A), transmission (B), perception (C) and modulation (D).

BOX 2.1

Inflammation and pain

- Tissue injury initiates an *inflammatory response*.
- The damaged cells release chemicals that are capable of activating and/or sensitising nociceptors (e.g. potassium, hydrogen ions, leukotrienes and prostaglandins).
- The inflammatory response is further enhanced by the release of mediators from inflammatory cells (such as histamine, serotonin, bradykinin) and nerve terminals (e.g. substance P).
- Many of these substances have specific receptor sites on nociceptors and can therefore initiate or lower the action potential threshold. In turn this causes *peripheral sensitisation (i.e. lower threshold and increased response to same level of stimulus)*.
- Inflammation increases local blood flow to produce local redness and warmth. In acute pain episodes this helps to promote healing by prompting us to protect and rest the affected area.

Source: Melzack and Wall (2008)

Sensitisation at the trauma/injury site is referred to as *primary hyperalgesia*. The sensitive area that extends beyond the area of tissue damage (i.e. *secondary hyperalgesia*) is the result of changes in spinal cord processing (Melzack and Wall 2008).

Transmission: Conveying impulses to the central nervous system

The transmission may occurs in three phases: via one of the ascending pathways -from the peripheral axon to the spinal cord, from the spinal cord to the brainstem and thalamus then on to the cerebral cortex.

Peripheral axon to spinal cord

The action potential initiated in nociceptors is carried toward the spinal cord along the axons of primary afferent nerve fibres: *A-delta fibres* and *C fibres* (see Table 2.4). Information about different nerve fibres and the impact of myelination is discussed in Box 2.2. Dermatomes are outlined in Box 2.3.

Spinal cord to brainstem and thalamus

For action potentials to continue once they reach the spinal cord they must be transmitted across the synapses between the primary afferent neurones and the second-

Table 2.4 Conduction speed of nerve fibres

Type of nerve fibre	Myelinated?	Conduction speed
A-alpha	Yes	80–120 m/sec
A-beta	Yes	35–90 m/sec
A-delta	Yes	5–40 m/sec
C	No	0.5–2 m/sec
Adapted from *The brain from top to bottom* (www.thebrain.mcgill.ca)		

BOX 2.2

Myelination and transmission speed

Myelin allows impulses to be transmitted more quickly, but transmission occurs even when there is no myelin. There are two sensations of pain: fast, sharp pain (via myelinated A-delta fibres), which is followed by slower, dull pain (via unmyelinated C fibres). Information about transmissions speeds can be found in Table 2.4.

The process of myelin production is not complete at birth. However, neonates are still capable of feeling pain and every effort should be made to ensure their pain is managed effectively (Loizzo et al. 2009).

BOX 2.3

Dermatomes

The human body is divided into zones known as dermatomes. A dermatome represents the area of the body served by a particular spinal nerve.

Knowledge of dermatomes assists in the management of *spinal* and *epidural analgesia*. This type of analgesia works by blocking transmission along a specific spinal nerve or group of nerves. Additional information about dermatomes and spinal/epidural analgesia can be found in Chapter 7.

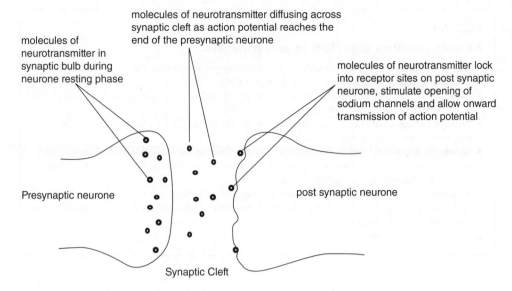

molecules of neurotransmitter diffusing across
synaptic cleft as action potential reaches the
end of the presynaptic neurone

molecules of
neurotransmitter in
synaptic bulb during
neurone resting phase

molecules of neurotransmitter lock
into receptor sites on post synaptic
neurone, stimulate opening of
sodium channels and allow onward
transmission of action potential

Presynaptic neurone

post synaptic neurone

Synaptic Cleft

Figure 2.2   Events at a simple synapse.

order neurones that ascend the spinal cord. The physiological events that occur at the synapse are summarised in Figure 2.2.

Once pain impulses succeed in overriding inhibitory mechanisms they are transmitted across the spinal cord to the anterolateral *spinothalamic tract*, which delivers pain impulses to the thalamus. In the thalamus, nociceptive fibres form synapses with other neurones that relay impulses to other areas of the brain (Clancy and McVicar 2009).

Fibres of the *spinoreticular tract* convey impulses from the dorsal horn of the spinal cord to the reticular formation in the brainstem before progressing to the cerebral cortex. This pathway is principally involved in our emotional or affective response to pain (Almeida et al. 2004).

Neurotransmitters used in transmission

Neurotransmitters are chemicals released in response to a nerve impulse reaching the presynaptic neurone (Figure 2.2). The neurotransmitters diffuse across the synaptic cleft and bind to receptor sites in postsynaptic neurones that depolarise the membrane and when the threshold is reached, an action potential is generated [convert the chemical signal back to an electrical signal] (Tortora and Derrickson 2012). Neurotransmitters interact with different receptors, which can result in either excitatory or inhibitory effects on nerve transmission.

Several excitatory and inhibitory neurotransmitters participate in nociception. The key neurotransmitters are identified in Box 2.4.

Endogenous opioids and gamma-aminobutyric acid (GABA)

Endogenous opioids and GABA act as neurotransmitters inhibiting (preventing) the excitation of postsynaptic neurones. Their action is considered under the heading *modulation*. The role of *serotonin* appears to be more complex as it can both inhibit and enhance the onward transmission of nociceptive impulses (Ossipov et al. 2010).

BOX 2.4

Neurotransmitters important in pain pathways

- **Gamma-aminobutyric acid (GABA)** causes *inhibition* of neuronal receptors in the CNS
- **Glutamate** causes *excitation* of neurones in the CNS
- **Substance P** causes *excitation* of neurones in the dorsal horn of the spinal cord and in the brain, enhances perception of pain
- **Noradrenaline** is concentrated in the brainstem and causes either *inhibition* or *excitation* of neurones depending on receptor subtype
- **Serotonin** is concentrated in the brainstem and is involved in the regulation of temperature, sensory perception, sleep and mood and depending on the receptor subtype it interacts with, can have inhibitory or facilitatory effects
- **Dopamine** is concentrated in the midbrain and is involved in the regulation of emotional responses and subconscious movements of the skeletal muscles and causes *inhibition* of neuronal receptors in dendrites

Adapted from Smith (2009)

Glutamate

Glutamate is a major excitatory neurotransmitter found in the CNS. When activated it is responsible for basal synaptic transmission and synaptic plasticity, such as those involved in learning and memory.

Noradrenaline

Noradrenaline is a key neurotransmitter for pain caused by disease or failure of an organ. Peripheral nociceptive stimuli activate noradrenergic brainstem projections to the spinal cord, resulting in antinociception and inhibition of spinal nociceptive neurones.

Substance P

Substance P is largely responsible for the transmission of pain from the periphery to the CNS (Clancy and McVicar 2009). Substance P enhances the perception of pain.

> The mechanisms by which many analgesic drugs act have yet to be established; there is increasing evidence that their actions imitate those of the neurotransmitters involved in descending inhibitory pathways.
> See Chapter 4 for more information about how analgesic drugs work.

Perception

Perception is essentially the point at which the individual becomes consciously aware of the existence of pain: its intensity, its nature and its location. Conscious awareness of any sensation is generally considered to involve the cortex. It has proven difficult to identify a precise point at which pain is perceived, but imaging techniques such as magnetic resonance imaging (MRI) and positron emission tomography (PET) have allowed researchers to 'track' the route taken by pain impulses. Such studies have revealed that:

- The processing of noxious information is complex and involves many areas of the brain (Latremoliere and Woolf 2009);
- Pain stimuli increase activity in several areas of the cerebral cortex (prefrontal cortex, primary and secondary somatosensory cortices, anterior cingulate cortex and insular cortex), the thalamus, basal ganglia and cerebellum (Schweinhardt and Bushnell 2010).

Table 2.5 Factors that influence the experience of pain

	Pharmacological	Physical	Psychological
Close the gate	Analgesic drugs Adjuvant analgesics	Counter-stimulation, e.g. massage, TENS, heat, acupuncture, acupressure Exercise Endogenous analgesics	Hypnosis/imagery Meditation Cognitive behavioural therapy (CBT) Suggestion of analgesic effect (placebo analgesics) Positive thoughts Relaxation Biofeedback Controlled breathing techniques Distraction
Open the gate		Severity of illness or injury Excessive activity Re-injury	Anxiety, fear or worry Tension or stress Depression Focusing on pain Catastrophising Anticipation of severe pain

Adapted from Smith (2009)

Modulation

The pain we experience can be influenced (*modulated*) by a host of biological, psychological and social factors (Table 2.5) known to affect our experience of pain. In essence, these factors inhibit or amplify nociceptive inputs. The multitude of modifying factors lends credence to the concept of the pain neuromatrix and to biopsychosocial models. (See Chapter 3 for additional information about the factors that affect children's behaviour when experiencing pain.)

Descending inhibition and modulation

Melzack and Wall's gate control theory (1965/2008) incorporated the suggestion that there were mechanisms by which activity originating in the brain could prevent the onward transmission of pain impulses by closing the spinal cord pain gate. They referred to this process as *descending inhibition* because it involves nerve impulses descending the spinal cord. Patel (2010) suggested that serotonin and norepinephrine are the principal neurotransmitters operating in the pathway that delivers descending inhibition. This may explain the analgesic properties of selective serotonin reuptake inhibitors (SSRIs) and tricyclic antidepressants, which are used for the management of chronic pain. There is evidence that descending inhibition is less efficient in adults who experience migraine headaches (Moulton et al. 2008).

The potential influence of suggestion or expectation on pain experience is illustrated in research by Goffaux et al. (2007) in a study that monitored descending inhibition in two groups of subjects under experimental conditions. One group of subjects were told that submerging their arm in cold water would reduce the intensity of a painful stimulus and the second group were told that it would enhance it. Individuals expecting an analgesic effect experienced less pain and reduced spinal reflex activity in response to the painful stimulus. This reduction was not seen in those who were told to expect an increase in pain.

Practice point

Expectations based on previous experiences and the confidence that children have in pain-reducing strategies influence naturally occurring anti-nociceptive stimuli (i.e. modify descending inhibition).

GABA is an important inhibitory neurotransmitter found extensively in the cerebral cortex and spinal cord (Patel 2010). GABA acts at synapses between the primary and secondary afferent neurone, inhibiting the release of chemicals that would otherwise stimulate the onward transmission of the pain stimulus (Melzack and Wall 2008).

Opioid neuropeptides
Endogenous opioids, such as endorphins and enkephalins, inhibit the release of substance P and other excitatory substances (those capable of transmitting an impulse across the synapse) from primary afferent neurones. These substances are natural analgesics that target opioid receptors, which inhibit transmitter release presynaptically and reduce excitability postsynaptically (Clancy and McVicar 2009). Opioid receptors are also used by opioid-based medicines to exert their analgesic effect (see Chapter 4).

The gate control theory
The *gate control theory* (Melzack and Wall 1965) helps conceptualise the mechanics of pain transmission. An overview of the gate control theory is presented in Figure 2.3. The crux of the theory is that there is a *gating mechanism* in the dorsal horn (substantia gelatinosa; SG) of the spinal cord where primary afferent neurones terminate. The theory proposes when the gate is closed, impulses from nociceptors cannot travel up the spinal cord. Melzack and Wall (1965) also hypothesised that impulses descending from the brain could operate the pain gate. Since the publication of this theory much of the physiological evidence required to support Melzack and Wall's proposals relating to events in the spinal cord has become available. However, the theory has been updated, leading Melzack (1999) to develop the *neuromatrix theory*. This helped make our understanding of the descending mechanisms clearer.

Additional information

More information about the gate control theory and how it relates to the neuromatrix theory can be found in Chapter 1 of Hadjistavropoulos, T. and Craig, K.D. (2004) *Pain: Psychological Perspectives*. Lawrence Erlbaum, Mahwah, NJ. Available at: www.federaljack.com/ebooks/ Illustrations that aid understanding of the gate control theory can be found at: http://science. howstuffworks.com/environmental/life/human-biology/pain4.htm

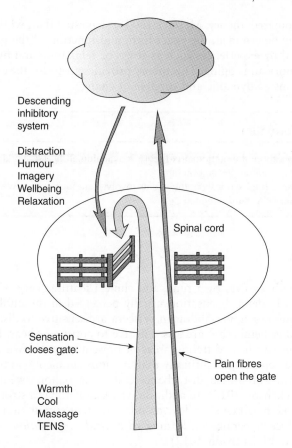

Figure 2.3   Explanation of the gate control theory.
Source: Eloise Carr and Eileen Mann, Pain, 2000, reproduced with permission from Palgrave Macmillan.

The neuromatrix theory of pain

Melzack (1999) noted that the gate control theory could not explain the existence of phenomena such as phantom limb pain. In the *neuromatrix theory* Melzack (1999) suggests that the mechanisms for interpreting and responding to pain are best viewed as a network of areas of the brain interacting with each other and with the gating mechanism in the spinal cord. Together these areas influence how we feel about a pain experience and how we interpret it, as well as determining our response. Collectively the areas that contribute to the pain neuromatrix also ensure that information received from nociceptors is combined with other sensory information, memory, emotions and arousal states; a notion consistent with viewing pain as a biopsychosocial process (see Chapter 3).

Ossipov et al. (2010) reviewed the research into the brain activity related to pain stimuli and pain perception. Much of the research is from studies using radiology imaging techniques that demonstrate a complex, integrated system involving diverse areas of the brain. The notion that there is a pain neuromatrix has been used to explain a wide range of phenomena that influence pain experience including placebo analgesics and the expectation/anticipation of pain (Ossipov et al. 2010; Eccleston et al. 2012).

Using the neuromatrix theory, Melzack (2005) suggested that, while pain responses may be genetically determined, the exact form and function of the pain neuromatrix may be modulated by experiences such as stress or relaxation and by cognitive functions such as memory and coping. This theory provides scope for the conceptualisation of pain mechanisms as dynamic and capable of change.

Additional information

Further information about the neuromatrix theory is available at: http://thebrain.mcgill.ca/flash/
i/i_03_cr/i_03_cr_dou/i_03_cr_dou.html
This video provides a brief synopsis of the events involved in nociception: www.youtube.com/
watch?v=n8y04SrkEZU&feature=related

Visceral Pain

Visceral pain usually evolves over time, and clinical features vary. The pain arises as a diffuse and poorly defined sensation usually perceived in the midline of the body, at the lower sternum or upper abdomen. Viscera are sensitive to distension (stretch), inflammation and ischemia, but are less sensitive to cutting or heat. Pain from different visceral organs can have differing areas of presentation, known as *referred pain*. Visceral pain is perceived more diffusely than noxious cutaneous stimulation and may be associated with autonomic disturbances, such as pallor, sweating and nausea (Sikandar and Dickenson 2012). In addition, visceral pain has a strong affective component, thus can be heightened by low mood. Persistent stimulation of visceral nociceptors can produce hyperalgesia, leading to *central sensitisation* and chronic pain states (Sikandar and Dickenson 2012).

Visceral organs do not have A-delta fibres but the C fibres carrying the pain information converge on the same area of spinal cord (substantia gelatinosa) where the A-delta fibres converge; thus the brain localises the pain as if it were originating from the peripheral area instead of the visceral organ.
This is known as *referred pain*. Referred pain also occurs in areas supplied by cranial nerves.
Source: Tortora and Derrickson (2012)

Additional information

Further information about referred pain can be found at:
www.patmedicalart.com/portfolio.html
http://antranik.org/visceral-sensory-neurons-and-referred-pain/

Physiology of Chronic and Neuropathic Pain

Chronic pain is considered to be pain that extends beyond the time normally required for healing to take place (Merskey and Bogduk 1994/2011). While this definition may seem imprecise and rather difficult to apply, it allows for the fact that different tissues and different injuries will require differing lengths of time to repair. Neuropathic pain is a term applied to pain that is caused by injury or disease affecting the somatosensory nervous system (Merskey and Bogduk 1994/2011). Neuropathic pain may be a component of acute pain following surgery or injury (Macintyre et al. 2010) and may therefore resolve once healing has taken place. However, neuropathic pain can progress to chronic pain as classified by the International Association for the Study of Pain (IASP).

Our understanding of persisting (chronic) pain states is improving, largely as a result of the development of imaging techniques. For example, brain imaging using functional MRI has detected a process referred to as *central sensitisation* or increased central neuronal responsiveness. Central sensitisation involves both a reduction in pain threshold and an amplification of the pain that is transmitted. It includes:

- pain hypersensitivity;
- allodynia;
- the perception of pain from tissue not affected by the injury or resulting inflammation;
- pain that continues after the pain stimulus has been removed and inflammatory chemicals have dissipated.

Central sensitisation is of interest to clinicians because:

- it helps illustrate the capacity of the nervous system to adapt to experience;
- it is used to provide potential insight into chronic pain states (Woolf 2011);
- sensitisation may account for the increased risk of chronic pain in children and adults who experience abdominal pain early in their lives (Walker et al. 2010).

As the term suggests, the mechanisms for central sensitisation have been attributed to processes that occur within the CNS and are distinct from peripheral sensitisation or primary hyperalgesia, which originates within the region of tissue injury. The lack of peripheral involvement in central sensitisation seems to be confirmed by the observation that *hyperalgesia* occurs even when tissues around the injury are infiltrated with local anaesthetic (Latremoliere and Woolf 2009).

Latremoliere and Woolf (2009) summarise the research that suggests there are a range of mechanisms that facilitate central sensitisation:

- Stimuli (that would not normally be painful) are transmitted on A-beta fibres, such that non-noxious stimuli are 'transferred' to the ascending *spinothalamic tract* and interpreted as pain.
- An increase in the excitability of postsynaptic neurones in the spinal cord (meaning less stimulation is required to open the gate).
- Greater excitation at synapses between neurones carrying pain impulses (thus more impulses pass through to be experienced as pain).
- Reduced inhibition in the spinal cord (meaning mechanisms that close the gate are not as effective).

There is a good deal of interest in determining the chemical mediators of chronic pain as this may prove useful in developing analgesics to prevent central sensitisation. Glutamate and its N-methyl-D-aspartate (NMDA) receptors appear to be key players; however, other chemicals such as bradykinin are also involved (Latremoliere and Woolf 2009).

Central sensitisation in chronic pain

Central sensitisation often features in acute pain experiences, most of which do not progress to chronic pain (Woolf 2011). However, structural changes may occur that most likely result in chronic, intractable pain (Kuner 2010). These changes include:

- a loss of grey matter resulting from the release of glutamate (Harris 2011);
- an increase in the number of connections that develop between synapses in pain pathways that are used repeatedly.

There is some evidence to suggest that structural adaptations facilitating central sensitisation are more likely to occur in early infancy when neural pathways are in the process of development (Johnson et al. 2011).

Additional information

More information about central sensitisation can be found at:
www.wellcome.ac.uk/en/pain/microsite/science4.html
http://juniorprof.wordpress.com/2008/07/07/what-is-central-sensitization/
www.youtube.com/watch?v=t5izZXxC9y4

Nervous System Development and Pain Sensation in Early Life

Plasticity relates to the shaping of the CNS by experience. The process challenges the common misconception that nervous system pathways are *hard-wired* and can only respond in predetermined ways. In reality, we develop sensitivity to things that we experience repeatedly and our nervous systems are then primed to perceive and respond to these experiences. This is particularly true of experiences that occur during periods of rapid nervous system development such as during infancy (Neill and Bowden 2004).

Additional information

A more detailed account of the development of pain mechanisms can be found in:
Anand, K.J.S., Stevens, B.J. and McGrath, P.J. (eds) (2007) *Pain in Neonates and Infants*, 3rd edition. Elsevier, Philadelphia.
The concept of plasticity is explored at:
http://thebrain.mcgill.ca/flash/d/d_07/d_07_cl/d_07_cl_tra/d_07_cl_tra.html
www.slideshare.net/vacagodx/infant-brain-development-2891731#btnNext
www.cirp.org/library/pain/anand4/

Mounting a response to pain involves a complex interaction between the nervous and endocrine systems, and the stress response it generates is not always appropriate or proportionate especially if pain exposure is prolonged. Repeated stimulation, levels of neurotransmitters and brain electrical signals change as neurones develop a 'memory' for responding to those signals. Frequent stimulation results in a stronger brain memory, so that the brain will respond more rapidly and effectively when experiencing the same stimulation in the future. The resulting changes in brain wiring and response are referred to as *nerve plasticity*. There is some evidence that early pain experience can reinforce pain pathways; however, research findings have not consistently demonstrated that infants who encounter severe or repeated pain early in life are at greater risk of hyperalgesia or an increased stress response to the pain they experience later in life (Taddio and Katz 2005; Vinall et al. 2012).

There is a wealth of literature which highlights that infants who experience chronic pain behavioural responses to painful events in early life are different from children who did not experience pain events in early life (Grunau et al. 2004). Premature infants in the neonatal intensive care unit (NICU) often experience multiple, painful procedures daily for routine monitoring, as well as any surgical interventions for their survival (Low and Schweinhardt 2012). Follow-up studies of ex-premature children provide compelling evidence for the long-term effects of early pain experiences:

- In a controlled study by Walker et al. (2009) on sensory sensitivity, extremely preterm infants born at less than 26 weeks gestation were followed through their childhood up to the age of 11 years. Walker et al. found established sensory thresholds in these children at age 11 and showed that these extremely preterm children had significantly decreased sensitivity to non-noxious mechanical and thermal stimuli compared to age- and sex-matched term children born from the controlled group.
- A similar result was seen in 9- to 12-year-old children who had previously experienced neonatal cardiac surgery; subjects were significantly less sensitive than the control group to non-noxious mechanical and thermal stimuli at both the previously operated site and non-injured areas (Schmelzle-Lubiecki et al. 2007).
- Other researchers suggest that there may be a period during development when the infant is particularly vulnerable to developing a long-lasting (perhaps life-long) sensitisation to pain (Bouza 2009; Loizzo et al. 2009).

The practice of protecting infants from pain must be based on the fundamental ethical principles of non-maleficence and beneficence (Beauchamp and Childress 2009) and managing their pain effectively must be based on research. The under-treatment of pain or not relieving pain in children is unethical as it results in suffering and causing harm. It is well established that the experience of pain during infancy may produce structural and functional reorganisation of developing nociceptive pathway which in turn may cause long-lasting alterations in pain processing that extend well into childhood and adulthood (Fitzgerald and Walker 2006). This adds weight to the need for effective understanding and management of pain in neonates, in order to minimise later consequences of early pain experience.

Summary

- Structures involved in pain perception include peripheral and central nervous system components that perceive a sensation and generate feelings about the experience as well as modulating incoming and outgoing impulses.
- The gate control theory remains useful in conceptualising nociceptive pain, but the neuromatrix theory provides a better framework for explaining the subjectivity of pain experiences and the development of chronic pain syndromes.
- Understanding the physiology of pain enables nurses and other healthcare professionals to appreciate the physical and psychological effects of pain and to gain insight into how pain management strategies work.
- Recent advances in the science of pain have established that neonates, even those born prematurely, have the capacity to feel pain and the potential to be adversely affected by it.

Acknowledgements

We would like to thank:

Dr Lynda Roderique from the Faculty of Health, Social Care and Education at Kingston University and St George's University of London for her work in editing the final version of this chapter.

Dr Suellen Walker from UCL Institute of Child Health and Great Ormond Street Hospital for Children for reviewing the chapter.

Zoe Clark from the Faculty of Health, Social Care and Education at Kingston University and St George's University of London for reviewing an earlier version of this chapter.

References

Almeida, T.F., Roizenblatt, S. and Tufik, S. (2004) Afferent pain pathways: A neuroanatomical review. *Brain Research* **1000**, 40–56.

Anand K.J.S., Al-Chaer, E.D., Bhutta A.T. and Hall R.W. (2007) Development of supraspinal pain processing. In: *Pain in Neonates and Infants* (eds K.J.S. Anand, B.J. Stevens and P.J. McGrath), 3rd edition, pp. 25–44. Elsevier, Philadelphia.

Beauchamp, T.L. and Childress, J.F. (2009) *Principles of Medical Ethics*, 6th edition. Oxford University Press, New York.

Beggs, S. and Fitzgerald, M. (2007) Development of peripheral and spinal nociceptive systems. In: *Pain in Neonates and Infants* (eds K.J.S. Anand, B.J. Stevens and P.J. McGrath), 3rd edition, pp. 11–24. Elsevier, Philadelphia.

Bouza, H. (2009) The impact of pain in the immature brain. *Journal of Maternal-Fetal and Neonatal Medicine* **22**(9), 722–753.

Carr, E.C.J. and Mann, E.M. (2000) *Pain: Creative Approaches to Effective Pain Management*. Macmillan Press, Basingstoke.

Charlton, J.E. (ed.) (2005) *Core Curriculum for Professional Education in Pain*, 3rd edition. IASP Press. Available from: www.iasp-pain.org/AM/Template.cfm?Section=IASP_Press_Books2& Template=/CM/HTMLDisplay.cfm&ContentID=10731 (accessed February 2013).

Clancy, J. and McVicar, A. (2009) *Physiology and Anatomy for Nurses and Health Care Practitioners: A Homeostatic Approach*. Hodder Arnold, London.

Eccleston, C., Fisher, E. A., Vervoort, T. and Crombez, G. (2012) Worry and catastrophizing about pain in youth: A reappraisal. *Pain* **153**, 1560–1562.

Fitzgerald, M. and Walker, S.M. (2006) Infant pain traces. *Pain* **125**(3), 204–205.

Goffaux, P., Redmond, W.J., Rainville, P. and Marchand, S. (2007) Descending analgesia: When the spine echoes what the brain expects. *Pain* **130**, 137–143.

Grunau, R., Weinberg, J. and Whitfield, M.F. (2004) Neonatal procedural pain and preterm infant cortisol response to novelty at 8 months. *Pediatrics* **114**(1), e77–e84.

Harris, R.E. (2011) Central pain states: A shift in thinking about chronic pain. *Journal of Family Practice* **60**(9) Suppl 2, S37–S42.

IASP (2011) Taxonomy. Available from: www.iasp-pain.org/Content/NavigationMenu/ GeneralResourceLinks/PainDefinitions/default.htm (accessed February 2013).

Johnson, C.C., Fernandes, A.M. and Campbell-Yeo, M. (2011) Pain in neonates is different. *Pain* **152**, S65–S73.

Kuner, R. (2010) Central mechanisms of pathophysiological pain. *Nature Medicine* **13**(11), 1258–1266.

Latremoliere, A. and Woolf, C.J. (2009) Central sensitization: A generator of pain by central neural plasticity. *Journal of Pain* **10**(9), 895–926.

Loizzo, A., Loizzo, S. and Capasso, A. (2009) Neurobiology of pain in children: An overview. *Open Biochemistry Journal* **3**, 18–25.

Low, L.A. and Schweinhardt, P. (2012) Early life adversity as a risk factor for fibromyalgia in later life. *Pain Research and Treatment* **2012**, 1–15.

Macintyre, P.E., Schug, S.A., Scott, D.A., Visser, E.J., Walker, S.M.; APM:SE Working Group of the Australian and New Zealand College of Anaesthetists and Faculty of Pain Medicine (2010) *Acute Pain Management: Scientific Evidence*, 3rd edition. ANZCA & FPM, Melbourne.

Melzack, R. (1999) From the gate to the neuromatrix. *Pain Supplement* 6, S121–126.

Melzack, R. (2005) Evolution of the neuromatrix theory of pain. The Prithvi Raj Lecture: presented at the Third World Congress of World Institute of Pain, Barcelona 2004. *Pain Practice* 5(2), 85–94.

Melzack, R. and Wall, R.D. (1965) Pain mechanisms: a new theory. *Science* 150, 971–979.

Melzack, R. and Wall, R.D. (2008) *The Challenge of Pain*, 2nd edition, Penguin, London.

Merskey, H. and Bogduk, N. (1994/2011) *Classification of Chronic Pain, 2nd edition.* IASP Task Force on Taxonomy (revised edition 2011 with new section III Pain Terms). Available from: www.iasp-pain.org/Content/NavigationMenu/Publications/FreeBooks/Classification_of_Chronic_Pain (accessed February 2013).

Moulton, E.A., Burstein, R., Tully, S., Hargreaves, R., Becerra, L. and Borsook, D. (2008) Interictal dysfunction of a brainstem descending modulatory centre in migraine patients. *PLoS ONE* 3(11), e3799.

Neill, S. and Bowden, L. (2004) Central nervous system development. In: *The Biology of Child Health: A Reader in Development and Assessment* (eds S. Neill and H. Knowles), pp 54–86. Palgrave Macmillan, Basingstoke, UK.

Ossipov, M.H., Dussor, G.O. and Porreca, F. (2010) Central modulation of pain. *Journal of Clinical Investigation* 120(11), 3779–3787.

Patel, N.B. (2010) Physiology of pain. In: *Guide to Pain Management in Low-Resource Settings* (eds A. Kopf and N.B. Patel), pp. 13–17. International Association for the Study of Pain, Seattle.

Schmelzle-Lubiecki, M.M., Campbell, K.A., Howard, R.A., Franck, L. and Fitzgerald, M. (2007) Long-term consequences of early infant injury and trauma upon somatosensory processing. *European Journal of Pain* 11(7), 799–809.

Schweinhardt, P. and Bushnell, M.C. (2010) Pain imaging in health and disease: How far have we come? *Journal of Clinical Investigation* 120(11), 3788–3797.

Sikandar, S. and Dickenson, A.H. (2012) Visceral pain: The ins and outs, the ups and downs. *Current Opinions in Supportive Palliative Care* 6(1), 17–26.

Smith, J. (2009) Anatomy and physiology of pain. In: *Managing Pain in Children: A Clinical Guide* (eds A. Twycross, S.J. Dowden, and E. Bruce), pp. 17–28. Wiley-Blackwell, Oxford.

Taddio, A. and Katz, J. (2005) The effects of early pain experience in neonates on pain responses in infancy and childhood. *Pediatric Drugs* 7(4), 245–257.

Taddio, A., Goldbach, M., Ipp, M., Stevens, B. and Koran, G. (1995) Effect of neonatal circumcision on pain responses during vaccination in boys. *Lancet* 345, 291–292.

Tortora, G.J. and Derrickson, B. (2012) *Principles of Anatomy and Physiology*, 13th edition. John Wiley & Sons, Chichester.

Vinall, J., Miller, S.P., Chau, V., Brummelte, S., Synnes, A.R. and Grunau, R.E. (2012) Neonatal pain in relation to postnatal growth in infants born very preterm. *Pain* 153, 1374–1381.

Walker, S.M., Franck, L.S., Fitzgerald, M., Myles, J. Stocks, J. and Marlow, N. (2009) Long-term impact of neonatal intensive care and surgery on somatosensory perception in children born extremely preterm. *Pain* 141(1–2), 79–87.

Walker, L.S., Dengler-Crish, C.M., Rippel, S. and Bruehl, S. (2010) Functional abdominal pain in childhood and adolescence increases risk for chronic pain in adults. *Pain* 150, 568–572.

Wall, P.D. and Melzack, R. (1989) *Textbook of Pain*. Churchill Livingstone, London.

Woolf, C.J. (2011) Central sensitization: Implications for the diagnosis and treatment of pain. *Pain* 152, S2–S15.

CHAPTER 3

Pain: A Biopsychosocial Phenomenon

Alison Twycross

Department for Children's Nursing and Children's Pain Management,
London South Bank University, United Kingdom

Anna Williams

Faculty of Health, Social Care and Education, Kingston University and
St George's University of London, United Kingdom

Introduction

Many factors influence the child's experience of and behaviour when in pain. These include age, level of cognitive development, culture, family learning, previous experiences of pain, and the child's personality and temperament. These can be classified as biological, psychological and social factors (Figure 3.1). This chapter will discuss each of these in turn. These factors are not, however, independent and interact in various ways to shape the child's experience of pain.

Biological Factors

Age

The effect of a child's age on their perception of pain has been examined in several studies. Children recognise at an early age that pain is unpleasant (McGrath and Hillier 2003). Their understanding and descriptions of pain depend on their age and also on their level of cognitive development and previous experiences of pain (McGrath and Hillier 2003). Several studies have examined children's experiences of procedural pain, which have demonstrated age-related differences in the pain intensity they report (Goodenough et al. 1999; McCarthy et al. 2010) and levels of behavioural distress during

Managing Pain in Children: A Clinical Guide for Nurses and Healthcare Professionals, Second Edition.
Edited by Alison Twycross, Stephanie Dowden, and Jennifer Stinson.
© 2014 John Wiley & Sons, Ltd. Published 2014 by John Wiley & Sons, Ltd.

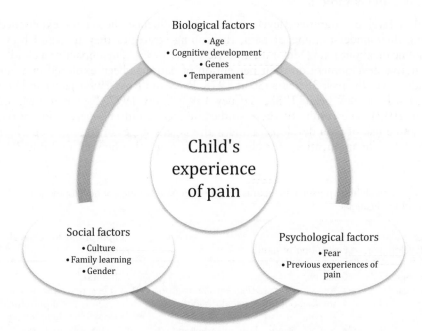

Figure 3.1 Pain as a biopsychosocial phenomenon.

procedures (McCarthy et al. 2010). Children's own ratings of pain and their levels of behavioural distress (as assessed by an observer) during painful procedures seem to decrease with age. This is attributable to several factors. Older children may have:

- a greater understanding of what is happening to them and thus feel less anxious;
- developed coping strategies and methods to distract themselves from procedural pain.

However, in relation to the effect of age on the experience of postoperative pain the research evidence is contradictory and inconclusive. No age-related differences were found by Gidron et al. (1995) among young people (*n* = 67), aged 13–20 years, undergoing oral surgery. However, Bennett-Branson and Craig (1993) found that for children (*n* = 60), aged 7–16 years, postoperative pain increased with age, as did pain with swallow after tonsillectomy in children aged 7–13 years (Crandall et al. 2009). Conversely, Palmero and Drotar (1996) found that for children (*n* = 28), aged 7–17 years, postoperative pain decreased with age.

In chronic pain, prevalence rates for most types of chronic pain tend to increase with age, with older children experiencing more headache, musculoskeletal, back, and nonspecific or general pain, but less abdominal pain than younger children (King et al. 2011).

Younger children may experience more procedure-related pain than older children.
In relation to postoperative pain it is unclear whether age influences children's perception of pain.
Prevalence rates for most types of chronic pain increase with age.

Cognitive development

A child's level of cognitive development may influence their pain experiences by shaping their understanding of pain, the coping strategies they use, and how they communicate about pain (McGrath and McAlpine 1993). The impact of a child's level of cognitive development on their perception of pain has been explored in a number of studies over the past 30 years (Scott 1978; Ross and Ross 1984; Jeans and Gordon 1981; Hurley and Whelan 1988; Gaffney 1993; Crow 1997; Esteve and Marquina-Aponte 2012). The results of these studies indicate children's perception about the cause and effect of pain develops in line with Piaget's stages of cognitive development (Table 3.1). The implications for clinical practice can also be seen in Table 3.1. It is

Table 3.1 How children perceive the cause and effect of pain at different developmental stages, and its clinical implications

Piaget's stage of development	Perception of pain	Implications for clinical practice
Preoperational (2–7 years)	Children: • focus on the physical sensations of pain • think about the magical disappearance of pain • are not able to distinguish between cause and effect of pain • often perceive pain as punishment for a wrongdoing or bad thought, particularly if the child did something they were told not to do immediately before they started experiencing pain • are more egocentric at this age; this may mean they hold someone else responsible for their pain and, therefore, are likely to strike out verbally or physically when they have pain • are apt to tell the clinician who gave them an injection, *you are mean*	Children: • need reassurance that pain is not a punishment • may *hate* the clinician who appears to be inflicting pain • cannot see the connection between treatment and relief of pain
Concrete operational (7–11 years)	Children: • relate to pain physically • are able to specify location in terms of body parts • have an increased awareness of their body and internal organs; their fear of bodily harm is a strong influence in their perception of painful events • have a fear of total annihilation (body destruction and death)	Children: • need reassurance about their fears regarding bodily annihilation • need appropriate explanations about their pain and treatment
Formal operational (12 years and above)	Children: • begin to solve problems • begin to understand the concept of *if . . . then* propositions • do not always have required coping mechanisms to facilitate consistent mature responses • imagine the sinister implications of pain	Children: • need opportunities to discuss their fears • need information about their condition and treatment

Source: Hurley and Whelan (1988); Twycross (1998)

important to note that a child's experiences of illness and hospitalisation may change their perception of and their ability to cope with pain; for example, they may regress to an earlier stage of development (Gaffney and Dunne 1986). In addition, children with cognitive impairment may function at a much earlier stage of development than their chronological age. Conversely, children with chronic illness often develop an understanding of concepts associated with a later stage of development.

Children develop an understanding about pain, which mirrors the stages of development described by Piaget.

Although his theories are widely accepted, Piaget is not without his critics. The area of most debate seems to be Piaget's preoperational stage. During this stage Piaget believes a child is not capable of conscious thought and is unable to grasp the concept of reality. However, in a review of the literature on cognitive development, Hauck (1991) suggests Piaget underestimates pre-school-age children's ability to think logically. Hauck cites research by other experts in the field of cognitive development that suggests if they are given information in the appropriate way children as young as 3 years are capable of greater logic than Piaget's theories suggest. These findings have important implications for healthcare professionals working with children (Hauck 1991). These implications become clearer with the results of Harbeck and Peterson's (1992) study where children as young as 3 years were interviewed. Even at this age children were able to describe their pain if the questions asked were appropriate to their level of understanding.

Genetics

Although genetic determinants of pain responses have been found, Mogil et al. (2000) argue it is unlikely that a simple genetic basis explains variation in pain sensitivity and responses. The results of one study, for instance, indicate that a single gene affects how people tolerate pain (Zubieta et al. 2003). This gene produces an enzyme, which regulates endorphin production in the body. Genes may also affect how people respond to different types of pain relief. Kleiber et al. (2007a) found that genotype predicted how effective topical anaesthetic was in children undergoing intravenous catheter insertion. Specifically, children who reported higher pain were more likely to have the EDNRA TT genotype, suggesting that variation in genes involved in peripheral nociception may mediate responses to topical anaesthetic.

Recent work explores the relationship between genes and pain, showing that genetic factors may play a role in pain perception.

Temperament

What is temperament?

Temperament refers to the general nature, behavioural style or characteristic mood of the individual (Chess and Thomas 1986).
Temperament is largely determined by an individual's genetic makeup, but is also considerably influenced by social and psychological factors.

Several studies have demonstrated that children of different temperaments behave differently when in pain (Box 3.1).

BOX 3.1

Summary of research about the effects of temperament on children's pain

Conte et al. *(2003)*

- Compared the influence of temperament, among other factors, in young people with juvenile primary fibromyalgia syndrome (JPFMS) against children with arthritis and healthy controls. Each group consisted of 16 children, aged 8–17 years.
- Children with JPFMS showed greater temperamental instability, in terms of lower mood, greater distractibility, irregularity of daily habits and low task orientation, as compared to both other groups. They also showed higher levels of anxiety and depression.
- Temperament is related to affective (emotional) responses and chronic pain but the relationship between the three is complex. Temperamental style may underlie psychological adjustment and influence pain coping strategies or it may increase sensitivity to pain, leading to poor adjustment.

Rocha et al. *(2003)*

- Explored factors (including temperament) predicting somatisation and pain reactivity in children ($n = 163$), aged 4½–5½ years, undergoing immunisations.
- Temperament was assessed using the *Behavioural Styles Questionnaire* (BSQ). The *Facial Action Coding System* (FACS) was used to develop an index of pain reflecting the child's reactivity to the procedure.
- Children described as being low in the temperament dimension of adjustment or adaptability showed higher pain reactivity.

Helgadottir and Wilson *(2004)*

- Examined the relationship between temperament (measured using BSQ) and pain intensity at home and in hospital for children ($n = 68$) aged 3–7 years undergoing tonsillectomy.
- Children rated their pain using the Wong-Baker Faces Pain Scale (see Chapter 6). Parents' assessed their child's pain behaviour at home using the *Post-operative Pain Measure for Parents* (Chambers et al. 1996).
- Children who rated high on the temperament dimensions of activity and negative mood reported more pain when in hospital. Children who were more distractible and had lower thresholds reported more pain when at home.

Kleiber et al. *(2007b)*

- Set out to describe the relationship between pain-sensitive temperament and self-report of pain intensity following surgery.
- Adolescents and young adults ($n = 59$) (average age 14 years) completed the *Sensitivity Inventory for Pain–Child Version* prior to admission.
- Pain intensity information was gathered from the computerised medical record.
- There was a small but significant correlation between the *perceptual sensitivity* and *reporting* subscales of the *Sensitivity Inventory for Pain* and pain intensity on the third postoperative day.

A child's temperament may influence how they behave when they are in pain (whether they cry and complain or withdraw and feign sleep), and the coping strategies they use. However, the proposed relationship between temperament and various aspects of the experience of pain is complex and multidimensional.

Additional information

For further information on the relationship between temperament and pain see:
Ranger, M. and Campbell-Yeo, M. (2008) Temperament and pain response: A review of the literature. *Pain Management Nursing* **9**(1), 2–9.

Psychological Factors

Fear

Fear has a huge impact on children's perception of pain. The International Association for the Study of Pain (1979) definition of pain, provided in Chapter 1, describes pain as both a *sensory* and an *emotional* experience. Fear and distress are common negative emotions experienced by children in pain. The greater the level of fear, the more likely a child is to feel pain and distress. Fear of pain is itself an important factor in the experience of children's pain (Huguet et al. 2011) and may predict responses to acute and longer-term pain. Fear may be associated with the avoidance of activity and consequent deconditioning and pain persistence (Wilson et al. 2011). A questionnaire developed to assess fear-avoidance beliefs is available, and has been used to show that greater fear-avoidance beliefs are associated with reduced activity and greater pain intensity (Wilson et al. 2011).

> Fear impacts on children's perceptions of pain.
> Treating only the sensory component of a painful and frightening procedure is rarely effective.
> The most effective interventions combine preparation and explanation and pharmacological, physical and psychological pain-relieving interventions.
> (See Chapter 4 for discussion about analgesic drugs, Chapter 5 for a discussion of physical and psychological methods of pain relief and Chapter 10 for information about managing procedural pain.)

Previous experiences of pain

Children's previous experiences of pain will influence how they react to subsequent painful events (see Chapter 1). Frequent exposure to painful stimuli does not desensitise the individual but increases their sensitivity to pain (Weisman et al. 1998; McGrath and Hillier 2003). The perception of pain is not a learned response (Anand and Craig 1996), but the experience of pain is modified by previous exposure to painful situations.

> How well a child's pain has been managed in the past affects their response to future painful experiences.
> Children experiencing frequent painful experiences become more sensitive to pain.
> This highlights the need to manage children's pain effectively from their first healthcare encounter.

Social Factors

Culture

> ### What is culture?
>
> Culture can be defined as the way of life of people. It consists of conventional patterns of thought and behaviour, including values, beliefs, rules of conduct, political organisation and economic activity, which are passed from one generation to the next by learning and not by inheritance (Hatch 1985).
> Culture is a framework for learning behaviour and communication, which might shape a child's perspective on health and illness (Craig 1986).

Given these definitions, a child's cultural background is likely to influence how they perceive and react to pain. The effect of culture on children's perception of and responses to pain is likely to be, at least in part, attributable to *social learning*. Social learning occurs when an individual learns something by observing another person doing it; in other words, it is learning by modelling (Bandura 1977). There is little conclusive evidence for differences in nociception, or the perception of pain itself, but studies suggest children's *expressions* of pain may be influenced by their cultural background (Finley et al. 2009). A recent systematic review of cross-cultural studies examining children's pain during medical procedures found cultural factors were associated with pain experience (Kristjansdottir et al. 2012). This review found that these cross-cultural differences were apparent specifically in relation to children's pain behaviour during painful procedures, their nonverbal expression of pain, and coping strategies used. Two studies exploring how children in a given culture perceive pain are outlined in Box 3.2.

BOX 3.2

Summary of research demonstrating how children's culture affects their perceptions of pain

Cheng et al. (2003)

- Explored hospitalised Taiwanese children's (*n* = 90) perceptions and experiences of acute pain using semi-structured interviews.
- Children based their definitions of pain on their own experiences and their observation of others in pain. Pain in others was identified through facial expressions or verbal reports.
- Findings were consistent with those of US studies. The few differences found related to how crying was interpreted and how parents talked to children about pain.

Jongudomkarn et al. (2006)

- Explored perceptions of pain among children in north-eastern Thailand.
- Two groups of children, aged 4–18 years, were included in the study: children in the community who had experienced pain during illness or after an accident (*n* = 17), and children who were chronically ill (*n* = 32). Participant and non-participant observation, drawings and semi-structured interviews were used to explore children's descriptions of pain.
- Children defined pain as dispiriting, as *torture* and as *suffering*. The expression of pain was influenced by cultural values of patience and endurance ('ot ton'). Children may refrain from overt expressions of pain, believing parents and family members will look after them and value endurance in the face of pain.

Culture has some impact on children's experience of pain, particularly in terms of how children express pain.

Family learning

The reaction of the family to a child in pain will teach them how to behave in a manner that is acceptable to their family. If the child receives minimal attention they will learn to cope with their pain. However, if the child receives a great deal of attention they will learn it is appropriate (and worthwhile) to express their pain. Indeed, children in families where one of the parents suffers from chronic pain are more likely to experience chronic and recurrent pain themselves (Aromaa et al. 2000; Saunders et al. 2007). Parents may reinforce particular behaviours through their own responses to their child's pain. In a study of children with juvenile idiopathic arthritis, parental 'protective' responses (such as increased parental presence and attention, or giving permission to avoid unwanted activities or responsibilities) were associated with child outcomes including decreased activity and decrease in positive mood (Connelly et al. 2010). These familial patterns can also be explained by Bandura's (1977) social learning theory, which emphasises the processes of observation, imitation and modelling, and the role of reinforcement and punishment in learning.

How a family responds to a child when they are in pain impacts on how the child behaves in future painful situations.

Gender

Research on the differences in pain perceptions and behaviour between boys and girls is contradictory and inconclusive. Some studies have found no gender difference in pain intensity during procedures (Bournaki 1997) or postoperatively (Hamers and Abu-Saad 2002; Crandall et al. 2009). Other studies have found gender differences in prevalence and response to pain as well as the use of coping strategies (Box 3.3). In chronic pain, prevalence rates for most types of pain are higher in girls than in boys (King et al. 2011), but mediating factors for the relationship between gender and pain are unclear.

Similar findings about gender and pain have been found in adults. A review of research on sex and gender differences in pain and analgesia suggests that differences do exist (Greenspan et al. 2007). The authors of this consensus report note that future efforts must be directed towards understanding the underlying mechanisms and clinical implications of these differences.

Gender differences in pain behaviours have in the past been attributed to social factors such as parents responding differently, in the same situation, depending on the gender of the child or to the fact it is more socially acceptable for girls to express pain than it is for boys. However, there is evidence that females may be more susceptible to pain

---

BOX 3.3

Summary of research about the effects of gender on children's pain experiences

Roth-Isigkeit et al. (2005)

- Explored the impact of pain on the everyday lives and activities of children and adolescents, and participants' perceptions of *triggers* for pain.
- The *Luebeck Pain-Screening Questionnaire* was used to gather information about the prevalence, characteristics and triggers of pain.
- For children (*n* = 749), aged 4–18 years, the prevalence of restrictions attributable to pain was significantly higher for girls than boys of the same age.
- Self-reported triggers also differed between girls and boys.

Lynch et al. (2007)

- Examined sex and age differences in coping strategies among children with chronic pain.
- Pain intensity (*Visual Analogue Scale*), pain coping strategies (*Pain Coping Questionnaire*) and coping efficacy were assessed in children, aged 8–12 years, and adolescents, aged 13–18 years, presenting to a paediatric chronic pain clinic (*n* = 272).
- Significant sex differences in coping strategies were found.
- Girls used social support-seeking more than boys, while boys used more behavioural distraction techniques.
- For girls, pain coping efficacy was also significantly negatively correlated with internalising/catastrophising.

Martin et al. (2007)

- Interviewed children (95 females; 48 males) three years after their last appointment at a paediatric pain clinic.
- They found females may be at higher risk for continuing pain and report greater use of healthcare, medication, physical and psychological pain-relieving strategies.

---

than males because of hormonal or neurobiological factors (Fillingim and Ness 2000; Kuba and Quinones-Jenab 2005). Both biological and psychosocial factors are, therefore, important to an understanding of sex differences in pain perception (Fillingim et al. 2009).

A child's gender may impact on how much pain they experience, how they express and cope with their pain, and how they respond to analgesic drugs or other pain relief interventions.

Additional information

For further information about the possible mechanisms underlying sex differences in pain, see: Fillingim, R.B., King, C.D., Ribeiro-Dasilva, M.C., Rahim-Williams, B. and Riley, J.L. (2009) Sex, gender, and pain: A review of recent clinical and experimental findings. *Journal of Pain* **10**(5), 447–485.

Summary

- Pain is a biopsychosocial phenomenon. Biological, psychological and social factors interact in shaping the child's experience of pain.
- A wide range of factors affect children's perception of pain and help to explain why different children behave differently when experiencing similar painful situations.
- Biological factors include the child's age, gender and genetic make-up.
- Psychological factors include fear, knowledge and previous experiences of pain.
- Social factors include culture and learning.
- Healthcare professionals must take all these factors into account when assessing and managing children's pain.

References

Anand, K.J.S. and Craig, K.D. (1996) New perspectives on the definition of pain. *Pain* 67, 3–6.

Aromaa, M., Sillanpaa, M., Rautava, P. and Helenius, H. (2000) Pain experience of children with headache and their families: A controlled study. *Pediatrics* 106(1), 270–275.

Bandura, A. (1977) *Social Learning Theory*. Prentice-Hall, New Jersey.

Bennett-Branson, S.M. and Craig, K.D. (1993) Postoperative pain in children: Developmental and family influences on spontaneous coping strategies. *Canadian Journal of Behavioral Sciences* 25, 355–383.

Bournaki, M-C. (1997) Correlates of pain-related responses to venipuncture in school-age children. *Nursing Research* 46(3), 147–154.

Chambers, C.T., Reid, G.J., McGrath, P.J. and Finley, G.A. (1996) Development and preliminary validation of a postoperative pain measure for parents. *Pain* 68(2–3), 307–313.

Cheng, S., Foster, R.L., Hester, N.O. and Huang, C. (2003) A qualitative inquiry of Taiwanese children's pain experiences. *Journal of Nursing Research* 11(4), 241–250.

Chess, S. and Thomas, A. (1986) *Temperament in Clinical Practice*. Guildford Press, New York.

Connelly, M., Anthony, K.K., Sarniak, R., Bromberg, M.H., Gil, K.M. and Schanberg, L.E. (2010) Parent pain responses as predictors of daily activities and mood in children with juvenile idiopathic arthritis: The utility of electronic diaries. *Journal of Pain and Symptom Management* 39(3), 579–590.

Conte, P.M., Walco, G.A. and Kimura, Y. (2003) Temperament and stress response in children with juvenile primary fibromyalgia syndrome. *Arthritis and Rheumatism* 48, 2923–2930.

Craig, K. (1986) Social modelling influences. In: *The Psychology of Pain* (ed. R.A. Strenbach), pp. 67–95. Raven Press Ltd, New York.

Crandall, M., Lammers, C., Senders, C. and Braun, J.V. (2009) Children's tonsillectomy experiences: Influencing factors. *Journal of Child Health Care* 13, 308–321.

Crow, C.S. (1997) Children's pain perspectives inventory (CPPI): Developmental assessment. *Pain* 72, 33–40.

Esteve, R. and Marquina-Aponte, V. (2012) Children's pain perspectives. *Child: Care, Health and Development* 3, 441–452.

Fillingim, R.B. and Ness, T.J. (2000) Sex-related hormonal influences on pain and analgesic responses. *Neuroscience & Biobehavioral Reviews* 24(4), 485–501.

Fillingim, R.B., King, C.D., Ribeiro-Dasilva, M.C., Rahim-Williams, B. and Riley, J.L. (2009) Sex, gender, and pain: A review of recent clinical and experimental findings. *Journal of Pain* 10(5), 447–485.

Finley, G.A., Kristjansdottir, O. and Forgeron, P.A. (2009) Cultural influences on the assessment of children's pain. *Pain Research and Management* 14, 33–37.

Gaffney, A. (1993) Cognitive development aspects of pain in school-age children. In: *Pain in Infants, Children and Adolescents* (eds N.L. Schechter, C.B. Berde and M. Yaster), pp. 75–86. Williams & Wilkins, Baltimore.

Gaffney, A. and Dunne, E.A. (1986) Developmental aspects of children's definitions of pain. *Pain* 26,105–117.

Gidron, Y., McGrath, P.J. and Goodday, R. (1995) The physical and psychosocial predictors of adolescents' recovery from oral surgery. *Journal of Behavioral Medicine* 18, 385–399.

Goodenough, B., Thomas, W., Champion, G.D., et al. (1999) Unravelling age effects and sex differences in needle pain: Ratings of sensory intensity and unpleasantness of venipuncture pain by children and their parents. *Pain* **80**, 179–190.

Greenspan, J.D., Craft, R.M., LeResche, L. et al.; the Consensus Working Group of the Sex, Gender, and Pain SIG of the IASP. (2007) Studying sex and gender differences in pain and analgesia: A consensus report. *Pain* **132**, S26–S45.

Hamers, J.P. and Abu-Saad, H.H. (2002) Children's pain at home following (adeno)tonsillectomy. *European Journal of Pain* **6**(3), 213–219.

Harbeck, C. and Peterson, L. (1992) Elephants dancing in my head: A developmental approach to children's concepts of specific pains. *Child Development* **63**, 138–149.

Hatch, E. (1985) Culture. In: *The Social Science Encyclopaedia* (eds A. Kuper and J. Kuper). Routledge & Kegan Paul, London.

Hauck, M. (1991) Cognitive abilities of preschool children: Implications for nurses working with young children. *Journal of Pediatric Nursing* **6**, 230–235.

Helgadottir, H.L. and Wilson, M.E. (2004) Temperament and pain in 3 to 7-year-old children undergoing tonsillectomy. *Journal of Pediatric Nursing* **19**(30), 204–213.

Huguet, A., McGrath, P.J. and Pardos, J. (2011) Development and preliminary testing of a scale to assess pain-related fear in children and adolescents. *Journal of Pain* **12**(8), 840–848.

Hurley, A. and Whelan, E.G. (1988) Cognitive development and children's perception of pain. *Pediatric Nursing* **14**(1), 21–24.

International Association for the Study of Pain (1979) Pain terms: A list with definitions and notes on usage. *Pain* **6**, 249–252.

Jeans, M.E. and Gordon, D. (1981) *Developmental characteristics of the concept of pain*. Paper presented at the 3rd world congress on pain, Edinburgh, Scotland.

Jongudomkarn, D., Aungsupakorn, N. and Camfield, L. (2006) The meanings of pain: A qualitative study of the perspectives of children living with pain in north-eastern Thailand. *Nursing and Health Sciences* **8**, 156–163.

King, S., Chambers, C.T., Huguet, A. et al. (2011) The epidemiology of chronic pain in children and adolescents revisited: A systematic review. *Pain* **152**, 2729–2738.

Kleiber, C., Schutte, D.L., McCarthy, A.M., Floria-Santos, M., Murray, J.C. and Hanrahan, K. (2007a) Predictors of topical anesthetic effectiveness in children. *Journal of Pain* **8**(2), 168–174.

Kleiber, C., Suwanraj, M., Dolan, L.A., Berg, M. and Kleese, A. (2007b) Pain-sensitive temperament and postoperative pain. *Journal of the Society of Pediatric Nursing* **12**(3), 149–158.

Kristjansdottir, O., Unruh, A.M., McAlpine, L. and McGrath, P.J. (2012) A systematic review of cross-cultural comparison studies of child, parent, and health professional outcomes associated with pediatric medical procedures. *Journal of Pain* **12**(3), 207–219.

Kuba, T. and Quinones-Jenab, V. (2005) The role of female gonadal hormones on behavioural sex differences in persistent and chronic pain: Clinical versus preclinical studies. *Brain Research Bulletin* **66**,179–188.

Lynch, A.M., Kashikar-Zuck, S., Goldschneider, K.R. and Jones, B.A. (2007) Sex and age differences in coping styles among children with chronic pain. *Journal of Pain and Symptom Management* **33**(2), 208–216.

Martin, A.L., McGrath, P.A., Brown, S.C. and Katz, J. (2007) Children with chronic pain: Impact of sex and age on long-term conditions. *Pain* **128**, 13–19.

McCarthy, A., Kleiber, C., Hanrahan, K., Zimmerman, M. B., Westhus, N. and Allen, S. (2010) Factors explaining children's responses to intravenous needle insertions. *Nursing Research* **59**(6), 407–416.

McGrath, P.J. and McAlpine, L. (1993) Psychologic perspectives on pediatric pain. *Journal of Pediatrics* **122**, S2–S8.

McGrath, P.A. and Hillier, L.M. (2003) Modifying the psychologic factors that intensify children's pain and prolong disability. In: *Pain in Infants, Children and Adolescents* (eds N.L. Schechter, C.B. Berde and M. Yaster), 2nd edition, pp. 85–127. Lippincott, Williams & Wilkins, Baltimore.

Mogil, J.S., Yu, L. and Basbaum, A.I. (2000) Pain genes? Natural variation and transgenic mutants. *Annual Review of Neuroscience* **23**, 777–811.

Palmero, T.M. and Drotar, D. (1996) Prediction of children's postoperative pain: The role of presurgical expectations and anticipatory emotions. *Journal of Pediatric Psychology* **21**, 683–698.

Rocha, E.M., Prkachin, K.M., Beaumont, S.L., Hardy, C.L. and Zumbo, B.D. (2003) Pain reactivity and somatization in kindergarten-age children. *Journal of Pediatric Psychology* **28**, 47–57.

Ross, D.M. and Ross, S.A. (1984) Childhood pain: the school-aged child's viewpoint. *Pain* 20,179–191.

Roth-Isigkeit, A., Thyen, U., Stoven, H., Schwarzenberger, J. and Schumaker, P. (2005) Pain among children and adolescents: Restrictions in daily living and triggering factors. *Pediatrics* 115(2), 152–162.

Saunders, K., Von Korff, M., LeResche, L. and Mancl, L. (2007) Relationship of common pain conditions in mothers and children. *Clinical Journal of Pain* 23(3), 204–213.

Scott, R. (1978) 'It hurts red': A preliminary study of children's perceptions of pain. *Perceptual and Motor Skills* 47, 787–791.

Twycross, A. (1998) Children's cognitive level and their perceptions of pain. In: *Paediatric Pain Management: A multi-disciplinary approach* (eds A. Twycross, A. Moriarty and T. Betts), pp 25–37. Radcliffe Medical Press, Oxford.

Weisman, S.J., Bernstein, B. and Schechter, N.L. (1998) Consequences of inadequate analgesia during painful procedures in children. *Archives of Pediatric Adolescent Medicine* 152,147–149.

Wilson, A.C., Lewandowski, A.S. and Palermo, T.M. (2011) Fear-avoidance beliefs and parental responses to pain in adolescents with chronic pain. *Pain Research and Management* 16(3),178–182.

Zubieta, J-K., Heitzeg, M.M., Smith, Y.R. et al. (2003) COMT val158met genotype affects [mu]-opioid neurotransmitter responses to a pain stressor. *Science* 299(5610), 1240–1243.

CHAPTER 4

Pharmacology of Analgesic Drugs

Stephanie Dowden

Paediatric Palliative Care, Princess Margaret Hospital for Children, Australia

Introduction

Understanding the pharmacology of analgesic drugs will enhance clinicians' pain management practice and thus improve management of pain in children. This chapter provides an overview of the pharmacology of commonly used analgesics and adjuvant medications. Misconceptions related to opioids will be discussed including addiction, tolerance and dependence. Finally the non-medical use of prescription opioids will be examined.

Most analgesic drugs are administered *off-label* (outside recommended guidelines for age, weight, indication or route) in children. There is limited data due to a lack of paediatric multicentre randomised controlled trials (RCTs), leaving clinicians to rely on best practice principles or recommendations from leading children's hospitals (World Health Organization [WHO] 2007, 2010a; Kimland and Odlind 2012). To address this issue, the European Union and the United States have introduced legislation to improve safety and to promote knowledge of medicines for children, but change is slow (Kimland and Odlind 2012).

While analgesic drugs have a significant role in pain management; combining their effect with physical and pharmacological strategies optimises pain management by integrating methods to block, reduce and modify pain responses (McGrath 2005; Association of Paediatric Anaesthetists [APA] 2012). These strategies are described in Chapter 5.

Misconceptions

The key misconceptions about using analgesic drugs for children are outlined in Table 4.1.

Managing Pain in Children: A Clinical Guide for Nurses and Healthcare Professionals, Second Edition.
Edited by Alison Twycross, Stephanie Dowden, and Jennifer Stinson.

Table 4.1 Misconceptions about using analgesic drugs for children

Misconception	Facts
Children are more sensitive to analgesic drugs than adults	• Children are not more sensitive to analgesic drugs than other adults, provided age-appropriate prescribing is followed
Children are at greater risk (than adults) of addiction from opioids	• The risk of opioid addiction in children has been exaggerated. with the incidence in the general population <3%
Opioids are unsafe for infants and children	• Safe opioid use for infants and children requires dose calculation according to their age, weight and medical condition

Source: Charlton (2005); McGrath (2005)

Table 4.2 Definitions of opioid terminology

Term	Definition
Tolerance	• Decreased effectiveness of a drug over time, thus a higher dose of the drug is needed to achieve the same effect • Tolerance develops to desired (analgesia) and undesired (sedation, pruritus [itch] etc.) effects of opioids at different rates
Physical dependence	• A physiological response to the abrupt discontinuation (or dose reduction or reversal) of a drug that leads to a withdrawal (abstinence) syndrome
Addiction	• Psychological dependence on drugs with aberrant drug seeking and drug using behaviour that is characterised by cravings, compulsion, loss of control and lack of concern for social or health consequences
Withdrawal syndrome	• A cluster of physiological signs and symptoms that occur following the abrupt discontinuation of an opioid
Pseudoaddiction	• Behaviours that may seem to be inappropriately drug-seeking but are a result of undertreatment of pain and resolve when pain relief is adequate

Source: Adapted from Macintyre et al. (2010)

Addiction, Tolerance and Dependence

Confusion exists among healthcare professionals about addiction, tolerance and physical dependence (Charlton 2005; Macintyre et al. 2010). Misinformation can be communicated to colleagues, patients and families, causing unnecessary anxiety and suboptimal pain management (Macintyre et al. 2010). To encourage uniformity of practice a number of professional organisations including the American Pain Society (APS), the American Academy of Pain Medicine (AAPM) and the American Society of Addiction Medicine (ASAM) have developed consensus statements and agreed definitions (AAPM 2001). Macintyre et al. (2010) provides a summary of these statements (Table 4.2).

Addiction risk

Fears of addiction related to the *short-term* use of opioids for severe pain are unsupported. The risk is considered no different to the risk of addiction in the general population, which is <3% (Ballantyne and LaForge 2007; Manchikanti et al. 2012a). There is no paediatric-specific data. There is some data suggesting higher incidence of addiction associated with *long-term* opioid use in adolescents and adults; the main at-risk groups are individuals with a history of substance abuse, risk-taking behaviours or depression (Fishbain et al. 2008; Carinci and Mao 2010; Manchikanti et al. 2012a).

Signs of both tolerance and physical dependence can occur in patients of all ages following administration of opioids and some other drugs (e.g. benzodiazepines and other sedatives) for more than 5–10 days (Anand et al. 2010). Importantly, *all* opioid-tolerant patients (taking opioids for medical *or* non-medical reasons) should be identified, with steps taken to ensure that their pain is appropriately managed and withdrawal syndrome is avoided (Box 4.1). Pseudo-addiction can be created due to clinicians with a poor understanding of the risk of addiction who withhold or minimise analgesia for patients with chronic or recurrent painful conditions. This, in turn, can lead to blaming and stigmatisation of the patient, rather than being prescribed effective analgesia or referral to pain specialists for ongoing management.

Opioid-induced hyperalgesia

Opioids paradoxically can *cause* pain. Opioid-induced hyperalgesia (OIH) presents as worsening pain despite increasing doses of opioids and usually occurs when high doses of opioids are given.

Management includes switching to another opioid or addition of adjuvant analgesics.
See www.eperc.mcw.edu/EPERC/FastFactsIndex/ff_142.htm

BOX 4.1

Pain management for opioid-tolerant patients

Who are opioid-tolerant patients?

- Patients with a history of non-medical opioid use or on a drug treatment (e.g. methadone) programme
- Patients with chronic cancer pain or non-cancer pain being treated with opioids
- Patients with acute opioid tolerance due to recent high opioid requirements, e.g. following surgery or major trauma

Key principles

- Ensure effective analgesia
- Be aware some patients may have or develop opioid-induced hyperalgesia (OIH)
- *Do not* withhold opioids (this places the patient at risk of acute opioid withdrawal)
- Usual opioid regimens should be continued and used as a starting point for other analgesia
- Adjuvant medications may assist with pain relief
- Opioid-tolerant patients may require higher doses of opioids, report higher pain scores and have lower levels of opioid adverse drug reactions than opioid-naïve patients
- Be alert to signs of opioid withdrawal, i.e. sweating, nausea and/or vomiting, agitation, diarrhoea, yawning, dilated pupils, anxiety, insomnia, tachycardia, hypertension and cramping abdominal pain

Source: Data from Macintyre et al. 2010

Opioid weaning protocols

Up to 60% of children who experience a critical illness requiring prolonged administration of analgesia and sedation develop *withdrawal syndrome*. This is due to opioids and benzodiazepines being stopped abruptly or weaned too fast (Anand et al. 2010). While this has been recognised since the 1990s, few hospitals managed this in a systematic way until recently (Birchley 2009). Weaning protocols and withdrawal screening tools have been developed based on tools used for infants with drug withdrawal (neonatal abstinence syndrome; NAS) (Birchley 2009).

Additional information

One screening tool that can be used for research or clinical practice in children is the Withdrawal Assessment Tool-1 [WAT-1]:

Franck, L.S., Harris, S., Soetenga, D., Amling, J. and Curley, M. (2008) The withdrawal assessment tool (WAT-1): Measuring iatrogenic withdrawal symptoms in pediatric critical care. *Pediatric Critical Care Medicine* **9**(6), 573–580. Available from: http://nursing.ucsf.edu/faculty/linda-franck

---

How Drugs Work

This section will summarise the main points relating to drugs and how they work, with particular emphasis on analgesic drugs. Additional reading of key pharmacology texts and Chapter 2 will assist in understanding the process of pain and how analgesic drugs affect and modify this.

- A drug is a bioactive molecule that is not normally a part of the body. It may be a therapeutic agent, a poison or a food component.
- The action of a drug is the chemical interaction between the drug and body tissue.
- Each drug affects the body in a specific way. However, no drug is completely specific in its action, which is why adverse drug reactions (*side effects*) can occur (Rang et al. 2012).
- The aim of drug therapy is to give the right dose of a drug, that is, enough to achieve a useful effect but not so much as to be toxic (Begg 2008).
- The two key pharmacological actions are pharmacodynamics (the study of drug action) and pharmacokinetics (the study of drug movement).

Commonly used pharmacology definitions are outlined in Table 4.3.

Pharmacodynamics

Pharmacodynamics is the mechanism of drug actions and their biochemical and physiological effects on body systems, that is, *what the drug does to the body* (Kanneh 2002a; Begg 2008).

- Drug molecules must be *bound* to a body substance to reach the target tissue and produce a physiological response (Rang et al. 2012).
- There are four types of substances to which drugs may be bound: receptors, ion channels, carriers and enzymes.

Table 4.3 Pharmacology definitions

Term	Definition
Adjuvant analgesics	Drugs that are not primarily analgesics but have independent or additive analgesic properties
Adverse drug reaction (ADR)	Undesired effect of the drug or consequences of the drug–receptor interaction occurring at usual or desired doses of the drug
Affinity	The attraction between the drug and the receptor (described as high or low)
Agonist	A drug that binds to a receptor and activates it (fully or partially)
Antagonist	A drug that binds to a receptor without activating it, but blocking agonist access
Bioavailability	The rate and extent of drug absorbed into systemic circulation after administration. Bioavailability is 100% after intravenous administration
Ceiling effect	When a higher dose of a drug will not produce a greater effect
Clearance	The rate at which a drug is eliminated from the body over time
Dose interval	Time needed between drug doses to keep the drug within the therapeutic index
Drug action	The action between the drug and receptor
Drug–drug interaction	When the effects of one drug are increased or decreased by another drug
Duration of action	Time the drug action lasts at an effective concentration
Enzymes	Proteins that regulate the rate of chemical reactions in the body
First-pass metabolism	Drugs that are taken orally enter the portal (hepatic) circulation and are partly metabolised prior to entering the systemic circulation
Half-life ($t^{1/2}$)	Time taken (in hours) for the drug concentration in blood to fall by one half its original value (due to metabolism or elimination)
Hormones	Chemical substances produced in the body by endocrine glands that initiate or regulate activity of some cells or organs
Ion channels	Pores in the cell membrane that allow passage of ions into and out of the cell
Loading dose	Administering a higher dose to achieve early therapeutic plasma levels
Maintenance dose	Dose required to maintain plasma drug levels at a steady state
Onset of action	Time it takes for the drug to begin working
Pro-drug	A drug that is metabolised in the body to another form before it becomes active
Receptors	Protein molecules activated by transmitters or hormones
Side effect	See *adverse drug reaction*
Steady state	The drug at a uniform level in the body, where the administration rate of the drug equals the elimination rate of the drug. Time to steady state is usually $4 \times t^{1/2}$
Therapeutic index (or 'therapeutic window')	The variance between the therapeutic dose and the toxic dose of a drug: Narrow or low therapeutic index drugs have a high risk of toxicity Wide or high therapeutic index drugs have a low risk of toxicity
Volume of distribution	How and where the drug is distributed around the body

Source: Kanneh (2002a, 2002b); Begg (2008); Neal (2012)

Receptors are proteins that perform an action in response to recognising another substance. Some drugs must combine with receptors to achieve an effect, like a key being inserted into a lock. Drugs bind to receptors in response to the concentration of the drug and their ability to bind (*affinity*) to a receptor. The higher the affinity of the drug, the lower the dose needed to produce an effect. Drugs can be *agonists* (that bind to receptors and activate them) or *antagonists* (that bind to receptors without activation or which block their usual action).

Morphine is a *full agonist* at the μ (mu) opioid receptor. It has strong *affinity* for the mu receptor, thus even a small dose will exert an effect. Morphine is a *partial agonist* at the δ (delta) and κ (kappa) opioid receptors.
Naloxone is an *antagonist* at the mu opioid receptor. This means it blocks the binding of morphine to the mu receptor, which in turn blocks the action of morphine.

Ion channels are pores in cell walls that allow passage of ions. Some ion channels require a receptor to be bound by an agonist before they open, with other ion channels being directly targeted by drugs (Rang et al. 2012).

Local anaesthetics (e.g. lignocaine [lidocaine], ropivicaine) directly target sodium ion channels in nerve fibres.
By blocking the sodium channels, conduction along the nerve fibre is prevented, thus blocking transmission of sensations such as pain and touch.

Carriers are protein molecules that help to *carry* or transport substances across cell membranes (Rang et al. 2012). Some carriers work at nerve terminals and are involved with the movement of neurotransmitters (e.g. serotonin, noradrenaline, γ-aminobutyric acid (GABA) and glutamate). These carriers are specifically targeted by some drugs, which can reduce or enhance the amount of neurotransmitter at the synapse.

Tramadol inhibits the reuptake of serotonin and noradrenaline from nerve synapses, thus leading to higher levels of these pain-modulating neurotransmitters.

Enzymes are biological catalysts that control the biochemical reactions of a cell (Bryant and Knights 2010). Some drugs can inhibit the action of an enzyme, thus altering the physiological response.

Nonsteroidal anti-inflammatory drugs (NSAIDs), such as ibuprofen and diclofenac, inhibit the action of the enzyme cyclo-oxygenase, which in turn stops the synthesis of prostaglandins and thus reduces pain and the inflammatory response.

Pharmacokinetics

Pharmacokinetics is the process of the movement of drugs through the body, involving absorption, distribution, metabolism and elimination (Kanneh 2002b). Begg (2008) describes pharmacokinetics more simply as *what the body does to the drug.*

Absorption involves entrance of the drug into the circulatory system from the site of entry. Absorption is dependent on factors such as the drug formulation, the route of administration, the blood flow at the site of administration and the surface area exposed to the drug (Kanneh 2002b).

Practice point

The rectal route of administration can lead to erratic drug absorption due to drug placement issues, rectal blood flow and faecal loading.
With the oral route of administration, liquid preparations are absorbed faster than tablet or capsule formulations.
Intravenous administration of drugs provides the fastest absorption.

Distribution of the drug around the body occurs once it enters the circulatory system and then reaches the target tissue. Drugs are mostly bound to plasma proteins and *piggy-back* on them to get to their destination. Drug distribution is affected by cardiac output, total amount of body water (infants and children have relatively more body water compared to adults) and the concentration of plasma proteins (decreased in infants compared to older children and adults) (Kanneh 2002b).

Metabolism is the process of breaking down drugs into active and/or inactive components (*metabolites*) prior to elimination. This process is mostly carried out by enzymes and occurs predominantly in the liver. The major enzyme group involved in metabolism of 70–80% of drugs is the cytochrome P450 enzymes (also known as *CYP enzymes*) (Begg 2008; Bryant and Knights 2010).

Practice point

The capacity for CYP enzymes to metabolise drugs has a genetic basis. Individuals can be poor metabolisers, intermediate metabolisers, extensive metabolisers or ultra-metabolisers of drugs. Thus, individual variations can range from no drug effect to serious adverse drug reactions (i.e. death).
In the future, screening to determine CYP phenotypes (pharmacogenetics) may allow for tailoring of analgesia specific to the individual's genetic makeup, thus reducing ADRs and allowing the smallest dose for the greatest effect.

The liver metabolises some drugs so efficiently that the amount reaching the systemic circulation is less than the amount first absorbed. This is known as *first-pass metabolism* and explains why larger doses are needed orally than by other routes. Morphine, which has a high first-pass effect, has a significant dosing difference when administered orally versus intravenously (IV), with the oral dose being two to three times greater than the intravenous dose.

Some drugs (pro-drugs) are inactive when administered and need to undergo metabolism to be converted from an inactive form to an active form (e.g. diamorphine and codeine are converted to morphine).

Elimination is the process of removal of the drug from the body. It occurs most commonly via renal excretion, with lesser amounts removed via the gastrointestinal system, expiration, saliva, sweat and tears. Drugs that are removed from the body primarily by renal excretion can cause toxicity when renal function is impaired (e.g. morphine or nonsteroidal anti-inflammatory drugs [NSAIDs]).

Practice point

If a patient has liver dysfunction they will have decreased rates of drug *metabolism*, thus increased systemic drug levels and an increased risk of toxicity.

If a patient has renal dysfunction they will have decreased drug *elimination* and thus increased systemic drug levels and an increased risk of toxicity.

Neonates have reduced liver and renal function due to *organ immaturity*.

Consequently, patients with liver and/or renal dysfunction and all neonates need lower drug doses, longer intervals between doses, or to be prescribed drugs with fewer liver or renal effects.

Routes of Drug Administration

The route of drug administration affects the speed of onset and the amount of therapeutic response (Bryant and Knights 2010). The effect that is desired from the drug will also influence the route chosen; for example, a topical route would be chosen for a drug that is required to act on the skin, but for a rapid systemic effect the parenteral or inhalation route would be more appropriate. There are four main routes of drug administration: enteral, parenteral, inhalation and topical/transmucosal (Table 4.4).

Other aspects to consider are the advantages and disadvantages of using different routes of analgesic drug administration, some of which are specific to children. All these factors need to be considered when deciding the best route to use (Table 4.5).

The oral route is the preferred route of administration for most analgesic drugs. For rapid analgesia with acute severe pain, titration using intermittent intravenous bolus doses is the most effective strategy (Macintyre et al. 2010; WHO 2012).

Selection of Analgesic Drugs

In addition to deciding the most appropriate *route* of administration it is also important to consider the most appropriate *type* of analgesic drug to give.

Practice point

For optimal analgesic drug selection:

- assess pain (see Chapter 6);
- identify the type and severity of pain (see Chapters 7, 8 and 9);
- select the most appropriate analgesic drug considering route, ADRs, benefits, risks and safety.

Table 4.4 Four main routes of drug administration

Route	Example
Enteral (via the gastrointestinal system) *This is the most common route of drug administration*	Oral (PO) Nasogastric (NG) Nasojejunal (NJ) Percutaneous endoscopic gastrostomy/gastric tube (PEG or G) or gastrostomy/jejunal tube (PEJ or GJ) Rectal (PR)
Parenteral (via injection)	Intra-articular Intravenous (IV) Intramuscular (IM) Subcutaneous (SC) Intrathecal (spinal) (IT) Epidural Intraosseous (IO)
Inhalation (via the respiratory system)	Gas Mist/aerosol Nebuliser/inhaler
Topical/transmucosal (via the skin and mucous membranes)	Skin Eyes Ears Transdermal (TD) Intranasal (IN) Sublingual/buccal

Source: Bryant and Knights (2010)

BOX 4.2

Two-step strategy for pain management

Step 1 (mild pain):

Paracetamol (acetaminophen) and/or ibuprofen

Step 2 (moderate to severe pain):

Strong opioid (morphine is recommended as first-line)
Adjuvant analgesics may be added at either step to enhance pain relief

Source: WHO (2012)

WHO analgesic ladder

The WHO *analgesic ladder* was developed as a model for providing guidelines to clinicians about cancer pain management (WHO 1996). It offered a three-step approach to pain management which suggested that, as pain increased, analgesia should be adjusted accordingly. The ladder was revised in 2012 to a two-step ladder (WHO 2012) (Box 4.2). The key aims of the new approach are:

- using a two-step strategy;
- dosing at regular intervals;
- appropriate route of administration;
- adapting treatment to the individual child.

Table 4.5 Advantages and disadvantages of the routes of analgesic drug administration

Route	Advantages	Disadvantages
Oral	Painless Large drug availability Preferred by children	Slow acting Problem if child is nauseated/vomiting Child may not be able to swallow Analgesics may have unpleasant taste First-pass metabolism Reliant on gut function
Nasogastric	Large drug availability Useful for high volume/unpleasant tasting medication	Slow acting Invasive/painful to insert NG tube Additional nursing care required Disliked by some children First-pass metabolism Reliant on gut function
Rectal	Useful if child is nauseated/vomiting Less first-pass metabolism Not reliant on gut function Useful if no IV, avoids IM injections	Unreliable bioavailability Slowest acting Limited drug choice Disliked by some children
Intravenous	Fast acting, allows rapid analgesia Avoids first-pass metabolism Useful for intermittent bolus, infusion and patient-controlled analgesia (PCA)	Invasive/painful to insert IV Additional nursing care required More ADR due to high drug bioavailability
Intramuscular	Easy insertion	Painful Disliked by children Slower onset Variability in drug levels/absorption
Subcutaneous	Easy insertion Avoids need for IV Useful in community settings Useful for intermittent bolus or infusion	Invasive/painful to insert Slower onset
Epidural	Fast acting Extremely effective, allows complete analgesia	Invasive, needs highly skilled clinicians Inserted under sedation/anaesthesia Additional nursing care required Risks/adverse effects of procedure
Transmucosal	Avoids first-pass metabolism Not reliant on gut function Fast acting and short acting Less invasive	Variable acceptability by children Limited drug availability
Topical	Least invasive route Painless	Very limited drug availability

Source: WHO (2010a, 2012)

Two-step strategy

The WHO 2012 guidelines were developed to provide *evidence-based recommendations* to improve pain management in children experiencing *persisting pain related to medical diseases*. The guidelines do not specifically apply to pain from trauma, surgery or procedures. WHO (2012) considers that in most situations adequate analgesia can be provided using this two-step approach. The *starting* step should be chosen according to current pain severity: step 1 for mild pain and step 2 for moderate to severe pain. Adjuvant analgesics are added as required according to the type and quality of the pain.

The strategy recognises that *weak* opioids have limited efficacy (e.g. codeine or dihydrocodeine [hydrocodone]) or lack evidence in children (e.g. tramadol) and thus little role in acute pain management. Instead, small doses of *strong* opioids should be titrated as they are more efficacious (WHO 2012). WHO (2012) recognises that these recommendations may not reflect current practice, and acknowledges that, as new data on safety and efficacy of different analgesics emerges, this approach may need to be revised. For optimal analgesia, combinations of analgesic drugs with different mechanisms of action can be given. This is known as *multi-modal analgesia* and is discussed in Chapter 7.

The following sections will provide details of the main analgesic drugs in three categories: non-opioids, opioids and adjuvant analgesic drugs. All drug doses described apply to children less than 50 kg. Once over 50 kg (approximately 12 years), adult dosing regimes apply.

Non-Opioid Analgesic Drugs

Paracetamol (acetaminophen)

Overview

Paracetamol:

- is the most commonly used analgesic drug for children;
- has antipyretic (fever reducing) activity, but minimal anti-inflammatory effects (unlike NSAIDs);
- is highly effective as a sole analgesic for mild pain with an excellent safety profile (Southey et al. 2009; Pierce and Voss 2010);
- enhances analgesia when used in combination with NSAIDs or tramadol (Remy et al. 2006);
- has opioid-sparing effects (reduces the amount of opioid required) of up to 20% in adults and children when given in combination with opioids (Remy et al. 2006; Hong et al. 2010a);
- has a greater opioid-sparing effect in children when combined with an opioid and NSAIDs (Hong et al. 2010b).

Action

- The mechanism of action is not fully understood. It is thought that paracetamol selectively inhibits prostaglandin synthesis (probably by inhibiting cyclo-oxygenase-3 [COX-3]) in the central nervous system (CNS), which is why it has antipyretic and analgesic actions but no anti-inflammatory effects or unwanted gastrointestinal effects (Chandrasekharan et al. 2002; Remy et al. 2006).

- Normal gastrointestinal function is required for oral paracetamol administration; thus if the child has an ileus the intravenous or rectal routes should be used (Anderson and Palmer 2006; APA 2012).

Metabolism/elimination

Paracetamol is metabolised in the liver; glucuronide and sulphate are the main metabolites, which are excreted via the kidneys. Another metabolite, N-acetyl-p-benzoquinone-imine (NAPQI) is responsible for the toxic effects of paracetamol. NAPQI is normally metabolised to a harmless compound by glutathione (an antioxidant enzyme). However, with excessive paracetamol levels (>150 mg/kg) glutathione is unable to metabolise NAPQI rapidly enough and liver toxicity results. In some clinical groups (nutritionally compromised, liver disease or abnormal gastrointestinal function) glutathione levels are depleted, leaving these patients at greater risk of paracetamol toxicity (Remy et al. 2006; Macintyre et al. 2010; Bryant and Knights 2010).

Practice point

Paracetamol toxicity is most likely to occur: (i) following a paracetamol overdose; (ii) with long-term paracetamol use; (iii) in patients who already have some degree of liver dysfunction; and (iv) in neonates.

Liver toxicity and subsequent fulminant liver failure present at least two to three days following a paracetamol overdose.

Unfortunately, early symptoms of paracetamol poisoning are nonspecific (nausea or vomiting, anorexia and abdominal pain). Thus if the paracetamol overdose is unsuspected or unreported, the consequences can be fatal.

With early intervention NAPQI is neutralised by administration of N-acetylcysteine to form a non-toxic compound that is excreted via the kidneys.

Adverse drug reactions

There are very low rates of ADRs with paracetamol, but the potential for hepatotoxicity still exists (Remy et al. 2006; Southey et al. 2009; Pierce and Voss 2010; Jones 2011). Acute hepatotoxicity is considered to be very unlikely when therapeutic dose regimes are followed. Minor ADRs from paracetamol are uncommon and include gastrointestinal upset and skin reactions.

Dose, onset time, peak effect and half-life

- Paracetamol can be administered via oral, rectal and intravenous routes (Table 4.6).
- For greatest efficacy a loading dose is suggested (in hospital settings only).
- Due to their immature liver function, neonates require reduced doses.

Nonsteroidal anti-inflammatory drugs

Overview

Nonsteroidal anti-inflammatory drugs:

- are used for the treatment of mild to moderate pain and have antipyretic and anti-inflammatory effects (APA 2012);
- have a high safety and efficacy profile and a significant opioid-sparing effect (Southey et al. 2009; Pierce and Voss 2010; APA 2012);

Table 4.6 Paracetamol (acetaminophen) doses for children (<50 kg)

Infant and child doses	Route	Dose	Onset/Peak/t1/2
	Oral	Loading dose: 20 mg/kg Then: 10–15 mg/kg 4- to 6-hourly (maximum dose: 60 mg/kg/day)	Onset time: 30–60 min Peak effect: 1–2 h t1/2: 1–3 h
	Rectal	Loading dose: 20–30 mg/kg Then: 20 mg/kg 6-hourly (maximum dose: 60 mg/kg/day)	Onset time and peak effect: variable (peak effect up to 2.5 h)
	IV	15 mg/kg 6-hourly (maximum dose: 40–60 mg/kg/day)	Onset time: 15–30 min Peak effect: 1 h t1/2: 1.5–3 h
Neonatal doses	**Route**	**Dose**	**Onset/Peak/t1/2**
Term neonates	Oral	5–10 mg/kg 6- to 8-hourly (maximum dose: 60 mg/kg/day)	Onset time: 30–60 min Peak effect: 1–3 h
	Rectal	20 mg/kg 8-hourly (maximum dose: 60 mg/kg/day)	Onset time and peak effect: variable (peak effect up to 2.5 h)
	IV	7.5 mg/kg 8-hourly (maximum dose: 30 mg/kg/day)	Onset time: 15–30 min Peak effect: 1 h

Source: Data from Anderson (2008); Palmer et al. (2008); Macintyre et al. (2010); Jones (2011); APA (2012); WHO (2012)

Note: Dosing guidelines vary between organisations and countries. The author has described doses or dose ranges based on the best available evidence at time of publication. Readers are advised to follow their own institution's guidelines.

- in children are used mainly in the postoperative setting, following trauma or for home-based pain and fever management and are also used for chronic pain and for bone pain caused by cancer (APA 2012);
- in combination with paracetamol are effective in the management of paediatric migraine (Damen et al. 2005);
- are first-line agents for persistent pain associated with juvenile idiopathic arthritis (Stinson et al. 2012).

Acetylsalicylic acid (aspirin) is indicated in the management of paediatric Kawasaki disease, rheumatic fever and juvenile arthritis (WHO 2010a).

Action

NSAIDs act by inhibiting the synthesis of prostaglandins by inhibiting the production of COX-1 (cyclo-oxygenase-1) and COX-2 (cyclo-oxygenase-2) enzymes. This in turn reduces inflammatory pain-inducing chemicals and thus decreases the response of peripheral and central pain receptors. Non-selective NSAIDs (e.g. ibuprofen, diclofenac, indomethacin, aspirin) block both COX-1 and COX-2, hence their higher incidence of ADRs. Selective NSAIDs (e.g. celecoxib, parecoxib) selectively block COX-2 in preference to COX-1. These are known as COX-2 inhibitors or coxibs. The effects of COX-1 and COX-2 enzymes are compared in Table 4.7.

Table 4.7 Comparing the effects of COX-1 and COX-2 enzymes

COX-1	COX-2
Present in most body tissues	Present in inflammatory cells when activated
Involved in cell/tissue homeostasis, maintain gastric acid balance, maintain protective mucous lining in gastrointestinal tract, maintain renal blood flow, platelet function and bronchodilation	Responsible for many mediators of inflammation leading to: vasodilation, oedema, hyperalgesia and pyrogenesis (fever production)
Blocking COX-1 causes gastric irritation/gastric ulceration, renal impairment or renal failure, platelet dysfunction (bleeding) and bronchospasm	Blocking COX-2 causes analgesia, anti-inflammatory and antipyretic actions

---

Practice point

When coxibs were introduced in the late 1990s it was thought that they would be safer than existing NSAIDs due to selective inhibition of COX-2 without affecting COX-1.

The level of selectivity was not as great as was first thought, with large numbers of adult patients suffering adverse cardiac and vascular events from some coxibs. Consequently, rofecoxib and valdecoxib were withdrawn from the market in 2004–2005.

Current recommendations suggest that both coxibs and nonselective NSAIDs should be used at their lowest effective dose, and long-term use avoided where possible.

Source: Conaghan (2012)

Metabolism/elimination
- Most NSAIDs undergo metabolism in the liver (Kokki 2003).
- Two-thirds of the drug or its metabolites are excreted via the kidneys, with the remainder excreted in the faeces (Kokki 2003).

Adverse drug reactions
- Due to their inhibition of COX-1 enzymes, NSAIDs have the potential for serious ADRs including: bleeding, gastric irritation, asthma and renal impairment.
- The risk of bleeding following surgery (mainly tonsillectomy) has been overstated but is still present (Kokki 2003; Anderson and Palmer 2006; APA 2012).
- NSAIDs may induce asthma in *aspirin/NSAID-sensitive asthmatics*, especially those with multiple allergies, severe eczema or nasal polyp disease (Anderson and Palmer 2006; APA 2012).
- Renal blood flow may be reduced and renal failure may result, particularly in children with pre-existing renal impairment, hypovolaemia or dehydration (APA 2012).
- NSAIDs should be avoided in children with liver failure (APA 2012).
- Concerns that NSAIDs slow bone healing, particularly following bone grafting, have not been demonstrated in human studies. The benefits of short-term use may outweigh the potential risks (Kokki 2003; APA 2012).
- Less serious ADRs include skin reactions, diarrhoea, nausea and vomiting.

Reye's syndrome

Use of aspirin in children with viral illnesses is associated with an increased risk of developing Reye's syndrome (acute encephalopathy with liver damage), although the degree of causality is questioned.

Thus it is not recommended that aspirin be used in children under 16 years in the UK (under 19 years in the USA) unless on the advice of a doctor.

This age recommendation varies in different countries.

Source: James (2004); Schror (2007)

Practice point

Adverse reactions to NSAIDs can occur with *all* routes of administration, not just the oral route.

NSAIDs should be avoided or used with caution in patients with:

- bleeding disorders or at risk of haemorrhage;
- renal or liver impairment;
- dehydration or hypovolaemia;
- moderate to severe asthma with nasal polyp disease;
- known aspirin or NSAID allergy or hypersensitivity;
- history of gastrointestinal ulceration or bleeding;
- planned major surgery (APA 2012).

NSAIDs are *not recommended* as analgesics for infants under the age of six months due to risk of renal toxicity and concerns they may interfere with cerebral and pulmonary blood flow (APA 2012).

Dose, onset time, peak effect and half-life

- NSAIDs can be administered via oral, rectal and IV routes (Table 4.8).
- Ibuprofen is the most studied NSAID in children, with more evidence of safety and efficacy than other NSAIDs (WHO 2012; APA 2012).

Practice point

Most non-opioid analgesic drugs have a *ceiling effect*, which means that doses higher than the recommended dose will not produce greater pain relief.

Most opioids (except codeine) do not have a ceiling effect other than that imposed by ADRs; therefore, larger doses can be given for increasing severity of pain.

Table 4.8 NSAID doses for children (<50 kg)

Drug	Route	Dose	Onset/Peak/t1/2
Ibuprofen	Oral	5–10 mg/kg 6- to 8-hourly (maximum 40 mg/kg/day)	Onset time: 20–30 min Peak effect: 1–2 h t1/2: 1–2 h
Celecoxib	Oral	10–25 kg: 50 mg 12-hourly >25 kg: 100 mg 12-hourly	Peak effect: 3 h t1/2: 3.7 h
Diclofenac	Oral or rectal	0.5–2 mg/kg 8- to 12-hourly (maximum 3 mg/kg/day)	Onset time: 20–30 min Peak effect: 1–2 h t1/2: 1–2 h
Ketorolac	Oral or IV	0.5 mg/kg 6- to 8-hourly (maximum 2 mg/kg/day) *IV = maximum 20 doses* *or 5 days duration*	Onset time: 20–30 min Peak effect: 1–2 h t1/2: 4–6 h (oral); 4 h (IV)
Naproxen	Oral	5–7.5 mg/kg 12-hourly (maximum 500 mg/dose)	Onset time: 20–30 min Peak effect: 2–4 h t1/2: 12–15 h

Source: Data from Stempak et al. (2002); Kokki (2003); Kraemer and Rose (2009); Standing et al. (2009); WHO (2010a); APA (2012)

Note: Dosing guidelines vary between organisations and countries. The author has described doses or dose ranges based on the best available evidence at time of publication. Readers are advised to follow their own institution's guidelines.

Opioid Analgesic Drugs

Overview
Opium:

- was discovered in pre-biblical times and is extracted from the opium poppy;
- was widely used from the Middle Ages in a medicine known as *tincture of opium* or laudanum;
- contains about 20 alkaloids (compounds), two of which, morphine and codeine, have analgesic action.

Opioid or opiate or narcotic?

Opioid: any substance with morphine-like actions including natural, semi-synthetic and synthetic opioids. *(This is the preferred term.)*

Opiate: any drug derived from the opium poppy (e.g. morphine), thus excluding synthetic opioids such as fentanyl.

Narcotic: an obsolete term for opioids because governments, law enforcement and media use the term to refer to drugs of addiction and other illicit drugs, thus it has no place in medical terminology about analgesic drugs.

Opioids:

- are used for treating moderate to severe pain;
- come in different levels of potency and efficacy. They are referred to as *weak opioids* (e.g. codeine, dihydrocodeine [hydrocodone], tramadol) or *strong opioids* (e.g. morphine, hydromorphone, fentanyl);
- can be given in reduced doses without loss of analgesic effect when used in combination with non-opioids such as paracetamol and NSAIDs.

Strong opioids have no ceiling dose for severe pain, with dosing only limited by ADRs.
  For acute pain management, one opioid is not superior over others; however, some opioids are better tolerated, thus some patients may benefit from changing to another opioid if they have adverse effects (Macintyre et al. 2010).

Action
- All opioids bind to opioid receptors located in the peripheral nervous system, central nervous system and spinal cord.
- Opioid receptors are distributed variably in the CNS with higher concentrations of receptors in areas most involved with nociception (e.g. the cerebral cortex, amygdala, thalamus and spinal cord).

There are three main opioid receptors:

1. **mu (μ)** primary action site for most opioid actions, except dysphoria;
2. **delta (δ)** contributes to spinal analgesia, reduced gut motility and dysphoria;
3. **kappa (κ)** contributes to peripheral analgesia, sedation and dysphoria.

The mu receptor has a principle role in analgesia:

- it is sub-typed into mu-1 and mu-2 receptors;
- the mu-1 receptor is responsible for analgesia;
- the mu-2 receptor is responsible for most opioid ADRs: respiratory depression, cardiovascular depression, decreased gastrointestinal motility, miosis (pupil constriction), sedation, euphoria, urinary retention and physical dependence;
- the opioid action of all known natural and synthetic opioids at mu receptors is *nonspecific*;
- no opioid has yet been found or developed that acts *only* on the mu-1 receptor.

There are two main cellular actions of opioid receptors:

1. They *close* calcium ion channels on presynaptic neurones, thus reducing the release of neurotransmitters that contribute to pain (e.g. substance P).
2. They *open* potassium ion channels, which inhibit postsynaptic neurones by reducing release of neurotransmitters that contribute to pain.

(Rang et al. 2012)

Metabolism/elimination
- Opioids are converted into metabolites (active and inactive) in the liver, then excreted via the renal system.
- All opioid metabolites may accumulate in patients receiving long-term opioids or in patients with renal impairment.

- Morphine has two main metabolites, morphine-3-glucuronide (M3G), which has no analgesic action, but causes neurotoxic effects (including myoclonus and tremor); and morphine-6-glucuronide (M6G), which is a powerful analgesic three to four times stronger than morphine.
- Hydromorphone has one main metabolite, hydromorphone-3-glucuronide (H3G), which can cause neurotoxic effects (including confusion, tremor and agitation).
- Pethidine (meperidine) has one main metabolite, *nor-pethidine*, which can cause neurotoxic effects (including nervousness, confusion, tremor and seizures). This metabolite rapidly accumulates when given as an infusion. Patients with renal dysfunction are at higher risk of nor-pethidine toxicity, as they clear the drug more slowly.
- Fentanyl has no active metabolites, although prolonged fentanyl infusions may result in drug accumulation and potential increase in ADRs. Fentanyl is the opioid of choice for children with renal impairment.
- Codeine and oxycodone are metabolised by the same P450 enzyme group.

Practice point

For years codeine was believed to be safer for children than other opioids. More recently, the inherited variation in the ability to metabolise codeine has been identified. Up to 40% of children are poor metabolisers, thus receive minimal or no analgesic effect from codeine.

There have been case reports of ADRs or death following therapeutic doses: breast-fed infants dying after maternal ingestion of codeine at normal doses and children dying following normal-for-age dosing of codeine. These deaths were due to the child or the mother being ultra-rapid metabolisers of codeine.

Many paediatric pain management specialists prefer to prescribe oral morphine or oxycodone as alternatives to codeine, with a number of children's hospitals' internationally no longer stocking codeine. This is also in line with the 2012 WHO recommendation.

Source: Food and Drug Administration (2007); Smith and Muralidharan (2010); Kelly et al. (2012); WHO (2012)

Adverse drug reactions

Most adverse reactions to opioids are dose-related (Table 4.9). By titrating the dose to the desired analgesic effect, ensuring vigilant observation (particularly in assessing sedation, see Chapter 7) and the use of opioid-sparing drugs (e.g. paracetamol and NSAIDs), most significant ADRs can be avoided (Macintyre et al. 2010).

It should also be noted that:

- *tolerance* develops to respiratory depression, sedation, euphoria, dysphoria, nausea, vomiting, pruritus and urinary retention;
- *minimal tolerance* develops to miosis and constipation.

Central nervous system effects

- The CNS effects of opioids (e.g. sedation, euphoria or dysphoria) are usually short-lived in duration and resolve within several days of commencing opioids.
- These effects may be dose-related, thus a dose reduction may resolve the symptoms.

Table 4.9 Opioid adverse drug reactions

Adverse reaction	Cause
Respiratory depression	Suppression of the brain stem respiratory centre leads to sedation, decreased tidal volume, reduced respiratory rate and reduced oxygen saturation, resulting in hypoxia and raised carbon dioxide levels, leading to further sedation and respiratory depression
Sedation	CNS effect but may be due to accumulation of metabolites in renal impairment or with high doses of opioids
Nausea and vomiting	Stimulation of the chemoreceptor trigger zone (vomiting centre) in the CNS, stimulation of the vestibular system (middle ear) and decreased gastric motility
Constipation	Decreased gastrointestinal motility, especially large intestine peristalsis
Miosis (pupil constriction)	CNS effect on the 3rd cranial nerve (oculomotor)
Euphoria	CNS effect causes altered perception of pain and a sense of wellbeing
Dysphoria	CNS effect, but may be due to accumulation of metabolites in renal impairment or with high doses of opioids
Urinary retention	Increased muscle tone of ureters, bladder and sphincter
Pruritus	Histamine release

Source: Rang et al. (2012)

- Switching to another opioid or adding adjuvant analgesia may assist.
- If the CNS effects are severe or do not resolve with opioid dose reduction, other causes may need to be considered, such as other medications, liver or renal dysfunction, electrolyte or metabolic abnormalities, or infection (Hain and Friedrichsdorf 2012).

Pethidine (meperidine) should be avoided in children due to the risk of *nor-pethidine toxicity*.

Dose, onset time, peak effect and half-life

- Opioids can be administered by almost all routes: oral, intravenous, subcutaneous, epidural and intrathecal, intranasal, inhaled, transmucosal and transdermal (Table 4.10).
- Requirements vary widely between individuals, thus the dose of opioids should *always* be titrated to effect.

(For details of opioid administration for acute pain, see Chapter 7. For details of opioid management in palliative care, see Chapter 9.)

Table 4.10 Opioid doses for children (<50 kg)

Drug	Route	Dose	Onset/Peak/t1/2
Weak opioids (not recommended by WHO)			
Codeine	Oral or PR	0.5–1 mg/kg 4-hourly (maximum 60 mg/dose)	Onset time: 15–20 min Peak effect: 30–60 min t1/2: 3 h
Dihydrocodeine (Hydrocodone)	Oral	0.5–1 mg/kg 4- to 6-hourly	Onset time: 30 min Peak effect: 30–60 min t1/2: 3 h
Tramadol	Oral or IV	1–2 mg/kg 4- to 6-hourly (maximum 100 mg/dose)	Onset time: 30–60 min (oral) Peak effect: 2 h t1/2: 6 h
Strong opioids (morphine, recommended as first line by WHO)			
Morphine	Oral IV	Oral: 0.2–0.4 mg/kg 3- to 4-hourly (immediate release) IV bolus: 0.05–0.1 mg/kg 2- to 4-hourly	Onset time: 2–5 min (IV) Peak effect: 30–60 min (oral) Peak effect: 5–20 min (IV) t1/2: 2–4 h
Buprenorphine	Oral/SL *(transdermal dosing, see Chapter 9)*	3–5 µg/kg 6- to 8-hourly	Onset time: 30 min Peak effect: 30–60 min t1/2: 3 h
Diamorphine (UK)	Intranasal IV	IN: 0.1 mg/kg (single dose) IV bolus: 25–100 µg/kg	Onset time: 20–30 min Peak effect: 30–45 min t1/2: 3 h
Fentanyl	Intranasal IV *(transdermal dosing, see Chapter 9)*	IN: 1.5 µg/kg (maximum 50 µg) (single dose) IV bolus: 0.5–1 µg/kg 1- to 2-hourly	Onset time: 1–3 min Peak effect: 10 min t1/2: 0.3–0.5 h
Hydromorphone	Oral or IV	Oral: 40–80 µg/kg 4-hourly IV bolus: 10–20 µg/kg 2- to 4-hourly	Onset time: 20 min (oral) Peak effect: 30–60 min (oral) t1/2: 3–4 h (oral)
Methadone	Oral *(IV, see Chapter 9)*	0.1–0.2 mg/kg 4- to 8-hourly	Onset time: 30–60 min Peak effect: 0.5–2 h t1/2: 15–80 h
Oxycodone	Oral	0.05–0.2 mg/kg 4-hourly (immediate release)	Onset time: 20–30 min Peak effect: 1–2 h t1/2: 3–4 h

Source: Data from Kraemer and Rose (2009); Macintyre et al. (2010); Mudd (2011); APA (2012); WHO (2012)
µg = microgram
Note: Dosing guidelines vary between organisations and countries. The author has described doses or dose ranges based on the best available evidence at time of publication. Readers are advised to follow their own institution's guidelines.

Opioid doses for infants

Neonates:

- require reduced doses of opioids due to their immature liver, renal and respiratory systems;
- have low drug clearance with a high volume of distribution, thus have a prolonged half-life;
- require opioid doses **25%** of child dose.

Infants from 1 month to 2 years:

- remain sensitive to opioids and at risk of apnoea for the first 3 months of life;
- have higher drug clearance but lower volume of distribution, thus need lower doses but increased dose frequency;
- require opioid doses starting at **25–50%** of child dose.

Source: Macintyre et al. (2010); APA (2012); WHO (2012)

Tramadol

Tramadol:

- has both opioid and non-opioid properties and is sometimes classified as a weak opioid;
- is used for mild to moderate pain;
- has a lower risk of respiratory depression and impairs gastrointestinal function less than other opioids at equi-analgesic doses (Macintyre et al. 2010);
- has an effect on both acute nociceptive and neuropathic pain.

Action

Tramadol is a partial agonist at the mu-opioid receptor but has no affinity for the delta or kappa opioid receptors (Bozkurt 2005). Its main action occurs centrally where it inhibits reuptake of the neurotransmitters noradrenaline and serotonin at the nerve synapse.

Adverse drug reactions

- Tramadol causes nausea and vomiting at similar or reduced rates to opioids (Bozkurt 2005).
- It has minimal effect on the cardiovascular or respiratory systems and does not cause sedation (Bozkurt 2005).
- Tramadol may have a reduced effect if given with codeine as it is partly metabolised by the same P450 enzyme system.
- Tramadol should be used with caution or avoided in patients with epilepsy, metabolic disorders or CNS infections or those taking psychotropic agents as it can lower the seizure threshold (Bozkurt 2005).
- *Serotonin syndrome* is a toxic state of excess serotonin activity in the CNS, most commonly caused by tramadol being co-prescribed with another serotonergic drug (e.g. pethidine, selective serotonin reuptake inhibitors [SSRIs] or monoamine oxidase inhibitor [MAOI] antidepressants) (Australian Medicines Handbook 2013).

Dose, onset time, peak effect and half-life

- Tramadol can be administered via oral or intravenous routes (Table 4.10).

Access to opioids

While it is recognised that opioid analgesics are indispensable for relieving pain, lack of access to opioids continues to be an issue for the majority of the world's population.
Barriers to opioid analgesic access include:

- limited medical knowledge;
- overly restrictive regulations and lack of enabling policies;
- supply challenges, especially in developing countries.

Source: WHO (2010b, 2012)

Practice point

A number of other opioids (e.g. ketobemidone, sufentanil, alfentanil, remifentanil) are used in paediatric practice (APA 2012).
However, as they are mainly used in very specialised situations (e.g. during anaesthesia or for intensive care) the doses are not discussed here.

Opioid antagonists

Naloxone
Naloxone:

- is a pure opioid antagonist, which occupies and displaces opioids from *all* opioid receptors;
- has the greatest affinity to the mu-opioid receptor;
- is used to manage opioid-induced ADRs (e.g. respiratory depression, sedation, nausea and vomiting, itch, and urinary retention);
- at high doses will reverse the analgesic effect of opioids and can induce acute withdrawal;
- is available in a sustained-release formulation combined with oxycodone to reduce gastrointestinal adverse effects of opioids without loss of analgesia.

(Power 2011)

Methynaltrexone
Methylnaltrexone:

- is a peripheral acting opioid antagonist that does not cross the blood–brain barrier, thus it does not reverse the effects of opioid analgesia or cause opioid withdrawal;
- is used to treat opioid-induced constipation;
- is not licensed for children, however since 2010 there have been a few case reports of its effectiveness in treating opioid-induced urinary retention, itch and constipation in infants and children.

(Miller and Hagemann 2011; Garten and Bührer 2012; Lee and Mooney 2012)

Table 4.11 Opioid antagonist doses for children (<50 kg)

Drug	Route	Dose	Onset/Peak/t1/2
Naloxone	IV	Pruritus/urinary retention: 0.25–1 µg/kg Sedation: 2–4 µg/kg Respiratory depression: 10–15 µg/kg Low-dose infusion for prevention of opioid-induced ADRs: 1–2 µg/kg/h	Onset time: 1–2 min Peak effect: 5 min t1/2: 1 h
Methynaltrexone	SC	0.15 mg/kg	Peak effect: 2–4 h t1/2: 8 h

Source: Data from Kraemer and Rose (2009); Portenoy et al. (2008); Miller and Hagemann (2011); Monitto et al. (2011)
µg = microgram
Note: Dosing guidelines vary between organisations and countries. The author has described doses or dose ranges based on the best available evidence at time of publication. Readers are advised to follow their own institution's guidelines.

Metabolism/elimination
- Naloxone is metabolised in the liver then excreted via the renal system.
- Methylnaltrexone is excreted mostly unchanged via the renal system.

Dose, onset time, peak effect and half-life
- Naloxone can be administered by a number of routes; however, the preferred route is intravenous (Table 4.11).
- Many patients achieve rapid reversal of opioid ADRs following very small doses of naloxone; thus doses should be titrated carefully to avoid inducing severe pain.
- The duration of action of naloxone is 45 minutes, which is shorter than most opioids, thus repeated intravenous bolus doses or an infusion may be required.
- Methylnaltrexone is usually administered via subcutaneous injection; however, there are reports of other routes being used (Portenoy et al. 2008).

(For details about managing opioid-induced respiratory depression see Chapter 7.)

Practice point

Opioid overdose can be caused by prescribing or administration error or with concurrent use of other sedating drugs (WHO 2012).

Adjuvant Analgesic Drugs

Adjuvant analgesic drugs or co-analgesics are drugs that work in a variety of ways to enhance analgesia (Knotkova and Pappagallo 2007; Khan et al. 2011), although many were originally developed for indications other than pain. Adjuvant analgesic drugs:

- work to assist analgesia (co-analgesics) (e.g. muscle relaxants or antispasticity drugs);
- may be used to counter the effect of an analgesic drug (e.g. laxatives or antiemetics);

- may be analgesics in their own right (e.g. ketamine, gabapentin or amitriptyline);
- have an analgesic response that is usually seen within hours to days and most adjuvant analgesics have a ceiling dose.

Local anaesthetics

Overview

- Local anaesthetics (LA) are drugs that *reversibly* block transmission of pain along nerve fibres (Neal 2012).
- Unlike most other analgesic drugs, local anaesthetics can give complete pain-relief without affecting conscious state.

Action

Local anaesthetics:

- work by blocking transmission in sensory, motor and autonomic nerve fibres (see Chapter 2);
- can be used topically (e.g. skin anaesthesia);
- can be administered by subcutaneous infiltration (e.g. wound infiltration);
- can be administered by intravenous infusion (lignocaine [lidocaine]) for neuropathic pain conditions (Nathan et al. 2005; Moulin et al. 2007);
- can be administered by direct injection to a peripheral nerve (e.g. ring block or femoral nerve block);
- can be injected adjacent to the spinal cord (e.g. caudal, epidural or intrathecal).

Smaller diameter nerve fibres (pain and autonomic) are more sensitive to local anaesthetics than larger diameter (motor and proprioceptive) nerve fibres.

When used in regional anaesthesia, local anaesthetics offer a range of benefits including decreased surgical stress response, reduced use of general anaesthesia, reduced need for postoperative ventilatory support, enhanced analgesia, reduced haemodynamic instability and earlier return of gut function (APA 2012; Bosenberg 2012).

Practice point

The degree, duration and efficacy of the LA block depends on the drug used, the dose administered and nature of the drug.

There are two main types of local anaesthetic: *amides* and *esters*.

Amides (e.g. lignocaine [lidocaine], prilocaine, bupivacaine, ropivacaine, levobupivacaine):

- are the most common *injected* anaesthetics;
- have longer duration of action;
- are metabolised by the liver;
- have a low incidence of allergy and more stable in solution.

Esters (e.g. amethocaine [tetracaine], cocaine, procaine, benzocaine):

- are the most common *topical* anaesthetics;
- have a shorter duration of action;

- are metabolised by tissue esterases;
- have a high incidence of allergy (including anaphylaxis).

Adverse drug reactions
- Most of the ADRs of LA are due to high plasma concentrations, which mainly affect the cardiac system and CNS, i.e. cardiac toxicity, vasodilation, hypotension and seizures.
- ADRs can be due to an individual's sensitivity to LA, the use of a high dose or (more commonly) due to an accidental injection of the LA into the general circulation.
- To avoid ADRs, maximum safe doses for age and weight are recommended and should be strictly followed (APA 2012).

Dose, onset time, peak effect and half-life
- Addition of vasoconstrictors (most often adrenaline) to the LA solution prolongs the effect by slowing the rate of absorption and metabolism, especially in single-shot regional anaesthesia techniques, e.g. caudal and limb blocks.
- Other drugs may be added to LAs for regional anaesthesia (e.g. epidural) to enhance analgesic effect: clonidine, ketamine or opioids (commonly fentanyl, morphine or hydromorphone).
- Longer-acting LAs (e.g. bupivacaine, ropivacaine or levobupivacaine) provide more effective analgesia for regional anaesthesia than short-acting LAs (e.g. lignocaine [lidocaine]).

(Macintyre et al. 2010; APA 2012)

(See Chapter 7 for a detailed discussion about regional anaesthesia.)

Topical local anaesthetics
- *Topical* LAs are extremely effective for the management of procedure-related pain in children, especially for venepuncture and intravenous cannulation (Murat et al. 2003; Zempsky 2008; Curtis et al. 2012).
- LA *gels* or *sprays* are used for surface anaesthesia prior to nasogastric tube or urinary catheter insertion or for painful conditions of the nose, mouth or throat (APA 2012).
- LA *creams, gel or liquids* may be applied to open wounds; however, these must be used with caution, as it is difficult to estimate the total dose given (APA 2012).
- Various drug combinations have been developed for surface anaesthesia. These include mixtures of lignocaine (lidocaine), adrenaline (epinephrine) and amethocaine (tetracaine) in liquid or gel. These are commonly used for laceration repair of face and scalp wounds (Murat et al. 2003; APA 2012).

Practice point

LA combinations *cannot* be used for end-arterial supplied areas (e.g. digits, genitalia, nose or ears) as adrenaline (epinephrine) can cause excessive vasoconstriction and tissue necrosis (APA 2012).

- Cocaine-containing LA preparations (e.g. lignocaine, adrenaline and cocaine [LAC]) are no longer recommended for use in children, as they have been associated with serious adverse drug reactions, including seizures and death (Murat et al. 2003).

The most common topical LAs used for children are:

- lignocaine (lidocaine)/prilocaine (EMLA®);
- amethocaine (tetracaine) (Ametop®, Pontocaine®, Dicaine® or AnGel®);
- 1% buffered lignocaine (lidocaine) (J-Tip®);
- 4% liposomal lignocaine (lidocaine) (ELA-Max®, *Maxilene®* or LMX₄®);
- lignocaine (lidocaine)/amethocaine (tetracaine) topical patch (Synera®).

Practice point

It is important that topical LA creams are left on for the correct amount of time, as children with a high level of anticipatory fear may become more distressed if the cream is left on for an insufficient time and they experience pain despite expecting (and being promised) anaesthesia (Lander et al. 2006).

The pharmacology of amethocaine (tetracaine) and EMLA® differs (Table 4.12). The vasodilatory effects, faster onset and prolonged duration of action make amethocaine (tetracaine) the topical anaesthetic drug of choice but, due to the higher rates of allergic reactions, some children require EMLA® instead.

Table 4.12 A comparison of the properties of amethocaine (tetracaine) and EMLA®

	Amethocaine (tetracaine) (Ametop®, AnGel®)	EMLA® (Eutectic Mixture of Local Anaesthetics)
Drug	4% tetracaine (amethocaine)	2.5% lignocaine (lidocaine) + 2.5% prilocaine
Route	Topical	Topical
Onset of action	Quick acting: Venepuncture: 30 min IV cannulation: 45 min	Slower acting: Venepuncture: 60–90 min IV cannulation: 90–120 min
Contact time	Remove after 1 h	Remove after 2–4 h
Duration of action after removal	Long acting: 4–6 h	Short acting: 1–2 h
Adverse drug reactions	Vasodilation Skin erythema (redness), itching, oedema Blistering if left in situ for too long	Vasoconstriction Skin blanching
Age	Licensed from 1 month of age	Licensed from 6 months of age

Source: Harvey and Morton (2007)

(The use of local anaesthetics for procedural pain management is detailed in Chapter 10.)

Ketamine

Overview

Ketamine is an anaesthetic drug that has powerful analgesic properties, even at very low doses. Ketamine:

- currently has three main paediatric applications: anaesthesia, procedural sedation and analgesia (Roelofse 2010);
- has significant non-opioid sparing effects but there is conflicting evidence of opioid-sparing properties (Macintyre et al. 2010; Dahmani et al. 2011).

There is a growing body of paediatric data, demonstrating efficacy as a sole agent or a co-analgesic for complex acute pain and cancer pain (Anderson and Palmer 2006; Roelofse 2010; Dahmani et al. 2011).

Action

- Ketamine is an *N*-methyl-D-aspartate (NMDA) receptor antagonist, therefore it blocks pain wind-up. (See Chapter 2 for details of windup and hyperalgesia.)
- Ketamine's main role is to reduce opioid-induced tolerance and hyperalgesia, thus it is probably most efficacious for escalating pain or for *opioid-resistant* pain (Macintyre et al. 2010).
- Single doses of ketamine are less effective than an infusion (in combination with opioid infusion/PCA or alone) as it has a very short half-life (Roelofse 2010).

Metabolism/elimination

Ketamine is metabolised in the liver with minimal drug remaining for renal excretion, thus it is useful to use for patients with renal or liver dysfunction.

Adverse drug reactions

- The main ADR related to ketamine is dysphoria, often accompanied by particularly vivid dreams and hallucinations. Dysphoria occurs in 10% of paediatric patients receiving ketamine and may be similar to the rates of dysphoria from opioids (Anderson and Palmer 2006).
- In contrast to opioids, respiratory depression and cardiovascular changes are minimal.
- When used at higher doses for procedural sedation, increased salivation, agitation and *emergence reactions* (imagery, hallucinations, delirium) have been reported.

Dose, onset time, peak effect and half-life

Routes of ketamine administration include intravenous, oral, intrathecal, epidural and subcutaneous (Table 4.13).

When used for procedural pain ketamine should be administered by a suitably trained clinician with advanced airway management skills (see Chapter 10 for further discussion).

Table 4.13 Ketamine doses for children (<50 kg)

Drug	Route	Dose	Onset/Peak/Duration
Ketamine (analgesia infusion)	IV	IV infusion: 0.05–0.2 mg/kg/h (as co-analgesic or sole agent)	Onset time: <1 min
Ketamine	Oral	5 mg/kg	Onset time: 10–20 min Peak effect: 20–30 min
Ketamine (procedural pain)	IV	IV bolus: 1–2 mg/kg	Onset time: <1 min Peak effect: 5–10 min t1/2: 2–3 h

Source: Data from Anderson and Palmer (2006); Morton (2008); Kraemer and Rose (2009); Roelofse (2010); APA (2012)
Note: Dosing guidelines vary between organisations and countries. The author has described doses or dose ranges based on the best available evidence at time of publication. Readers are advised to follow their own institution's guidelines.

Nitrous oxide

In children, nitrous oxide is primarily used for anaesthesia and procedural pain management. The use of nitrous oxide for procedural pain management is discussed in Chapter 10.

Other adjuvant analgesic drugs

Limited paediatric data exists about other adjuvant analgesic drugs, with the majority of publications being case studies or case series with small patient numbers, lacking controls and with limited follow-up (Walco et al. 2010). Many drug treatments are extrapolated from adult studies with insufficient evidence other than consensus to guide practice. Although there is some evidence of their efficacy in adults, clinicians caution against direct transfer of treatments and strategies from adults to children (Walco et al. 2010). As these drugs are being used increasingly for children with complex or chronic pain, a brief overview is included (Table 4.14).

The use of antiemetics and laxatives are discussed in Chapter 7, the use of radiotherapy is discussed in Chapter 9 and the use of sucrose is discussed in Chapter 10.

Table 4.14 Adjuvant analgesic drugs

Drug class	Description/Evidence
Alpha-2 agonists (e.g. clonidine, dexmedetomidine)	Alpha-2 agonists work by reducing central sympathetic output. They reduce anaesthetic and opioid requirements and have sedative and analgesic properties (Buck 2006; Macintyre et al. 2010). Alpha-2 agonists are used in children as sedatives, anxiolytics and analgesics and to control symptoms of opioid and benzodiazepine withdrawal (Kraemer and Rose 2009; APA 2012). Clonidine is administered via oral, IV, transdermal and epidural routes in children (APA 2012). Dexmedetomidine reduces opioid use by 50% when used in the ICU setting (Macintyre et al. 2010).

Continued

Table 4.14 Continued

Drug class	Description/Evidence
	Dexmedetomidine is an alternative to benzodiazepines for sedation in the paediatric ICU setting and for procedural sedation in children (Buck 2006, Mason and Lerman 2011). Combining ketamine with dexmedetomidine provides good procedural sedation in children without airway compromise (Tobias 2012).
Antiepileptic drugs (AEDs) (e.g. carbamazepine, gabapentin, lamotrigine, oxcarbazepine, phenytoin, pregabalin, topiramate)	AEDs work by reducing neuronal excitability (Knotkova and Pappagallo 2007). The mechanisms of pain and epilepsy are similar, which is why AEDs are effective analgesic agents. Carbamazepine is effective in the treatment of adult neuropathic pain; however, it has more ADRs and is used less frequently since gabapentin became available (Wiffen et al. 2011a). Gabapentin, pregabalin, carbamazepine, phenytoin are effective for the management of adult neuropathic pain (Moulin et al. 2007; Dworkin et al. 2010). Gabapentin and pregabalin are licensed for use in adult neuropathic pain, and although not licensed in children, both are used (Walco et al. 2010). Gabapentin has been reported to be effective in single case studies of children with complex regional pain syndrome (CRPS) (Tong and Nelson 2000; Wheeler et al. 2000), a case series of neuropathic pain in five adolescents (Butkovic et al. 2006), and in a study of seven children with phantom limb pain (Rusy et al. 2001). Gabapentin was successful in reducing severe irritability and distress in children with severe neurologic impairment (Hauer et al. 2007). Lamotrigine is ineffective for the treatment of neuropathic pain in adults. This may be due to its different mechanism of action compared to other AEDs (Wiffen et al. 2011b). Oxcarbazepine was reported to be effective in a single case study of an adolescent with therapy-resistant CRPS (Lalwani et al. 2005). Topiramate is approved for migraine prophylaxis in adults and children (Golden et al. 2006; British National Formulary for Children 2012). Despite the frequent use of AEDs for pain in children, there is insufficient data regarding their efficacy in children and adolescents (Golden et al. 2006).
Antispasticity drugs (e.g. baclofen, botulinum toxin)	Baclofen is an effective antispasticity agent, which acts on GABA receptors at the spinal cord level. In children, baclofen is administered orally or intrathecally for the treatment of severe spasticity and dystonia associated with cerebral palsy and progressive neurological conditions (Albright and Ferson 2006; Bonouvrié et al. 2012). Botulinum toxin is effective in the treatment of spasticity in children, reducing spasticity, improving function and increasing range of movement (Tickner et al. 2012). When given prior to orthopaedic surgery in children, botulinum toxin alleviates postoperative pain by reducing muscle tone and spasticity (Ramachandran and Eastwood 2006). There is inconclusive data to suggest botulinum toxin may be effective for neuropathic pain (Dworkin et al. 2010).

Table 4.14 Continued

Drug class	Description/Evidence
Benzodiazepines (e.g. clonazepam, diazepam, lorazepam, midazolam)	Benzodiazepines relieve skeletal muscle spasms and reduce muscle tone, thus reducing pain, particularly following orthopaedic surgery in children (Kraemer and Rose 2009; Chung et al. 2011). Diazepam reduces muscle spasm and hypertonia in children with cerebral palsy (Mathew et al. 2005). Benzodiazepines may be used as adjunct analgesic drugs to systemic or regional analgesics (Kraemer and Rose 2009).
Bisphosphonates (e.g. alendronate, etidronate, pamidronate)	Bisphosphonates inhibit bone resorption (breakdown) thus slowing bone loss. Their use in children was limited until recent years due to concerns about long-term effects (Sebestyen et al. 2012). Bisphosphonates are effective in treating childhood conditions that involve bone loss, e.g. osteogenesis imperfecta, osteoporosis, soft-tissue calcification, metabolic bone diseases, hypercalcaemia and bony metastases (Sebestyen et al. 2012; Winston et al. 2012). Use of bisphosphonates reduces pain, improves function, decreases fracture rates and increases bone strength (Sebestyen et al. 2012). Pamidronate resulted in resolution of pain and MRI documented inflammation in children ($n = 9$) with chronic recurrent multifocal osteomyelitis (Miettunen et al. 2009).
Cannabinoids (e.g. dronabinol, nabilone)	Cannabinoids work by activating cannabinoid receptors and are used to treat pain and nausea (Grotenhermen and Muller-Vahl 2012). There is evidence that cannabinoids are safe and effective for chronic non-cancer pain in adults (Lynch and Campbell 2011). Bottorff et al. (2009) interviewed adolescents ($n = 20$) who used marijuana for therapeutic reasons, including five who used it for pain-relief of injuries, burns, and headache. There have been case reports of dronabinol use in children for neuropathic pain, spasticity and dystonia (Rudich et al. 2003; Lorenz 2004).
Corticosteroids (e.g. dexamethasone, methylprednisolone, prednisolone)	Corticosteroids are effective for neuropathic pain, cancer pain and headache (associated with raised intracranial pressure) in children (Association of Paediatric Palliative Medicine [APPM] 2012). Due to their high rate of ADRs the lowest possible dose should be given with consideration of steroid *pulses* (short bursts of treatment) rather than continual use (APPM 2012).
Selective serotonin reuptake inhibitors (SSRIs) (e.g. citalopram, fluoxetine, paroxetine, sertraline)	There is limited evidence that SSRIs are better than placebo for treating neuropathic pain in adults and their use in children is not recommended (Moulin et al. 2007; Saarto and Wiffen 2010).
Serotonin and noradrenaline reuptake inhibitors (SNRIs) (e.g. duloxetine, venlafaxine)	SNRIs work by selectively inhibiting serotonin and noradrenaline with less sedation and fewer ADRs than TCAs or SSRIs (Gronow 2011). Venlafaxine is as effective as TCAs for treating adult neuropathic pain (Saarto and Wiffen 2010). Duloxetine is effective for diabetic peripheral neuropathy in adults (Gronow 2011). Duloxetine has been effective in two children with severe depression associated with chronic pain (Meighen 2007).

Continued

Table 4.14 Continued

Drug class	Description/Evidence
Topical drugs (e.g. capsaicin, clonidine, local anaesthetics, NSAIDs)	A number of medications have an analgesic effect when applied topically to the skin. They also have fewer ADRs, as they are not taken systemically (McCleane 2007; Gronow 2011). Capsaicin is extracted from chilli peppers and works by inactivating C-fibres and depleting nerve endings of substance P. It is used for the treatment of neuropathies and other neuropathic pain. Long-term benefits of capsaicin remain unclear (Derry et al. 2009; Dworkin et al. 2010; Gronow 2011). Clonidine can have both a central and peripheral action when administered topically. It reduces hyperalgesia in sympathetically maintained pain (McCleane 2007). Topical 5% lignocaine (lidocaine) is effective for peripheral neuropathy in adults (Gronow 2011). Topical NSAIDs provide good pain-relief equivalent to oral NSAIDs in hand and knee osteoarthritis in adults with fewer ADRs (Derry et al. 2012).
Tricyclic antidepressants (TCAs) (e.g. amitriptyline, nortriptyline, imipramine, desipramine)	TCAs work by blocking the re-uptake of serotonin and noradrenaline at the nerve synapse. TCAs have analgesic actions in addition to their antidepressant properties. Their additional effects of improved sleep and mood elevation may also improve pain (Jackson et al. 2010). TCAs are more effective than SSRIs for neuropathic pain in adults (Saarto and Wiffen 2010). TCAs are effective for neuropathic pain especially in cases where sleep is disturbed (Macintyre et al. 2010; Jackson et al. 2010). There is evidence that TCAs can substantially reduce pain from migraine, tension-type headaches and mixed headaches (Jackson et al. 2010). For preventative treatment of childhood migraine, amitriptyline is preferred due to its once daily dosing and minimal ADRs (O'Brien et al. 2012).
Triptans (e.g. naratriptan, sumatriptan, zolmitriptan)	Triptans (serotonin receptor agonists) work by constricting cerebral blood vessels by acting selectively at serotonin receptors. For migraine/headaches in children not responsive to simple analgesics, triptan or combination NSAID/triptan therapy is recommended (O'Brien et al. 2012).

Managing and Minimising the Non-Medical Use of Opioids

In the last two decades there has been a dramatic increase in opioid prescribing and both medical and non-medical use of prescription opioids (NMUPO) with corresponding high rates of morbidity and mortality in adolescents and adults (Carinci and Mao 2010; Ling et al. 2011; Manchikanti et al. 2012a, McCabe et al. 2012a).

- McCabe et al. (2012a) studied the prevalence of medical and non-medical use of opioids in senior high school students (mean age 18 years) in the USA (*n* = 7374). 17.6% reported lifetime medical use of prescription opioids, while 12.9% reported non-medical use. Approximately 80% reporting NMUPO obtained their opioids from leftover medication.

- In another study, McCabe et al. (2012b) reviewed prevalence and behaviours associated with co-ingestion of opioids and other drugs in senior high school students (mean age 18 years) in the USA (n = 12,441). The prevalence of NMUPO was 12.3%, but 70% of those who reported NMUPO co-ingested opioids and other drugs.
- Nakawaki and Crano (2012) studied a large cohort (n = 126,764) of US adolescents (aged 12–17 years) to predict the non-medical use of opioids and stimulants. They found that persistent use of common illicit substances; especially marijuana and inhalants, was the greatest predictor of non-medical use of prescription opioids.

Practice point

Prior to prescribing opioids in the community setting, reviewing an adolescent's history of prescription opioid use and substance use behaviours is important because concurrent use of alcohol and illicit substances increases the risk of NMUPO.
Careful monitoring of quantities and refills of prescribed opioids are key to minimising NMUPO. Parents need to be educated about the risks of leftover medication.

Source: McCabe et al. (2012a)

The difficult task faced by prescribers is the need to balance pain relief and harm minimisation while being mindful of risk factors that predispose people to NMUPO. Although opioids have been shown to have some efficacy in adult neuropathic pain (Moulin et al. 2007), there is a lack of evidence of the long-term usefulness of opioids for persistent pain (Carinci and Mao 2010; Ling et al. 2011; Kotalik 2012). To address all these issues a number of strategies have been implemented (Box 4.3).

BOX 4.3

Practices to reduce NMUPO

Regulatory restrictions

- Restriction of opioid access
- Monitoring of prescribers
- Increased regulation and monitoring of prescriptions

Clinical practice changes

- Pre-prescribing screening of all patients who will be prescribed long-term opioids in the community
- Urine drug testing
- Establishing treatment goals of opioid therapy
- Treatment agreements/opioid contracts
- Best-practice based prescribing
- Information and education

Source: Manchikanti (2012c)

The evidence of efficacy for these strategies is variable. The American Society of Interventional Pain Physicians (ASIPP) released a number of documents reviewing current evidence and guiding practice. However, ASIPP acknowledge these are not a standard of care as the evidence is evolving (Manchikanti 2012a; Manchikanti 2012b; Manchikanti 2012c).

Additional information

Here are useful references about safe opioid prescribing.
Family Education Sheet on Opioid Treatment, Children's Hospital, Boston (2012): www .childrenshospital.org/patientsfamilies/Site1393/Documents/Opioidtreatment.pdf
CS Mott Children's Hospital, Ann Arbor (2013): http://mottnpch.org/reports-surveys/parents-numb-misuse-narcotic-pain-medicines-youth
American Academy of Pain Medicine (AAPM) Safe prescribing practice for chronic opioid therapy: www.painmed.org
American Society of Interventional Pain Physicians (ASIPP): www.asipp.org
National Pain Center, McMaster University, Canada: http://nationalpaincentre.mcmaster.ca/opioidmanager/
Opioids for persistent pain: Good practice (A consensus statement prepared on behalf of the British Pain Society, the Faculty of Pain Medicine of the Royal College of Anaesthetists, the Royal College of General Practitioners and the Faculty of Addictions of the Royal College of Psychiatrists) (2010): www.britishpainsociety.org
The Royal Australasian College of Physicians, Prescription Opioid Policy: Improving management of chronic non-malignant pain and prevention of problems associated with prescription opioid use, Sydney 2009: www.racp.edu.au/download

---

Summary

- Many analgesic drugs have not been tested in children or are administered *off-label*.
- Misconceptions about analgesic drugs, particularly opioids, contribute to the under-treatment of pain in children.
- Confusion about opioid terminology leads to anxiety in families and healthcare professionals and suboptimal pain management practice.
- Combining analgesic drugs with non-drug strategies ensures better pain management outcomes.
- Healthcare professionals need to be aware of their patient's liver and renal function and the need for reduced doses of analgesic drugs if these are impaired.
- The route of drug administration affects the onset and efficacy of a drug. There are advantages and disadvantages with different administration routes, which should be considered prior to analgesic selection.
- Analgesic drugs should be selected using a step-wise approach based on the type and severity of pain, onset and peak effect of the drug, benefits, risks and adverse drug reactions.
- The main analgesic drugs fall into three categories: non-opioids, opioids and adjuvant drugs.
- Limited data exists on efficacy of adjuvant analgesics in children.
- Non-medical use of prescription opioids is a growing cause of significant morbidity and mortality in adolescents and adults. Careful consideration of risks should occur before prescribing long-term opioids in the community setting.

Additional information

Australia:
National Health and Medical Research Council: www.nhmrc.gov.au/guidelines/publications/
subject/Pain%20Management
UK:
British Pain Society: www.britishpainsociety.org/
Anaesthesia UK: www.frca.co.uk/sectioncontents.aspx?sectionid=148#
USA:
Department of Pain Medicine and Palliative Care, Beth Israel Medical Center: www.stoppain
.org
Medline Plus information about pain management: www.nlm.nih.gov/medlineplus/pain.html
Parent and child pain information: www.med.umich.edu/yourchild/topics/pain.htm
Special Interest Group on Pain in Childhood (IASP): http://childpain.org/
Pain treatment topics: http://pain-topics.org/

References

American Academy of Pain Medicine, American Pain Society and American Society of Addiction Medicine (2001) Consensus statement from the American Academy of Pain Medicine, the American Pain Society and the American Society of Addiction Medicine: Definitions related to the use of opioids for the treatment of pain. Available from: www.painmed.org/search.aspx?f=80ands=definitions (accessed January 2013).

Albright, A.L. and Ferson, S.S. (2006) Intrathecal baclofen therapy in children. *Neurosurgical Focus* **21**(2), E3, 1–6.

Anand, K.J., Willson, D.F., Berger, J. et al. (2010) Tolerance and withdrawal from prolonged opioid use in critically ill children. *Pediatrics* **125**(5), e1208–1225.

Anderson, B.J. (2008) Paracetamol (acetaminophen): Mechanisms of action. *Paediatric Anaesthesia* **18**(10), 915–921.

Anderson, B.J. and Palmer G.M. (2006) Recent developments in the pharmacological management of pain in children. *Current Opinion in Anaesthesiology* **19**, 285–292.

Association of Paediatric Palliative Medicine (APPM) (2012) *APPM Master Formulary*, 2nd edition. Available from: www.act.org.uk (accessed January 2013).

Association of Paediatric Anaesthetists of Great Britain and Ireland (APA) (2012) *Good Practice in Postoperative and Procedural Pain*, 2nd edition. Available from: http://onlinelibrary.wiley.com/doi/10.1111/j.1460-9592.2012.03838.x/pdf (accessed January 2013).

Australian Medicines Handbook (2013) *Australian Medicines Handbook 2013*. Australian Medicines Handbook Pty Ltd, Adelaide.

Ballantyne, J.C. and LaForge, K.S. (2007) Opioid dependence and addiction during opioid treatment of chronic pain. *Pain* **129**, 235–255.

Begg, E.J. (2008) *Instant Clinical Pharmacology*, 2nd edition. John Wiley & Sons, Chichester.

Birchley, G. (2009) Opioid and benzodiazepine withdrawal syndromes in the paediatric intensive care unit: a review of recent literature. *Nursing in Critical Care* **14**(1), 26–37.

Bonouvrié, L.A., van Schie, P.E., Becher, J.G., van Ouwerkerk, W.J. and Vermeulen, R.J. (2012) Intrathecal baclofen for progressive neurological disease in childhood. *European Journal of Paediatric Neurology* **16**(3), 279–284.

Bosenberg, A. (2012) Benefits of regional anesthesia in children. *Pediatric Anesthesia* **22**, 10–18.

Bottorff, J.L., Johnson, J.L., Moffat, B.M. and Mulvogue, T. (2009) Relief-oriented use of marijuana by teens. *Substance Abuse Treatment Prevention and Policy* **4**, 7.

Bozkurt, P. (2005) Use of tramadol in children. *Pediatric Anesthesia* **15**, 1041–1047.

British National Formulary for Children (BNFC) (2012) BMJ Publishing Group, RPS Publishing, RCPCH Publications, London.

Bryant, B. and Knights, K. (2010) *Pharmacology for Health Professionals*, 3rd edition. Elsevier (Australia) Pty Ltd.

Buck, M.L. (2006) Dexmedetomidine for sedation in the pediatric intensive care setting. *Pediatric Pharmacotherapy* **12**(1), 1–4.

Butkovic, D., Toljan, S. and Mihovilovic-Novak, B. (2006) Experience with gabapentin for neuropathic pain in adolescents: Report of 5 cases. *Paediatric Anaesthesia* **16**(3), 325–329.

Carinci, A.J. and Mao, J. (2010) Pain and opioid addiction: What's the connection? *Current Pain and Headache Reports* **14**, 17–21.

Chandrasekharan, N.V., Dai, H., Roos. K.L. et al. (2002) COX-3, a cyclooxygenase-1 variant inhibited by acetaminophen and other analgesic/antipyretic drugs: Cloning, structure, and expression. *Proceedings of the National Academy of Sciences of the United States of America* **99**(21), 13926–13931.

Charlton, J.E. (ed.) (2005) *Core Curriculum for Professional Education in Pain,* 3rd edition. IASP Task Force on Professional Education, IASP Publications, Seattle.

Chung, C.Y., Chen, C.L. and Wong, A.M. (2011) Pharmacotherapy of spasticity in children with cerebral palsy. *Journal of the Formosa Medical Association* **110**(4), 215–222.

Conaghan, P.G. (2012) A turbulent decade for NSAIDs: Update on current concepts of classification, epidemiology, comparative efficacy, and toxicity. *Rheumatology International* **32**(6), 1491–1502.

Curtis, S., Wingert, A. and Ali, S. (2012) The Cochrane Library and procedural pain in children: An overview of the reviews. *Evidence-Based Child Health* **7**, 1363–1399.

Dahmani, S., Michelet, D., Abback, P. et al. (2011) Ketamine for perioperative pain management in children: A meta-analysis of published studies. *Pediatric Anesthesia* **21**, 636–652.

Damen, L., Bruijn, J.K., Verhagen, A.P., Berger, M.Y., Passchier. J. and Koes, B.W. (2005) Symptomatic treatment of migraine in children: A systematic review of medication trials. *Pediatrics* **116**(2), e295–302.

Derry, S., Lloyd, R., Moore, R.A. and McQuay, H.J. (2009) Topical capsaicin for chronic neuropathic pain in adults. *Cochrane Database of Systematic Reviews* issue 4.

Derry, S., Moore, R.A. and Rabbie, R. (2012) Topical NSAIDs for chronic musculoskeletal pain in adults. *Cochrane Database of Systematic Reviews* issue 9.

Dworkin, R.H., O'Connor, A.B., Audette, J. et al. (2010) Recommendations for the pharmacological management of neuropathic pain: An overview and literature update. *Mayo Clinic Proceedings* **85**(3), S3–S14.

Fishbain, D.A., Cole, B., Lewis, J., Rosomoff, H.L. and Rosomoff, R.S. (2008) What percentage of chronic nonmalignant pain patients exposed to chronic opioid analgesic therapy develop abuse/addiction and/or aberrant drug-related behaviors? A structured evidence-based review. *Pain Medicine* **9**(4), 444–459.

Food and Drug Administration (FDA) (2007) *Warning for Nursing Mothers taking Codeine.* Available from: www.fda.gov/ForConsumers/ConsumerUpdate (accessed January 2013).

Garten, L. and Bührer, C. (2012) Reversal of morphine-induced urinary retention after methylnaltrexone. *Archives of Disease in Childhood: Fetal and Neonatal Edition* **97**(2), F151–F153.

Golden, A.S., Haut, S.R. and Moshe, S.L. (2006) Nonepileptic uses of antiepileptic drugs in children and adolescents. *Journal of Pediatric Neurology* **34**(6), 421–432.

Gronow, D.W. (2011) The place of pharmacological treatment of chronic pain. *Anaesthesia and Intensive Care Medicine* **12**(2), 39–41.

Grotenhermen, F. and Muller-Vahl, K. (2012) The therapeutic potential of cannabis and cannabinoids. *Deutsches Arzteblatt International* **109**(29–30), 495–501.

Harvey, A.J. and Morton, N.J. (2007) Management of procedural pain in children. *Archives of Disease in Childhood: Education and Practice Edition* **92**, ep2–ep26.

Hain, R.D. and Friedrichsdorf, S.J. (2012) Pharmacological approaches to pain. 1: 'By the ladder' – the WHO approach to management of pain in palliative care. In: *Oxford Textbook of Palliative Care in Children* (eds A. Goldman, R. Hain and S. Liben), 2nd edition, pp. 218–233. Oxford University Press, Oxford.

Hauer, J.M., Wical, B.S. and Charnas, L. (2007) Gabapentin successfully manages chronic unexplained irritability in children with severe neurologic impairment. *Pediatrics* **119**(2), e519–522.

Hong, J.Y., Kim, W.O., Koo, B.N., Cho, J.S., Suk, E.H. and Kil, H.K. (2010a) Fentanyl-sparing effect of acetaminophen as a mixture of fentanyl in intravenous parent-/nurse-controlled analgesia after pediatric ureteroneocystostomy. *Anesthesiology* **113**(3), 672–677.

Hong, J.Y., Won Han, S., Kim, W.O. and Kil, H.K. (2010b) Fentanyl sparing effects of combined ketorolac and acetaminophen for outpatient inguinal hernia repair in children. *Journal of Urology* **183**(4), 1551–1555.

Jackson, J.L., Shimeall, W., Sessums, L. et al. (2010) Tricyclic antidepressants and headaches: Systematic review and meta-analysis. *BMJ* **20**, 341:c5222.

James, S. (2004) *Review of Aspirin/Reye's syndrome warning statement*. Therapeutic Goods Administration, Department of Health and Ageing. Australian Government, Woden (ACT) Available from: www.tga.gov.au/pdf/archive/review-aspirin-reyes-syndrome-0404.pdf (accessed January 2013).

Jones, V.M. (2011) Acetaminophen injection: A review of clinical information. *Journal of Pain and Palliative Care Pharmacotherapy* **25**, 340–349.

Kanneh, A. (2002a) Paediatric pharmacological principles: An update. Part 1 Drug development and pharmacodynamics. *Paediatric Nursing* **14**(8), 36–42.

Kanneh, A. (2002b) Paediatric pharmacological principles: An update. Part 2 Pharmacokinetics: absorption and distribution. *Paediatric Nursing* **14**(9), 39–43.

Kelly, L.E., Rieder, M., van den Anker, J. et al. (2012) More codeine fatalities after tonsillectomy in North American children. *Pediatrics* **129**, e1343–e1347.

Khan, M.I., Walsh, D. and Brito-Dellan, N. (2011) Opioid and adjuvant analgesics: Compared and contrasted. *American Journal of Hospice and Palliative Care* **28**(5), 378–383.

Kimland, E. and Odlind, V. (2012) Off-label drug use in pediatric patients. *Clinical Pharmacology and Therapeutics* **91**(5), 796–801.

Knotkova, H. and Pappagallo, M. (2007) Adjuvant analgesics. *Medical Clinics of North America* **91**, 113–124.

Kokki, H. (2003) Nonsteroidal anti-inflammatory drugs for postoperative pain: A focus on children. *Pediatric Drugs* **5**(2), 103–123.

Kotalik, J. (2012) Controlling pain and reducing misuse of opioids. *Canadian Family Physician* **58**, 381–385.

Kraemer, F.W. and Rose, J.B. (2009) Pharmacologic management of acute pediatric pain. *Anesthesiology Clinics* **27**(2), 241–268.

Lalwani, K., Shoham, A., Koh, J.L. and McGraw, T. (2005) Use of oxcarbazepine to treat a pediatric patient with resistant complex regional pain syndrome. *Journal of Pain* **6**(10), 704–706.

Lander, J.A., Weltman, B.J. and So, S.S. (2006) EMLA and amethocaine for reduction of children's pain associated with needle insertion. *Cochrane Database of Systematic Reviews* **issue 3**.

Lee, J.M. and Mooney, J. (2012) Methylnaltrexone in treatment of opioid-induced constipation in a pediatric patient. *Clinical Journal of Pain* **28**(4), 338–341.

Ling, W., Mooney, L. and Hillhouse, M. (2011) Prescription opioid abuse, pain and addiction: Clinical issues and implications. *Drug and Alcohol Review* **30**, 300–305.

Lorenz, R. (2004) On the application of cannabis in paediatrics and epileptology. *Neuro Endocrinology Letters* **25**(1–2), 40–44.

Lynch, M.E. and Campbell, F. (2011) Cannabinoids for treatment of chronic non-cancer pain: A systematic review of randomized trials. *British Journal of Clinical Pharmacology* **72**(5), 735–744.

Manchikanti, L., Helm, S. 2nd, Fellows, B., Janata, J.W. Pampati, V. Grider, J.S. and Boswell, M.V. (2012a) Opioid epidemic in the United States. *Pain Physician* **15**, ES9–ES38.

Manchikanti, L., Abdi, S., Atluri, S. et al. and American Society of Interventional Pain Physicians (2012b) *American Society of Interventional Pain Physicians (ASIPP) Guidelines for responsible opioid prescribing in chronic non-cancer pain: Part 1 Evidence Assessment*. *Pain Physician* **15**, S1–S66.

Manchikanti, L., Abdi, S., Atluri, S. et al. and American Society of Interventional Pain Physicians (2012c) American Society of Interventional Pain Physicians (ASIPP) *Guidelines for responsible opioid prescribing in chronic non-cancer pain: Part 2 Guidance*. *Pain Physician* **15**, S67–S116.

Mason, K.P. and Lerman, J. (2011) Dexmedetomidine in children: Current knowledge and future applications. *Anesthesia and Analgesia* **113**, 1129–1142.

Mathew, A., Mathew, M.C., Thomas, M. and Antonisamy, B. (2005) The efficacy of diazepam in enhancing motor function in children with spastic cerebral palsy. *Journal of Tropical Pediatrics* **51**, 109–113.

McCabe, S.E., West, B.T., Teter, C.J. and Boyd, C.J. (2012a) Medical and nonmedical use of prescription opioids among high school seniors in the United States. *Archives of Pediatric and Adolescent Medicine* **166**(9), 797–802.

McCabe, S.E., West, B.T., Teter, C.J. and Boyd, C.J. (2012b) Co-ingestion of prescription opioids and other drugs among high school seniors: Results from a national study. *Drug Alcohol Dependence* **126**(1–2), 65–70.

McCleane, G. (2007) Topical analgesics. *Medical Clinics of North America* **91**, 125–139.

McGrath, P.A. (2005) Children – not simply 'little adults'. In: *The Paths of Pain: 1975–2005* (eds H. Merskey, J.D. Loeser and R. Dubner), pp, 433–446. IASP Press, Seattle.

Macintyre PE, Schug SA, Scott DA, Visser EJ, Walker SM. APM: SE Working Group of the Australian and New Zealand College of Anaesthetists and Faculty of Pain Medicine (2010) *Acute Pain Management: Scientific Evidence,* 3rd edition. Available at: www.fpm.anzca.edu.au/resources/books-and-publications.

Meighen, K.G. (2007) Duloxetine treatment of pediatric chronic pain and co-morbid major depressive disorder. *Journal of Child and Adolescent Psychopharmacology* 17(1), 121–127.

Miettunen, P.M., Wei, X., Kaura, D., Reslan, W.A., Aguirre, A.N. and Kellner, J.D. (2009) Dramatic pain relief and resolution of bone inflammation following pamidronate in 9 pediatric patients with persistent chronic recurrent multifocal osteomyelitis (CRMO). *Pediatric Rheumatology Online Journal* 7, 2.

Miller, J.L. and Hagemann, T.M. (2011) Use of pure opioid antagonists for management of opioid-induced pruritus. *American Journal of Health-System Pharmacy* 68, 1419–1425.

Monitto, C.L., Kost-Byerly, S., White, E. et al. (2011) The optimal dose of prophylactic intravenous naloxone in ameliorating opioid-induced side effects in children receiving intravenous patient-controlled analgesia morphine for moderate to severe pain: A dose finding study. *Anesthesia and Analgesia* 113, 834–842.

Morton, N.S. (2008) Ketamine for procedural sedation and analgesia in pediatric emergency medicine: A UK perspective. *Pediatric Anesthesia* 18, 25–29.

Moulin, D.E., Clark, A.J., Gilron, I. et al. and Canadian Pain Society. (2007) Pharmacological management of chronic neuropathic pain: Consensus statement and guidelines from the Canadian Pain Society. *Pain Research and Management* 12(1), 13–21.

Mudd, S. (2011) Intranasal fentanyl for pain management in children: A systematic review of the literature. *Journal of Pediatric Health Care* 25(5), 316–322.

Murat, I., Gall, O. and Tourniaire, B. (2003) Procedural pain in children, evidence-based best practice and guidelines. *Regional Anesthesia and Pain Medicine* 28, 561–572.

Nakawaki, B. and Crano, W.D. (2012) Predicting adolescents' persistence, non-persistence, and recent onset of nonmedical use of opioids and stimulants. *Addictive Behaviors* 37(6), 716–721.

Nathan, A., Rose, J.B., Guite, J.W., Hehir, D. and Milovcich, K. (2005) Primary erythromelalgia in a child responding to intravenous lidocaine and oral mexiletine treatment. *Pediatrics* 115(4), e504–e507.

Neal, M.J. (2012) *Medical Pharmacology at a Glance,* 7th edition. John Wiley & Sons Ltd, Chichester.

O'Brien, H.L., Kabbouche, M.A. and Hershey, A.D. (2012) Treating pediatric migraine: An expert opinion. *Expert Opinion on Pharmacotherapy* 13(7), 959–966.

Palmer, G.M., Atkins, M., Anderson, B.J. et al. (2008) I.V. acetaminophen pharmacokinetics in neonates after multiple doses. *British Journal of Anaesthesia* 101(4), 523–530.

Pierce, C.A. and Voss, B. (2010) Efficacy and safety of ibuprofen and acetaminophen in children and adults: A meta-analysis and qualitative review. *Annals of Pharmacotherapy* 44(3), 489–506.

Portenoy, R.K., Thomas, J., Moehl Boatwright, M.L. et al. (2008) Subcutaneous methylnaltrexone for the treatment of opioid-induced constipation in patients with advanced illness: A double-blind, randomized, parallel group, dose-ranging study. *Journal of Pain and Symptom Management* 35, 458–468.

Power I. (2011) An update on analgesics. *British Journal of Anaesthesia* 107(1), 19–24.

Ramachandran, M. and Eastwood, D.M. (2006) Botulinum toxin and its orthopaedic applications. *Journal of Bone and Joint Surgery British Volume* 88(8), 981–987.

Rang H.P., Dale M.M., Ritter J.M., Flower, R.J. and Henderson, G. (2012) *Pharmacology,* 7th edition. Elsevier/Churchill Livingstone, Edinburgh.

Remy, C., Marret, E. and Bonnet, F. (2006) State of the art of paracetamol in acute pain therapy. *Current Opinion in Anesthesiology* 19, 562–565.

Roelofse, J.A. (2010) The evolution of ketamine applications in children. *Paediatric Anaesthesia* 20(3), 240–245.

Rudich, Z., Stinson, J., Jeavons, M. and Brown, S.C. (2003) Treatment of chronic intractable neuropathic pain with dronabinol: Case report of two adolescents. *Pain Research and Management* 8(4), 221–224.

Rusy, L.M., Troshynski, T.J. and Weisman, S.J. (2001) Gabapentin in phantom limb pain management in children and young adults: Report of seven cases. *Journal of Pain and Symptom Management* 21(1), 78–82.

Saarto, T. and Wiffen, P.J. (2010) Antidepressants for neuropathic pain. *Cochrane Database Systematic Reviews* **issue 4**.

Schror, K. (2007) Aspirin and Reye syndrome: A review of the evidence. *Pediatric Drugs* **9**(3), 191–200.

Sebestyen, J.F., Srivastava, T. and Alon, U.S. (2012) Bisphosphonates use in children. *Clinical Pediatrics* **51**(11), 1011–1024.

Smith, M.T. and Muralidharan, A. (2010) Pharmacogenetics. *Pain Clinical Updates* **18**(8), 1–8.

Southey, E.R., Soares-Weiser, K. and Kleijnen, J. (2009) Systematic review and meta-analysis of the clinical safety and tolerability of ibuprofen compared with paracetamol in paediatric pain and fever. *Current Medical Research and Opinion* **25**(9), 2207–2222.

Standing, J.F., Savage, I., Pritchard, D. and Waddington, M. (2009) Diclofenac for acute pain in children. *Cochrane Database of Systematic Reviews* **issue 4**.

Stempak, D., Gammon, J., Klein, J., Koren, G. and Baruchel, S. (2002) Single-dose and steady-state pharmacokinetics of celecoxib in children. *Clinical Pharmacology and Therapeutics* **72**(5), 490–497.

Stinson, J.N., Luca, N.J. and Jibb, L.A. (2012) Assessment and management of pain in juvenile idiopathic arthritis. *Pain, Research and Management* **17**(6), 391–396.

Tickner, N., Apps, J.R., Keady, S. and Sutcliffe, A.G. (2012) An overview of drug therapies used in the treatment of dystonia and spasticity in children. *Archives of Disease in Childhood, Education and Practice Edition* **97**(6), 230–235.

Tobias, J.D. (2012) Dexmedetomidine and ketamine: An effective alternative for procedural sedation? *Pediatric Critical Care Medicine* **13**(4), 423–427.

Tong, H.C. and Nelson, V.S. (2000) Recurrent and migratory reflex sympathetic dystrophy in children. *Pediatric Rehabilitation* **4**(2), 87–89.

Walco, GA., Dworkin, R.H., Krane, E.J., LeBel, A.A. and Treede, R.D. (2010). Neuropathic pain in children: Special considerations. *Mayo Clinic proceedings* **85**(3 suppl), S33–S41.

Wiffen, P.J., Derry, S., Moore, R.A. and McQuay, H.J. (2011a) Carbamazepine for acute and chronic pain in adults. *Cochrane Database of Systematic Reviews* **issue 1**.

Wiffen, P.J., Derry, S. and Moore, R.A. (2011b) Lamotrigine for acute and chronic pain. *Cochrane Database of Systematic Reviews* **issue 2**.

Winston, M.J., Srivastava, T., Jarka, D. and Alon, U.S. (2012) Bisphosphonates for pain management in children with benign cartilage tumors. *Clinical Journal of Pain* **28**(3), 268–272.

Wheeler, D.S., Vaux, K.K. and Tam, D.A. (2000) Use of gabapentin in the treatment of childhood reflex sympathetic dystrophy. *Pediatric Neurology* **22**(3), 220–221.

World Health Organization (1996) *Cancer Pain Relief*, 2nd edition, World Health Organization, Geneva.

World Health Organization (2007) *Promoting safety of medicines for children*, World Health Organization, Geneva.

World Health Organization (2010a) *Model Formulary for Children*, World Health Organization, Geneva.

World Health Organization (2010b) *Medicines: Access to controlled medicines (narcotic and psychotropic substances)*, Fact sheet No. 336. World Health Organization, Geneva.

World Health Organization (2012) *Persisting pain in children: WHO guidelines on the pharmacological treatment of persisting pain in children with medical illnesses*. World Health Organization, Geneva.

Zempsky, W.T. (2008) Pharmacologic approaches for reducing venous access pain in children. *Pediatrics* **122** (Suppl 3), S140–S153.

CHAPTER 5

Physical and Psychological Methods of Pain Relief in Children

Alison Twycross

Department for Children's Nursing and Children's Pain Management,
London South Bank University, United Kingdom

Jennifer Stinson

Chronic Pain Programme, The Hospital for Sick Children;
Lawrence S. Bloomberg Faculty of Nursing, University of Toronto, Canada

Introduction

This chapter will provide an overview of the most commonly used physical and psychological methods available to aid the relief of pain in children. Methods used to relieve pain in infants are also discussed. For each method, relevant research will be summarised and further reading suggested. Psychological preparation and play are discussed in Chapter 10.

Physical Pain-Relieving Methods

Acupuncture

What is acupuncture?

- Acupuncture is a system of ancient medicine, healing and Eastern philosophy originating in China.
- Acupuncture is based on the theory that energy (*chi*) flows through the body along channels known as *meridians*, which are connected by acupuncture points.
- If the flow of energy is obstructed, pain results.
- The energy flow is restored by inserting needles at acupuncture points along the meridians involved, which eliminates or reduces pain.
- Acupuncture should only be carried out by a trained practitioner.

Managing Pain in Children: A Clinical Guide for Nurses and Healthcare Professionals, Second Edition.
Edited by Alison Twycross, Stephanie Dowden, and Jennifer Stinson.
© 2014 John Wiley & Sons, Ltd. Published 2014 by John Wiley & Sons, Ltd.

Research evidence: Acupuncture and acute pain

- A randomised controlled trial (RCT) to evaluate the effectiveness of acupuncture to control pain and agitation after bilateral myringotomy tube placement in children ($n = 60$) found that acupuncture provided significant benefit in pain and agitation reduction (Lin et al. 2009). The time to first postoperative analgesic administration was significantly shorter in the control group. The number of patients who required analgesia was considerably less in the acupuncture group. No adverse effects related to acupuncture were observed.
- Wu et al. (2009) examined the acceptability and feasibility of acupuncture for postoperative pain control in hospitalised children ($n = 20$), aged 7 months to 18 years. Patients received two 10- to 15-minute sessions of acupuncture 24–48 hours apart. Acupuncture was well tolerated by patients, without adverse events. In follow-up interviews, 70% of parents and patients believed acupuncture helped the child's pain. Children's pain scores were significantly reduced 4 hours after treatment.

Research evidence: Acupuncture and chronic pain

- In Lin et al.'s (2002) study, children ($n = 243$) received acupuncture over a 6-week period. Pain intensity scores decreased significantly. Children's overall feelings of wellbeing improved and the study also reported increased attendance at school, improved sleep patterns, and the ability to take part in more extracurricular activities. No side-effects or complications were reported.
- A combined acupuncture and hypnotherapy package was used by Zeltzer et al. (2002) for children ($n = 31$) with chronic pain. Ninety percent of patients completed the 6-week course. No adverse effects were reported and both children and parents reported significant improvements in children's pain and functioning.
- In Gottschling et al.'s (2008) study, 43 children with migraine or tension-type headache were randomised to low-level laser acupuncture (one treatment per week) or placebo in the control group. The intervention group had significantly fewer headaches per month, lower headache severity and fewer monthly hours of headaches compared to the control group.

Additional information

A review of the use of acupuncture as a pain-relieving intervention for children can be found in:

Kundu, A. and Berman, B. (2007) Acupuncture for pediatric pain and symptom management. *Pediatric Clinics of North America* **54**, 885–899.

Research summary

The research evidence suggests that acupuncture is an effective treatment for chronic pain.
Most children find acupuncture an acceptable treatment for chronic pain.
There is some evidence that acupuncture enhances the effectiveness of pain medications for acute pain.
Further research is needed in this area.

Heat and cold

> Topical sources of heat and cold can be applied to a painful area and are useful for pain relief or comfort.
> However, the underlying mechanism of pain relief from heating and cooling are uncertain.

Research evidence: Heat and cold as pain-relieving interventions

In the past 10 years two studies have explored the link between cold therapy and pain relief in children:

- Hasanpour et al. (2006) studied the effect of local cold therapy and distraction in pain relief for children ($n = 90$), aged 5–12 years, receiving an intramuscular penicillin injection. Pain intensity was significantly higher in the control group receiving neither cold therapy nor distraction.
- Movahedi and colleagues (2006) undertook a quasi-experimental study to explore the impact of applying an ice bag to the injection site for 3 minutes prior to venepuncture for children ($n = 8$), aged 6–12 years, in the emergency department. Children were divided into two groups (control and test). There were no differences between the groups in relation to physiological responses but behavioural responses during and after the procedure and subjective responses after the procedure were significantly lower in the test group.

There are no paediatric studies about the use of heat to manage pain.

Contraindications for heat and cold therapy

Heat and cold therapy should not be used:

- on skin which has an absence of sensation caused by vascular disorders, burns, wounds, oedema, dermatological conditions, areas treated with radiation, grafted tissue, and with epidural/local anaesthesia blocks;
- with patients unable to move away from the heat or cold source;
- with patients who are unable to communicate that the heat or cold source has become uncomfortable.

(Lane and Latham 2009)

Cold therapy may also increase pain in some situations such as muscle spasm, musculoskeletal injuries, nerve root irritation and arthritis (Lane and Latham 2009).

Additional information

A discussion of some of the issues that need considering when using heat and cold in practice can be found in: Lane, E. and Latham, T. (2009) Managing pain using heat and cold therapy. *Paediatric Nursing* **21**(6), 14–16.

Research summary

No studies have explored the use of heat as a physical method of pain relief in children.
Two studies have explored the use of cold as a pain-relieving intervention.
Cold therapy appears to reduce the pain associated with injections and venepuncture.

Massage

What is massage?

Massage therapy involves manipulation of the body by combining tactile and kinaesthetic stimulation performed in purposeful sequential application (Tsao 2007).
The precise mechanism of action is not known.

Research evidence: Massage as a pain-relieving intervention

- The efficacy of massage therapy was examined in children ($n = 57$) presenting to a chronic paediatric pain clinic for pain management (Suresh et al. 2008). After massage therapy, patients reported significant improvement in their levels of distress, pain, tension, discomfort and mood compared with their pre-massage ratings.
- In children with cancer ($n = 17$), massage was more effective than quiet time at reducing heart rate, anxiety and parental anxiety (Post-White et al. 2009). There were no significant changes in blood pressure, cortisol, pain, nausea, or fatigue. Children reported that massage helped them feel better, lessened their anxiety, and had longer-lasting effects than quiet time.
- Lemanek et al. (2009) undertook an RCT to investigate the effects of massage on young people ($n = 34$) with sickle cell disease (SCD). Participants were assigned to a massage therapy or an attention control group. Parents were trained in massage in their homes and instructed to provide nightly massages. Young people receiving massage showed higher levels of functional status and lower levels of depression, anxiety and pain. However, parents in the massage therapy group reported higher levels of depression and anxiety following the intervention. Health service utilisation rates were unchanged.

Additional information

Tsao (2007) has undertaken a review of the effectiveness of massage in the management of chronic pain, available from: www.ncbi.nlm.nih.gov/pmc/articles/PMC1876616/
A discussion paper about the use of massage in paediatric palliative care has been written by Buttle, D.G., McMurtry, C.M. and Marshall, S. (2011) *Pediatric Pain Letter* **13**(3). The paper is available from: http://childpain.org/ppl/issues/v13n3_2011/v13n3_mcmurtry.pdf

Research summary

The primary effect of massage appears to be change in mood (affect) rather than pain.
There is some evidence to support the use of massage for children with chronic pain.
Massage may help children cope with burns dressings better than children receiving pain medications alone.
For children with cancer, massage made them feel better but did not reduce their pain scores.
There is some evidence that massage helps children with SCD cope with their pain.
Research is needed to explore the use of massage in paediatric palliative care.

Transcutaneous electric nerve stimulation

What is transcutaneous electric nerve stimulation (TENS)?

TENS is a method for stimulating nerves through electrodes applied to the skin.
TENS is a safe, non-invasive pain-relieving strategy for partially or completely blocking the pain sensation.
The analgesic effect of TENS has been explained by the gate control theory, which suggests that stimulation of the large-diameter afferent nerve fibres can close the gate. (See Chapter 2 for more information about the gate control theory.)

Research evidence: TENS as a pain-relieving intervention

Only one study has examined the use of TENS to relieve children's pain:

- TENS significantly reduced venepuncture pain in a blinded placebo-controlled trial of school children ($n = 514$) aged 5–17 years (Lander and Fowler-Kerry 1993).

Additional information

The following websites provide additional information about TENS:
http://emedicine.medscape.com/article/325107-overview
www.cancer.org/Treatment/TreatmentsandSideEffects/ComplementaryandAlternativeMedicine/ManualHealingandPhysicalTouch/transcutaneous-electrical-nerve-stimulation
www.webmd.com/pain-management/tc/transcutaneous-electrical-nerve-stimulation-tens-topic-overview

Research summary

The only study looking at the use of TENS in children was published 20 years ago.

Psychological Pain-Relieving Methods

Biofeedback

What is biofeedback?

Biofeedback is a technique that trains people to control bodily processes that normally occur involuntarily, such as heart rate, blood pressure, muscle tension and skin temperature.
Electrodes attached to the skin measure these processes and display them on a monitor. With training from a biofeedback therapist, children can learn to alter their heart rate or blood pressure. At first the monitor is used by children to watch their progress, but eventually they will be able to achieve success without a monitor.
Types of biofeedback include thermal, electro-encephalography (EEG), muscle electromyography (EMG) and temporal pulse biofeedback. (See below for additional sources of information.)
Children should be taught biofeedback by a trained practitioner.

Research evidence: Biofeedback and chronic pain

- Hermann and Blanchard (2002) reviewed 15 studies using *thermal biofeedback* alone or with other treatments. They found that two-thirds of paediatric migraine sufferers had a 50% reduction in symptoms.
- Hermann and Blanchard (2002) also reviewed three studies using *electromyography biofeedback* to treat children with tension headaches; there was an 80–90% success rate in these studies.
- Scharff et al. (2002) compared *thermal biofeedback* (hand-warming) to an attention placebo (hand-cooling) and a waiting-list group. Children (*n* = 36) with migraine and their parents were randomly assigned to three groups. Children in the hand-warming group were more likely to achieve clinical improvement in migraine. These differences were still evident 6 months after the study.
- Myrvik and colleagues (2012) explored the use of *thermal biofeedback* assisted relaxation training (BART) with children (*n* = 10) with sickle cell disease. Reductions in patient-reported pain frequency were found after completing one session. Some small improvements were noted in health-related quality of life and pain-related disability.

Additional information

The following websites provide additional information about biofeedback:
www.umm.edu/altmed/articles/biofeedback-000349.htm
www.biofeedbacktherapyinfo.com/

Research summary

Biofeedback reduces the pain associated with headache and migraine.
There is some evidence that biofeedback helps children with SCD cope with pain.
Biofeedback may have a place in the treatment of other types of chronic pain in children.

Cognitive behavioural therapy

What is cognitive behavioural therapy?

Cognitive behavioural therapy (CBT) is a type of psychotherapy (or 'talk therapy') based on the theory that psychological symptoms are related to the interaction of thoughts, behaviours and emotions. In CBT, the therapist and patient work on identifying and directly changing negative thoughts and behaviours that may be maintaining symptoms.
CBT aims to improve the way a child manages and copes with their pain through the use of techniques such as education, distraction, relaxation and biofeedback. The aim is for the child to use and apply healthy adaptive behaviours (e.g. those that assist in managing and coping with pain).
CBT should only be carried out by a trained practitioner.

Research evidence: CBT and chronic pain
- In Eccleston et al.'s (2003) study adolescents ($n = 57$) with chronic pain and an accompanying adult ($n = 57$) completed a 3-week residential programme of group CBT. Immediately after treatment adolescents reported significant improvements in relation to disability and physical function. Three months post-treatment adolescents maintained physical improvements and reduced anxiety, disability and somatic awareness. Participants also had improved school attendance with 40% having returned to full-time education.
- A systematic review looking at the evidence relating to the use of psychological therapies found that CBT is effective in reducing the severity and frequency of chronic headache, recurrent abdominal pain and fibromyalgia (Eccleston et al. 2012).

Research evidence: CBT and sickle cell disease pain
A systematic review exploring the use of psychological interventions for the management of pain in people with sickle cell disease looked at the effectiveness of CBT (Anie and Green 2012). One study found that CBT reduced the affective (emotional) component of pain but not the sensory component. Another study evaluating CBT reported inconclusive results for the assessment of coping strategies, and showed no difference between groups assessed on health service use. There is a need for further research.

Additional information

An insight into what CBT comprises can be gained from a video on this website: www.nhs.uk/conditions/cognitive-behavioural-therapy/Pages/Introduction.aspx
Anie and Green's (2012) and Eccleston et al.'s (2012) systematic reviews are available from: www.thecochranelibrary.com/view/0/index.html

---

Research summary

CBT is a useful pain-relieving strategy, particularly for children with chronic pain such as headaches, recurrent abdominal pain and fibromyalgia.
More research is needed to explore the use of CBT to help children cope with pain related to medical conditions.

Distraction

What is distraction?

Distraction is a way of helping a child cope with a painful or difficult procedure. It aims to take the child's mind off the procedure by concentrating on something else. There are various methods of distraction therapy – some are very simple to do; others need more practice.
The effectiveness of distraction can be explained by the *gate control theory* (see Chapter 2). The use of distraction techniques closes the *gate* because pain is put at the periphery of awareness, with attention being focused on the distracter rather than on the pain.
Distraction is a relatively easy strategy for healthcare professionals to use to help children cope with pain.

Research evidence: Distraction and needle-related pain

- A systematic review of psychological interventions for the management of needle-related pain found *distraction* to be a particularly effective way of reducing children's pain in this context (Uman et al. 2010).
- McMurtry et al. (2010) examined 100 children (40 boys, 60 girls), aged 5–10 years, and the responses of their parents (86 mothers, 14 fathers) during venepuncture. They found that when an adult provided reassurance (e.g. 'it's okay') this increased the child's distress, whereas distraction helped them cope with the venepuncture pain.

Research evidence: Distraction and other types of pain

- Distraction techniques were found to be a useful addition to analgesic drugs for children (*n* = 24) with musculoskeletal pain in the emergency department (Tanabe et al. 2002). Children who were distracted had significantly less pain than those who only received analgesic drugs.
- Sinha et al. (2006) found the use of distraction techniques reduced the sensory and affective (emotional) components of pain among children (*n* = 240), aged 6–18 years, undergoing laceration repair in the emergency department.

Additional information

A review of distraction techniques for children undergoing procedures can be found at: Koller, D. and Goldman, R. (2011) Distraction techniques for children undergoing procedures: A critical review of pediatric research. *Journal of Pediatric Nursing* **27**(6), 652–681.

This website provides useful information about distracting children: www.gosh.nhs.uk/medical-conditions/procedures-and-treatments/distraction-therapy/

Uman et al.'s (2010) systematic review is available from: www.thecochranelibrary.com/view/0/index.html

---

Using distraction techniques in practice

To determine an effective distraction strategy the healthcare professional should involve the child and parents in identifying what is particularly interesting to the child. The characteristics of an effective distraction technique are outlined in Box 5.1. The method chosen needs to be relevant to the child's age and developmental stage; examples are given in Table 5.1.

BOX 5.1

Characteristics of effective distraction strategies for brief episodes of pain

The distraction technique must be:

1. Interesting to the child
2. Consistent with the child's energy level and ability to concentrate
3. Stimulate at least one of the major senses:
   - Hearing
   - Vision
   - Touch
   - Movement
4. Capable of providing a change in stimuli when the pain changes, e.g., increasing stimuli as pain increases

Table 5.1 Distraction techniques for children of different ages

Pre-school children	School-aged child	Teenager
Blowing bubbles	Games and puzzles	Listening through headphones to stories or music
Windmill toys	Listening through headphones to stories or music	Watching television or a video
Singing	Watching television or a video	Playing interactive computer games
Reading pop-up books	Playing interactive computer games	Reading their favourite novel
Blowing an imaginary feather off the doctor's nose	Blowing an imaginary candle to make it flicker	Breathing out/controlled breathing
Playing with a kaleidoscope	Breathing out/controlled breathing	Playing their favourite video or computer game
Playing with finger puppets	Looking in a mirror to see the view through a nearby window	Listening to their favourite music
Singing along	Singing along	

Virtual reality as a distraction technique

Several studies explore the use of virtual reality (VR) as a distraction technique. This involves using a computer and a visual simulation game. These studies focus predominately on children receiving cancer treatments and burns dressings.

Studies relating to children receiving cancer treatments:

- Gershon et al. (2004) tested the use of VR distraction to reduce anxiety and pain in children with cancer ($n = 59$), aged 7–19 years, whose treatment involved access to subcutaneous ports. Reductions in pain and anxiety were found for children using the virtual reality distraction.
- VR distraction was also shown to reduce distress during (central venous) port access procedures in children ($n = 20$), aged 7–14 years, with oncology conditions (Wolitzky et al. 2005).

Studies relating to children receiving attention to burns dressings:

- A VR game combined with analgesic drugs was found to be more effective at reducing children's ($n = 9$) pain during burns dressings than analgesic drugs alone (Das et al. 2005).
- Schmitt et al. (2011) carried out an RCT that found VR in combination with analgesic drugs is an effective pain reduction technique in the paediatric burn population undergoing painful rehabilitation therapy. The magnitude of the analgesic effect was clinically meaningful and was maintained with repeated use.
- Kipping and colleagues (2012) used an RCT to explore the use of VR for adolescents ($n = 41$) undergoing burns dressings. Nursing staff reported a significant reduction in pain scores during dressing changes and significantly fewer rescue doses of Entonox® for participants receiving VR.

Additional information

Pictures of VR equipment and images can be seen at: www.hitl.washington.edu/projects/vrpain/

Involving parents in distraction

Parents can help with distraction activities but need guidance from healthcare professionals as to how to best help their child. When parents are taught how to distract their child during a painful procedure, children experience less anxiety and pain (Walker et al. 2006; McMurtry et al. 2010). Teaching parents distraction techniques for their child has a two-fold effect:

- It reduces parental feelings of helplessness;
- It benefits the child by reducing their distress.

Parents may need to be guided to select a distraction technique appropriate for their child (Box 5.1 and Table 5.1).

Additional information

A YouTube video discussing how to prepare parents for their role in distracting their child during a painful procedure is available at: www.youtube.com/watch?v=NOx93bimNG8

Research summary

Distraction appears to be a useful tool for reducing children's pain during needle-related procedures.
Distraction may be useful for other types of short-lasting pain.
The effectiveness of distraction as a pain-relieving strategy is influenced by the method used.
Active methods of distraction appear to be more helpful than passive methods.
Virtual reality has also been shown to be an effective distraction technique for children having burns dressings; cancer treatment; and IV cannulas inserted.

Hypnosis

What is hypnosis?

Hypnosis is an artificially induced altered state of consciousness, characterised by heightened suggestibility and receptivity to direction.
This altered state of consciousness, occurring within a relaxed physical state, allows a trance that is different from both the normal state of being awake and any of the stages associated with sleep.
Through hypnosis children can be helped to focus their attention away from pain and towards an imaginative experience they view as comforting, safe, fun or intriguing.

Within this section the term *hypnosis* will be used to encompass both hypnosis and guided imagery. (The terms hypnosis and guided imagery are often used interchangeably but the methods used within research papers are not always comparable. The reader is advised to check the original papers for details of the method used.)

Research evidence: Hypnosis and postoperative pain

- In Huth et al.'s (2004) study, children, aged 7–12 years, admitted for tonsillectomy and/or adenoidectomy were randomly assigned to two groups. Children ($n = 36$) in the experimental group watched a video on the use of hypnosis and listened to a 30-minute audiotape about hypnosis a week before surgery. Children ($n = 37$) in the attention-control group received an equal amount of preoperative time from the investigator. The children who received hypnosis training had significantly lower pain scores in the first 4 hours postoperatively.
- In Pölkki et al.'s (2008) study the efficacy of hypnosis and relaxation in hospitalised children's postoperative pain relief was tested. Children ($n = 60$), aged 8–12 years, undergoing appendectomy or upper/lower limb surgery were randomly assigned to listen to a hypnosis CD-ROM. Children ($n = 30$) in the experimental group reported significantly less pain.

Research evidence: Hypnosis and procedural pain

- In Butler et al.'s (2005) study, children undergoing a voiding cystogram (cystourethrogram) were randomised to receive hypnosis ($n = 21$) or standard care ($n = 23$). Procedure times were significantly shorter for children receiving hypnosis (by an average of 14 minutes). Children in the hypnosis group also demonstrated fewer pain behaviours, and their parents reported the procedure was significantly less traumatic.
- Liossi et al. (2006) compared the effectiveness of a local anaesthetic cream (EMLA®) and self-hypnosis with the use of EMLA® alone, or the use of EMLA® with attention (from the researcher). Children ($n = 45$), aged 6–16 years, were randomised into the three groups. Children in the group receiving EMLA cream and self-hypnosis demonstrated less anticipatory anxiety and less procedural pain and anxiety.
- Richardson and colleagues (2006) carried out a systematic review of eight studies ($n = 313$) comparing hypnosis with other cognitive and cognitive behavioural interventions for the management of procedural pain in children with cancer. They concluded that hypnosis appears to reduce procedure-related pain and distress in cancer patients, but further research is required.

Research evidence: Hypnosis and recurrent abdominal pain

- Children ($n = 10$) with recurrent abdominal pain (RAP) were trained in relaxation and hypnosis. Pain diaries were completed at 0, 1 and 2 months and demonstrated a significant (67%) decrease in pain over the period of the study (Ball et al. 2003).
- Similar findings were obtained in a study by Weydert et al. (2006) with children ($n = 22$) aged 5–18 years.
- Van Tilburg et al. (2009) explored the effectiveness of a home-based hypnosis programme. Children ($n = 34$) aged 6–15 years with RAP were randomly assigned to receive standard care +/– hypnosis for 2 months. The children who received hypnosis had significantly reduced scores for treatment pain and disability.

Additional information

A useful summary of the studies relating to hypnosis and pain can be found in:
Wood, C. and Bioy, A. (2008) Hypnosis and pain in children. *Journal of Pain and Symptom Management* **35**(4), 437–446.
Butler et al.'s (2005) paper is available from:
http://pediatrics.aappublications.org/search?fulltext=Hypnosis+reduces+distress+and+duration+of+an+invasive+medical+procedure+for+children&submit=yes&x=37&y=10)
Van Tilburg et al.'s (2009) paper is available from:
http://pediatrics.aappublications.org/content/124/5/e890.full.pdf+html?sid=43650bae-3f87-43df-b487-611543c723d7

Research summary

Hypnosis has been used in conjunction with pain medications to enhance children's pain care postoperatively.
Hypnosis can be used to help children cope with painful procedures such as venepuncture, IV cannulation, cardiac catheterisation and lumbar punctures.
Hypnosis in combination with relaxation appears to be an effective strategy for managing recurrent abdominal pain.

Music therapy

What is music therapy?

Music therapy can be either active or passive.
Active music therapy is when a music therapist is involved and music is used as a method of interactive communication.
Passive music therapy is when someone listens to music without the involvement of a music therapist.

Research evidence: Music therapy and painful procedures

- Klassen et al. (2008) carried out a systematic review of the effect of active and passive music therapy for pain and anxiety in children undergoing painful procedures. They concluded that music significantly reduces pain and anxiety in children undergoing medical and dental procedures.
- Caprilli and colleagues (2007) carried out an RCT to determine whether active music therapy reduced pain and anxiety in children, aged 4–13 years, undergoing venepuncture. Children (*n* = 54) were assigned to the music group and 54 others were assigned to a control group where they received support from their parent. Results demonstrated that distress and pain intensity were significantly reduced for children in the intervention group.
- Yu et al. (2009) undertook an RCT of music on anxiety and pain in 60 children with cerebral palsy receiving acupuncture. They found that music significantly reduced anxiety but not pain.

- Nguyen and colleagues (2010) conducted an RCT in 40 children, aged 7–12 years, with leukaemia undergoing a lumbar puncture. Children were randomised to a music or control group. Children in the music group had significantly lower pain scores and lower heart and respiratory rates during and after lumbar puncture compared to the control group.
- Kristjansdottir and Kristjansdottir (2011) carried out an RCT with children, aged 14 years, undergoing a routine immunisation. Participants were randomly assigned to three groups: musical distraction with headphones ($n = 38$), musical distraction without headphones ($n = 41$) and standard care ($n = 39$). Adolescents receiving music therapy were less likely to report pain compared to the control group. Listening to music without headphones was most effective.

Research evidence: Music therapy and postoperative pain

- Nilsson and colleagues (2009) tested the effect of postoperative music on morphine consumption, pain, distress and anxiety with children ($n = 80$), aged 7–16 years, undergoing day surgery. Children in the music group received less morphine in the recovery room and had significantly lower facial affective scores. There were no significant differences in pain scores or vital signs. Children reported the music as calming and relaxing.

Research evidence: Music therapy and palliative care

- Lindenfelser et al. (2012) carried out an exploratory study in the use of music therapy in paediatric palliative care. Parents ($n = 14$) were interviewed and described music therapy as resulting in physical improvements in their child as well as providing comfort and stimulation. They also described music therapy as being a positive experience for the whole family.

Research summary

Music therapy appears to be an effective method of relieving the pain and anxiety associated with painful procedures.
Music therapy may be a useful adjunct to pain medications for postoperative pain.
Music therapy might be a useful strategy in paediatric palliative care.
There are differences in the way music therapy is defined in different studies. This needs taking into account when considering the generalisability of the findings.

Relaxation

What is relaxation?

Relaxation encompasses several techniques that promote stress reduction, the elimination of tension throughout the body, and a calm and peaceful state of mind.
For a young child relaxation may simply consist of being held in a comfortable well-supported position or being rocked in a wide rhythmical arc. For older children it involves actively teaching them to engage in progressive relaxation of the muscle groups.
The effectiveness of relaxation can also be explained by the *gate control theory* (see Chapter 2). As the child relaxes the *gate* is closed.

Research evidence: Relaxation and chronic pain

- The results of seven RCTs conducted with adolescents ($n = 288$) over a 20-year period were examined by Larsson et al. (2005). Therapist-assisted relaxation was

found to be an effective treatment for adolescents suffering from recurrent tension headaches or migraine.
- A systematic review found good evidence that relaxation is effective in reducing the severity and frequency of chronic headache, recurrent abdominal pain and fibromyalgia in children (Eccleston et al. 2012).

Additional information

This video provides an example of how a relaxation session could be carried out: www.youtube.com/watch?v=LFHzThaj7r4

Eccleston et al.'s (2012) systematic review is available from the Cochrane library at: www.thecochranelibrary.com/view/0/index.html

---

Research summary

Relaxation appears to be an effective pain-relieving intervention for chronic headaches, recurrent abdominal pain and fibromyalgia.

Physical Methods of Pain Relief for Neonates

Unwell neonates are exposed to multiple painful procedures during their time in hospital, with the most common being the heel-stick for blood sampling. Some painful procedures are still carried out without analgesic drugs being administered (Harrison et al. 2009). Physical methods should be used in combination with analgesic drugs to manage procedural pain in neonates.

Breastfeeding

How does breastfeeding work as a pain-relieving strategy?

The exact mechanism of how breast milk and breastfeeding work is not known. However, the initial hypotheses suggested by Blass and colleagues are the most probable:

- Presence of a comforting person (mother) (Blass et al. 1995);
- Physical sensation (skin to skin contact with comforting person) (Blass et al. 1995);
- Diversion of attention (Gunnar 1984);
- Sweetness of breast milk (Blass and Shide 1995).
- Compared to infant formulas, breast milk contains a higher concentration of tryptophan (Heine 1999), a precursor of melatonin. Melatonin has been shown to increase the concentration of beta-endorphins (Barrett et al. 2000) and so could be one of the mechanisms for the nociceptive effects of breast milk.
- Levels of cholecystokinin, a neuropeptide and gut hormone associated with calming effects in animal models (Blass and Shide 1993), have been reported to be elevated in neonates 30 and 60 minutes after breastfeeding, due to the presence of milk in the intestines (Uvnas-Moberg et al. 1993).
- Preterm neonates incapable of direct breastfeeding from the mother may benefit (through some of the mechanisms listed above) from placement of breast milk on the tongue or breast milk administered orally or via a nasogastric tube (supplemental breast milk).

Research evidence: Breastfeeding and procedural pain
The results of a systematic review by Shah et al. (2012) concluded:

- if available, breastfeeding or breast milk should be used to relieve procedural pain in neonates undergoing a single procedure;
- breastfeeding is more effective than swaddling or the use of a dummy (pacifier);
- breastfeeding was as effective as the administration of glucose/sucrose;
- breast milk alone was not as effective as breastfeeding or sweet taste;
- further research is needed to explore the effectiveness of breast milk for repeated painful procedures, and the mechanism of action.

However, a more recent RCT found no improvement in pain scores where infants ($n = 57$) born at 30–36 weeks gestational age were randomised to breastfeeding or a dummy during venepuncture (Holsti et al. 2011).

Comparing the efficacy of breast milk and sweet taste (sucrose or glucose)
Several studies have compared the efficacy of breast milk and sucrose in relation to managing heel-stick pain in neonates.

- One study has reported that breastfeeding may be superior to sucrose. Codipietro et al. (2008) examined full-term infants ($n = 101$) randomised to sucrose or breast-feeding undergoing heel-stick for metabolic screening. Infants in the breastfeeding group had lower pain (PIPP; see Chapter 6) scores, cried less and had fewer adverse changes in heart rate and oxygen saturation levels.
- More recently, one RCT concluded that breast milk is better than sucrose for late preterm infants (Simonse et al. 2012). However, the results of another RCT suggest the opposite (Bueno et al. 2012).

Additional information

Shah et al.'s (2012) systematic review is available from the Cochrane library at: www.thecochranelibrary.com/view/0/index.html

---

Research summary

Breastfeeding or feeding with supplemental breast milk reduces pain and distress behaviours.
Breastfeeding or breast milk should be used to reduce procedural pain in neonates having single painful procedures.
Breast milk alone, although helpful, is less effective than breastfeeding or sweet taste.
Breastfeeding is more effective than swaddling or the use of a dummy, and has a similar efficacy to the administration of sucrose, although further research is needed in this context.
More research is needed on the effect of repeated breastfeeding or supplemental breast milk as a pain-relieving intervention.

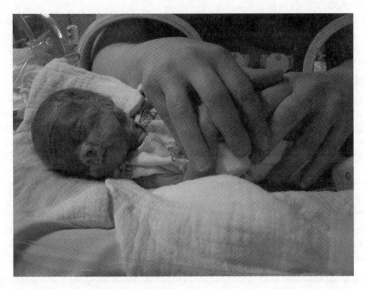

Figure 5.1 Facilitated tucking. Used with the kind permission of the Neonatal Intensive Care Unit, University Hospital Inselspital, Bern, Switzerland.

Facilitated tucking (or containment)

What is facilitated tucking?

Facilitated tucking (FT) involves holding a neonate's body so that the limbs are in close proximity to the trunk.

FT involves the infant being held in a side-lying, flexed position using both touch and position (Figure 5.1).

FT is thought to give the infant the chance to control their own body, which may increase their ability to control pain (Axelin et al. 2006).

FT differs from swaddling because the neonate is held in position by a parent or healthcare professional.

Research evidence: Facilitated tucking and procedural pain

- A systematic review suggests that FT may be beneficial to preterm infants during painful procedures (Obeidat et al. 2009).
- Another systematic review concluded there was sufficient evidence to recommend FT as a pain-relieving intervention for neonates (Pillai Riddell et al. 2012).
- Liaw et al. (2012) carried out an RCT with infants ($n = 34$) to compare the effectiveness of non-nutritive sucking (NNS) and FT. Both interventions reduced pain scores more than routine care during heel-stick procedures. NNS reduced pain scores more than FT. However, FT supported infants' physiological and behavioural stability more.
- Cignacco and colleagues (2012) conducted a multicentre RCT to compare the effectiveness of oral sucrose, FT and a combination of both interventions in 71 preterm infants (24–32 weeks) during heel-stick procedures. FT alone was significantly less effective in relieving procedural pain compared to sucrose. There is some evidence that FT in combination with sucrose has an additive benefit.

- Another RCT explored whether or not parents could carry out FT and concluded this was a safe and effective pain management method during suction treatment of preterm infants ($n = 20$) (Axelin et al. 2006).

The clinical utility of FT
The clinical utility of FT has been explored in one study (Cignacco et al. 2010). FT using two nurses could increase workload and may not be as efficacious as other physical pain-relieving strategies. This requires further research, particularly given the effectiveness of parents conducting FT. Parents could perhaps be involved in implementing FT with one nurse.

Additional information

Pillai Riddell et al.'s (2012) systematic review is available from the Cochrane library at: www.thecochranelibrary.com/view/0/index.html

---

Research summary

Facilitated tucking appears to be an effective method for reducing procedural pain in neonates such as suctioning or heel-stick.
Facilitated tucking may be best used as an adjuvant therapy in combination with other strategies. More research is needed.
Parents can safely carry out facilitated tucking.

Kangaroo care (skin-to-skin contact)

What is kangaroo care?

Kangaroo care (KC) involves a neonate being taken out of the incubator or cot (undressed) and laid on the bare skin of their mother or father (Cignacco et al. 2007).
The baby is held upright at a 40–60 degree angle and covered by the parent's blouse or shirt; additional coverings are added if needed (Tsao et al. 2008).

Research evidence: Kangaroo care and procedural pain
To date there have been 18 clinical trials (RCTs or randomised cross-over design) examining the effect of kangaroo care provided to neonates delivered at term or preterm, undergoing common painful procedures in the NICU. Duration of the kangaroo care prior to the procedure ranged from 2 minutes to 3 hours, with the majority being less than 30 minutes. Fourteen of the trials examined heel-stick, three intramuscular injections, and one included venepuncture and heel-stick. Although outcomes varied across the studies, findings were consistently positive, indicating lower composite pain scores, shortened cry duration, faster recovery, less heart rate variability, lower cortisol response and less alteration in heart rate and oxygen saturations.
    The results of individual studies found:

- With preterm neonates ($n = 74$), aged over 32 weeks gestation, KC produced a reduction in the pain response to a heel-stick procedure compared to neonates in a control group at 30, 60 and 90 seconds post-procedure (Johnston et al. 2003).

- Preterm neonates ($n = 61$) between 28 and 32 weeks gestational age were included in Johnston et al.'s (2008) RCT comparing KC with remaining in an incubator swaddled in the prone position. Pain scores 90 seconds post heel-stick were significantly lower in the KC group. Time to recovery was also significantly shorter.
- Chermont et al. (2009) compared the efficacy of oral 25% dextrose treatment and/or KC in term neonates ($n = 640$) during an intramuscular injection. Neonates were randomly assigned to four groups (no analgesia [routine]; oral 25% dextrose; skin-to-skin contact; and a combination of oral dextrose and skin-to-skin contact). Oral 25% dextrose reduced the duration of procedural pain. KC decreased both the response to injection pain and the duration. The combination of the two measures was more effective than either measure separately for term neonates.
- Cong et al. (2009) carried out an RCT to determine if KC resulted in improved balance in autonomic responses (i.e. less change in infants' behavioural state, heart rate and heart rate variability) to heel-stick pain than when infants remained in an incubator for the heel-stick. Infants ($n = 14$) aged 30–32 weeks gestation were included in the study. Infants experienced better autonomic balance in response to KC than remaining in the incubator.

A systematic review concluded there was sufficient evidence to recommend KC as a pain-relieving intervention for neonates (Pillai Riddell et al. 2012).

Is kangaroo care as effective if carried out by fathers?
One study has compared paternal ($n = 62$) versus maternal ($n = 62$) KC to reduce pain from heel-stick (Johnston et al. 2011a). Mothers were slightly more effective than fathers in decreasing pain response.

Additional information

This YouTube video provides an understanding of what KC comprises: www.youtube.com/watch?v=8hLo4_4ksAI

Pillai Riddell et al.'s (2012) systematic review is available from the Cochrane library at: www.thecochranelibrary.com/view/0/index.html

Chermont et al.'s (2009) paper is available from: http://pediatrics.aappublications.org/content/124/6/e1101.full.pdf+html

Johnston et al.'s (2008) paper is available from: www.biomedcentral.com/content/pdf/1471-2431-8-13.pdf

---

Research summary

Kangaroo care appears to be a useful strategy for managing needle-stick pain in term and preterm neonates.

Kangaroo care appears slightly more effective when carried out by mothers rather than fathers; however, more research is needed in this area.

Non-nutritive sucking

What is non-nutritive sucking?

Non-nutritive sucking (NNS) refers to the using a dummy with an infant to promote sucking without breast or infant formula (Cignacco et al. 2007).

Research evidence: NNS and procedural pain

Most of the studies relating to NNS compare its efficacy with other pain-relieving interventions.

- Gibbins et al. (2002) carried out an RCT to compare the efficacy and safety of three interventions for relieving procedural pain associated with heel-sticks in preterm and term neonates ($n = 190$). Significant differences in pain response existed among treatment groups ($p < 0.001$), with the lowest mean pain scores in the sucrose and NNS groups.
- Boyle et al. (2006) undertook an RCT to explore the effectiveness of sucrose and NNS to relieve pain when screening for retinopathy of prematurity. Neonates ($n = 40$) in two NICUs were randomised to four groups (sterile water, sucrose solution, sterile water with dummy, sucrose with dummy). Neonates using a dummy had significantly lower pain scores than those receiving sterile water alone or glucose.
- Liu et al. (2010) carried out an RCT to compare the efficacy of NNS and a glucose solution as a pain-relieving intervention for neonates undergoing venepuncture. Neonates ($n = 105$) were randomly assigned to three groups (NNS, glucose, control). The NNS and glucose groups had significantly lower pain scores than the control group during the procedure and the recovery phase. Neonates receiving NNS also had significantly lower pain scores than those receiving glucose.
- Liaw et al. (2012) carried out an RCT with infants ($n = 34$) to compare the effectiveness of NNS and FT. Both interventions reduced pain scores more than routine care during heel-sticks. NNS reduced pain scores more than FT. However, FT supported infants' physiological and behavioural stability (i.e. these infants demonstrated lower stress-related behaviours and less changes in heart rate and oxygen saturation) more than NNS.

Research summary

Non-nutritive sucking appears to relieve neonates' pain when experiencing needle-related pain. It may not be effective for other types of pain such as testing for retinopathy of prematurity.
Most studies have shown that NNS has a synergistic effect when given with sucrose.
Some studies suggest that NNS is more effective than the administration of sucrose for needle-related pain. This finding needs further study.
The combination of sucrose and NNS was the most efficacious intervention for single heel-sticks.

Sucrose

Sucrose as a pain-relieving intervention

The administration of sucrose in dosages of 0.5–2.0 ml of 12.5% solution approximately two minutes prior to a single heel-stick is effective in providing pain relief to both term and preterm infants (Murki and Subramanian 2011).
Sucrose is administered orally using a syringe.
Sucrose is thought to reduce the effect of pain by providing taste stimulation to the cellular membrane receptors in the brain, where the endogenous opioid system is located (Blass and Hoffmeyer 1991).

Research evidence: Sucrose and procedural pain

A systematic review of the efficacy of sucrose suggests it is a safe and effective method of reducing procedural pain from one-off events (Stevens et al. 2010). Information about the optimum dose of sucrose remains inconclusive.

Issues related to the use of sucrose in neonates

The use of sucrose on consecutive days needs further exploration (Johnston et al. 2011b):

- One study reported poorer neurodevelopmental scores with more frequent (repeated) administration of sucrose during the first week of life (Johnston et al. 2002).
- However, following further analysis this was found to only be the case for neonates who had received 10 or more doses in a 24-hour period (Johnston et al. 2008).
- Another study examined the use of sucrose over a 4-week period and found no higher incidence of adverse events (Stevens et al. 2005). This needs further research, particularly as sucrose is a common intervention in the management of neonatal pain.
- The need for additional research is further supported by the findings of an RCT that suggested giving sucrose solution to infants ($n = 29$ received sucrose; $n = 30$ received sterile water) dulled their behavioural responses to pain rather than relieving it (Slater et al. 2010).

Additional information

A review on the use of sucrose for procedural pain management in infants can be found in: Harrison, D., Beggs, S. and Stevens, B. (2012) Sucrose of procedural pain management in infants. *Pediatrics* **130**(5), 918–925.
The WHO Reproductive Health Library have published a review on sucrose for analgesia in newborn infants undergoing painful procedures. This is available from: http://apps.who.int/rhl/newborn/cd001069_murkis_com/en/index.html
Stevens et al.'s (2010) systematic review is available from the Cochrane library at: www.thecochranelibrary.com/view/0/index.html

---

Research summary

The administration of sucrose is proven to be an effective method for managing procedural pain in infants.
Further research is needed about the optimum dose as well as the safety and efficacy with repeated use over time and in older infants.
Longitudinal studies are needed to address long-lasting neurodevelopmental outcomes.

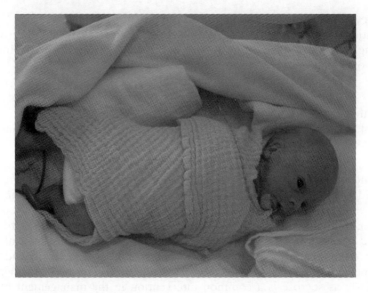

Figure 5.2　Swaddling. Used with the kind permission of the Neonatal Intensive Care Unit, University Hospital Inselspital, Bern, Switzerland.

Swaddling

What is swaddling?

Swaddling involves (firmly) wrapping the infant in a cloth or blanket to make them feel secure (Figure 5.2).

In contrast to facilitated tucking, with swaddling the infant is not touched.

Research evidence: Swaddling and procedural pain

- In a meta-analysis of 108 term and preterm neonates, Prasopkittikun and Tilkskul-chai (2003) concluded that positive effects (reduced pain scores and less change in heart rate and oxygen saturation) from swaddling were present in all the neonates but lasted a significantly shorter time in younger neonates.
- Huang et al. (2004) compared the effects of FT and swaddling. Premature infants ($n = 32$) were randomly assigned to FT or swaddling while undergoing two heel-stick procedures. Pain responses to heel-stick under swaddling were lower, but significant differences between the two interventions were only found at the 3rd and 7th minute. There was little difference between swaddling and FT in reducing changes in infants' heart rate and oxygen saturation.

Research summary

Swaddling has been shown to be effective in reducing procedural pain in neonates.

Additional information: Neonatal physical and psychological pain-relieving methods

Two review papers have been published that can be downloaded free and provide a useful summary of research on physical and psychological pain-relieving methods for neonates:

Tsao, J.C.I., Evans, S., Meldrum, M., Altman, T. and Zeltzer, L.K. (2008a) A review of CAM for procedural pain in infancy: Part I. Sucrose and non-nutritive sucking. *Evidence Based Complementary and Alternative Medicine* **5**(4), 371–381. Available from: www.ncbi.nlm.nih.gov/pmc/articles/PMC2586318/?tool=pubmed

Tsao, J.C.I., Evans, S., Meldrum, M., Altman, T. and Zeltzer, L.K. (2008b) A review of CAM for procedural pain in infancy: Part II. Other interventions. *Evidence Based Complementary and Alternative Medicine* **5**(4), 399–407. Available from: www.ncbi.nlm.nih.gov/pmc/articles/PMC2586313/?tool=pubmed

Other useful sources of information include:

Campbell-Yeo, M., Fernandes, A. and Johnston, C. (2011) Procedural pain management for neonates using nonpharmacological strategies: Part 2: Mother-driven interventions. *Advances in Neonatal Care* **11**(5), 312–318.

Fernandes, A., Campbell-Yeo, M. and Johnston, C.C. (2011) Procedural pain management for neonates using non-pharmacological strategies Part 1: Sensorial Interventions. *Advances in Neonatal Care* **11**(4), 235–241.

Johnston, C.C., Fernandes, A.M. and Campbell-Yeo, M. (2011) Pain in neonates is different. *Pain* **52**(3 Suppl), S65–S73.

Summary

- Acupuncture appears to be an effective pain-relieving intervention for chronic pain and is effective and acceptable to children, and may enhance the effectiveness of medications for acute pain.
- Cold therapy appears to reduce the pain associated with injections and venepuncture.
- Massage appears to improve mood (affect) rather than reducing pain, and may benefit children with chronic pain and children having burns dressings.
- Biofeedback reduces the pain associated with headache and migraine and may have a place in the treatment of other types of chronic pain in children, such as sickle cell disease.
- Cognitive behavioural therapy (CBT) is a useful pain-relieving strategy, particularly for children with chronic pain such as headaches, recurrent abdominal pain and fibromyalgia.
- Distraction appears to be a useful tool for reducing children's pain during needle-related procedures and for other types of short-lasting pain. Active methods of distraction appear to be more helpful than passive methods.
- Virtual reality is an effective distraction technique for children undergoing painful procedures.
- Hypnosis has been used in conjunction with pain medications to enhance children's pain care post-operatively, and can help children cope with painful procedures.
- Hypnosis in combination with relaxation appears to be an effective strategy for managing recurrent abdominal pain.
- Music therapy appears to be effective in relieving the pain and anxiety associated with painful procedures and may be a useful adjunct to medications for postoperative pain.
- Relaxation appears to be an effective pain-relieving intervention for chronic headaches, recurrent abdominal pain and fibromyalgia.

- Breastfeeding or feeding with supplemental breast milk reduces pain and distress behaviours and should be used to reduce procedural pain in neonates having single painful procedures. Breast milk alone, although helpful, is less effective than breast-feeding or sweet taste.
- Breastfeeding is more effective than swaddling or the use of a dummy, and has a similar efficacy to the administration of sucrose.
- Facilitated tucking (FT) appears to be effective for reducing procedural pain in neonates such as suctioning or heel-stick. It may be best used as an adjuvant therapy.
- Kangaroo care (KC) is useful for managing needle-stick pain in term and preterm neonates and appears slightly more effective when carried out by mothers rather than fathers.
- Non-nutritive sucking (NNS) appears to relieve neonates' needle-related pain. It may not be effective for other types of pain such as testing for retinopathy of prematurity. The combination of sucrose and NNS was the most efficacious intervention for single heel-sticks.
- The administration of sucrose is proven to be an effective method for managing procedural pain in infants.
- Swaddling has been shown to be effective in reducing procedural pain in neonates.

Acknowledgements
We would like to thank Dr Marsha Campbell-Yeo from IWK Health Centre and Dalhousie University, Halifax, Canada for reviewing the neonatal section of this chapter.

References

Anie, K.A. and Green, J. (2012) Psychological therapies for sickle cell disease and pain. *Cochrane Database of Systematic Reviews* **issue** 2.

Axelin, A., Salantera, S. and Lehtonen, L. (2006) 'Facilitated tucking by parents' in pain management of preterm infants – a randomized crossover trial. *Early Human Development* **82**, 241–247.

Ball, T.M., Shapiro, D.E., Monhelm, C.J. and Weydert, J.A. (2003) A pilot study of the use of guided imagery for the treatment of recurrent abdominal pain in children. *Clinical Pediatrics* **42**(6), 527–532.

Barrett, T., Kent, S. and Voudoris, N. (2000) Does melatonin modulate beta-endorphin, corticosterone, and pain threshold? *Life Sciences* **66**, 467–476.

Blass, E.M. and Hoffmeyer, L.B. (1991) Sucrose as an analgesic for newborn infants. *Pediatrics* **87**, 215–218.

Blass, E.M. and Shide, D.J. (1993) Endogenous cholecystokinin reduces vocalization in isolated 10-day-old rats. *Behavioral Neuroscience* **107**(3), 488–492.

Blass, E.M.,and Shide, D.J., Zaw-Mon, C. and Sorrentino, J. (1995) Mother as shield: Differential effects of contact and nursing on pain responsivity in infant rats – evidence for nonopioid mediation. *Behavioral Neuroscience* **109**, 342–353.

Boyle, E.M., Freer, Y., Khan-Orakzai, Z. et al. (2006) Sucrose and non-nutritive sucking for relief of pain in screening for retinopathy of prematurity: A randomised controlled trial. *Archives of Disease in Childhood: Fetal and Neonatal Edition* **91**(3), F166–168.

Bueno, M., Stevens, B., de Camargo, P.P., Toma, E., Krebs, V.L. and Kimura, A.F. (2012) Breast milk and glucose for pain relief in preterm infants: A noninferiority randomized controlled trial. *Pediatrics* **129**(4), 664–670.

Butler, L.D., Symons, B.K., Henderson, S.L., Shortliffe, L.D. and Spiegel D. (2005) Hypnosis reduces distress and duration of an invasive medical procedure for children. *Pediatrics* **115**(1), e77–85.

Caprilli, S., Anastasi, F., Grotto, R.P., Scollo Abeti, M. and Messeri, A. (2007) Interactive music as a treatment for pain and stress in children during venipuncture. *Journal of Development and Behavioral Pediatrics* **28**(5), 399–403.

Chermont, A.F., Falcao, L.F.M., de Souza Silva, E.H.L., Balda, R.C. and Guinsberg, R. (2009) Skin-to-skin contact and/or oral 25% dextrose for procedural pain relief for term newborn infants. *Pediatrics* **124**(6), 1101–1107.

Cignacco, E., Axelin, A., Stoffel, L., Sellam, G., Anand, K. and Engberg, S. (2010) Facilitated tucking as a non-pharmacological intervention for neonatal pain relief: Is it clinically feasible? *Acta Pediatrics* **99**(12), 1763–1765.

Cignacco, E., Hamers, J.P.H., Stoffel, L. et al. (2007) The efficacy of non-pharmacological interventions in the management of procedural pain in preterm and term neonates: A systematic literature review. *European Journal of Pain* **11**, 139–152.

Cignacco, E., Sellam, G., Stoffel, L. et al. (2012) Oral sucrose and 'facilitated tucking' for repeated pain relief in preterms: A randomized controlled trial. *Pediatrics* **129**(2), 299–308.

Codipietro, L., Ceccarelli, M. and Ponzone, A. (2008) Breastfeeding or oral sucrose solution in term neonates receiving heel lance: A randomized controlled trial. *Pediatrics* **122**(3), e716–e721.

Cong, X., Ludington-Hoe, S.M., McCain, G. and Fu, P. (2009) Kangaroo care modifies preterm infant heart rate variability in response to heel stick pain: Pilot study. *Early Human Development* **85**, 561–567.

Das, D.A., Grimmer, K.A., Sparnon, A.L., McRae, S.E. and Thomas, B.H. (2005) The efficacy of playing a virtual reality game in modulating pain for children with acute burn injuries: A randomised controlled trial. *BMC Pediatrics* **5**(1), 1–10.

Eccleston, C., Malleson, P.N., Clinch, J., Connell, H. and Sourbut, C. (2003) Chronic pain in adolescents: Evaluation of a programme of interdisciplinary cognitive behaviour therapy. *Archives of Disease in Childhood* **88**, 881–885.

Eccleston, C., Palermo, T.M., Williams, A.C.D.C., Lewandowski, A. and Morley, S. (2012) Psychological therapies for the management of chronic and recurrent pain in children and adolescents. *Cochrane Database of Systematic Reviews* **issue 12**.

Gershon, J., Zimand. E., Pickering, M., Rothbaum, B.O. and Hodges, L. (2004) A pilot and feasibility study of virtual reality as a distraction for children with cancer. *Journal of the American Academy of Child and Adolescent Psychiatry* **43**(10), 1243–1249.

Gibbins, S., Stevens, B., Hodnett, E., Pinelli, J., Ohlsson, A. and Darlington, G. (2002) Efficacy and safety of sucrose for procedural pain relief in preterm and term neonates. *Nursing Research* **51**(6), 375–382.

Gottschling, S., Meyer, S., Gribova, I. et al. (2008) Laser acupuncture in children with headache: A double-blind, randomized, bicenter, placebo-controlled trial. *Pain* **37**(2), 405–412.

Gunnar, M. (1984) The effects of a pacifying stimulus on behavioural and adrenocortical responses to circumcision in the newborn. *Journal of the American Academy of Child and Adolescent Psychiatry* **23**, 34–38

Harrison, D., Loughnan, P., Manias, E. and Johnston, L. (2009) Analgesics administered during minor painful procedures in a cohort of hospitalized infants: A prospective clinical audit. *Journal of Pain* **10**(7), 715–722.

Hasanpour, M., Tootoonchi, M., Aein, F. and Yadegarfar, G. (2006) The effects of two non-pharmacologic pain management methods for intramuscular injection pain in children. *Acute Pain* **8**(1), 7–12.

Heine, W.E. (1999) The significance of tryptophan in infant nutrition. *Advances in Experimental Medicine and Biology* **467**, 705–710.

Hermann, C. and Blanchard, E.B. (2002) Biofeedback in the treatment of headache and other childhood pain. *Applied Psychophysiology and Biofeedback* **27**(2), 143–162.

Holsti, L., Oberlander, T.F. and Brant, R. (2011) Does breastfeeding reduce acute procedural pain in preterm infants in the neonatal intensive care unit? A randomized clinical trial. *Pain* **152**(11), 2575–2581.

Huang, C.M., Tung, W.S., Kuo, L.L. and Chang, Y.J. (2004) Comparison of pain responses of premature infants to heelstick between containment and swaddling. *Nursing Research* **12**, 31–40.

Huth, M.M., Broome, M.E. and Good, M. (2004) Imagery reduces children's post-operative pain. *Pain* **110**, 439–448.

Johnston, C.C., Filion, F., Snider, L. et al. (2002) Routine sucrose analgesia during the first week of life in neonates younger than 31 weeks postconceptual age. *Pediatrics* **110**, 523–528.

Johnston, C.C., Stevens, B.. Pinelli, J. et al. (2003) Kangaroo care is effective in diminishing pain response in preterm neonates. *Archives of Pediatrics and Adolescent Medicine* **157**(11), 1084–1088.

Johnston, C.C., Campbell-Yeo, M. and Filion, F. (2011a) Paternal vs maternal kangaroo care for procedural pain in preterm neonates: A randomized crossover trial. *Archives of Pediatric and Adolescent Medicine* **165**(9), 792–796.

Johnston, C.C., Fernandes, A.M. and Campbell-Yeo, M. (2011b) Pain in neonates is different. *Pain* **52**(3 Suppl), S65–S73.

Johnston, C.C., Filion, F., Campbell-Yeo, M. et al. (2008) 'Kangaroo' mother care diminishes pain from heel lance in very pre-term neonates: A crossover trial. *BMC Pediatrics* 8(13), 1–9.

Kipping, B., Rodger, S., Miller, K. and Kimble, R.M. (2012) Virtual reality for acute pain reduction in adolescents undergoing burn wound care: A prospective randomized controlled trial. *Burns* 38(5), 650–657.

Klassen, J.A., Liang, Y., Tjosvold, L., Klassem, T.P. and Hartling, L. (2008) Music for pain and anxiety in children undergoing medical procedures: A systematic review of randomized controlled trials. *Ambulatory Pediatrics* 8(2), 117–128.

Kristjansdottir, O. and Kristjansdottir, G. (2011) Randomized controlled trial of musical distraction with and without headphones for adolescents' immunization pain. *Scandinavian Journal of Caring Sciences* 25(1): 19–26.

Lander, J. and Fowler-Kerry, S. (1993) TENS for children's procedural pain. *Pain* 52(2), 209–216.

Lane, E. and Latham, T. (2009) Managing pain using heat and cold therapy. *Paediatric Nursing* 21(6),14–16.

Larsson, B., Carlsson, J., Fichtel, A. and Melin, L. (2005) Relaxation treatment of adolescent headache sufferers: Results from a school-based replication series. *Headache* 45, 692–704.

Lemanek, K.L., Ranalli, M. and Lukens, C. (2009) A randomized controlled trial of massage therapy in children with sickle cell disease. *Journal of Pediatric Psychology* 34(10), 1091–1096.

Liaw, J.J., Yang, L., Wang, K.W., Chen, C.M., Chang, Y.C. and Yin, T. (2012) Non-nutritive sucking and facilitated tucking relieve preterm infant pain during heel-stick procedures: A prospective, randomised controlled crossover trial. *International Journal of Nursing Studies* 49(3), 300–309.

Lin, Y., Bioteau. A. and Lee, A. (2002) Acupuncture for the treatment of pediatric pain: A pilot study. *Medical Acupuncture* 14(1), 45–46.

Lin, Y.C., Tassone, R.F., Jahng, S. et al. (2009) Acupuncture management of pain and emergence agitation in children after bilateral myringotomy and tympanostomy tube insertion. *Paediatric Anaesthesia* 19(11), 1096–1101.

Lindenfelser, K.J., Hense, C. and McFerran, K. (2012) Music therapy in pediatric palliative care: Family-centered care to enhance quality of life. *American Journal of Hospice and Palliative Medicine* 29(3), 219–222.

Liossi, C., White, P. and Hatira, P. (2006) Randomized clinical trial of local anesthetic versus a combination of local anesthetic with self-hypnosis in the management of pediatric procedure-related pain. *Health Psychology* 25(3), 307–315.

Liu, M.F., Lin, K.C., Chou, Y.H. and Lee, T.Y. (2010) Using non-nutritive sucking and oral glucose solution with neonates to relieve pain: A randomised controlled trial. *Journal of Clinical Nursing* 19(11–12), 1604–1611.

McMurtry, C.M., Chambers, C.T., McGrath, P.J., and Asp, E. (2010) When 'don't worry' communicates fear: Children's perceptions of parental reassurance and distraction during a painful medical procedure. *Pain* 150(1), 52–58.

Movahedi, A.F., Rostami, S., Salsadi, M., Keikhaee, B. and Moradi, A. (2006) Effect of local refrigeration prior to venipuncture on pain-related responses in school age children. *Australian Journal of Advanced Nursing* 24(2), 51–55.

Murki, S. and Subramanian, S. (2011) *Sucrose for analgesia in newborn infants undergoing painful procedures: RHL commentary*. The WHO Reproductive Health Library. World Health Organization, Geneva.

Myrvik, M.P., Campbell, A.D. and Butcher, J.L.J. (2012) Single-session biofeedback-assisted relaxation training in children with sickle cell disease. *Journal of Pediatric Hematology/Oncology* 34(5), 340–343.

Nguyen, T.N, Nilsson, S., Hellstrom, A.L. and Bengtson, A. (2010). Music therapy to reduce pain and anxiety in children with cancer undergoing lumbar puncture: A randomized controlled trial. *Journal of Pediatric Oncology Nursing* 27, 146–155.

Nilsson, S., Kolinsky, E., Nilsson, U., Sidenvall, B. and Enskar, K. (2009) School-aged children's experiences of post-operative music medicine on pain, distress, and anxiety. *Paediatric Anaesthesia* 19(12), 1184–1190.

Obeidat, H., Kahalaf, I., Callister, L.C. and Froelicher, E.S. (2009) Use of facilitated tucking for nonpharmacological pain management in preterm infants: \a systematic review. *Journal of Perinatal and Neonatal Nursing* 23(4), 372–377.

Pillai Riddell, R.R., Racine, N.M., Turcotte, K. et al. (2012) Non-pharmacological management of infant and young child procedural pain. *Cochrane Database of Systematic Reviews* issue 5.

Pölkki, T., Pietilä, A.M., Vehviläinen-Julkunen, K., Laukkala, H. and Kiviluoma, K. (2008) Imagery-induced relaxation in children's postoperative pain relief: A randomized pilot study. *Journal of Pediatric Nursing* 23(3), 217–224.

Post-White, J., Fitzgerald, M., Savik, K., Hooke, M.C., Hannahan, A.B. and Spencer, S.F. (2009) Massage therapy for children with cancer. *Journal of Pediatric Oncology Nursing* 26(1), 16–28.

Prasopkittikun, T. and Tilkskulchai, F. (2003) Management of pain from heel stick in neonates: An analysis of research conducted in Thailand. *Journal of Perinatal and Neonatal Nursing* 7, 304–312.

Richardson, J., Smith, J.E., McCall, G. and Pilkington, K. (2006) Hypnosis for procedure-related pain and distress in pediatric cancer patients: A systematic review of effectiveness and methodology related to hypnosis interventions. *Journal of Pain and Symptom Management* 31(3), 70–84.

Scharff, L., Marcus, D.A. and Masek, B.J. (2002) A controlled study of minimal-contact thermal biofeedback treatment in children with migraine. *Journal of Pediatric Psychology* 27(2), 109–119.

Schmitt, Y.S., Hoffman, H.G., Blough, D.K. et al. (2011) A randomized, controlled trial of immersive virtual reality analgesia, during physical therapy for pediatric burns. *Burns* 37(1), 61–68.

Shah, P.S., Aliwalas, L.L. and Shah, V.S. (2012) Breastfeeding or breast milk for procedural pain in neonates. *Cochrane Database of Systematic Reviews* issue 12.

Simonse, E., Mulder, P.G. and van Beek, R.H. (2012) Analgesic effect of breast milk versus sucrose for analgesia during heel lance in late preterm infants. *Pediatrics* 129(4), 657–663.

Sinha, M., Christopher, N.C., Fenn, R. and Reeves, L. (2006) Evaluation of nonpharmacologic methods of pain and anxiety management for laceration repair in the pediatric emergency department. *Pediatrics* 117(4), 1162–1168.

Slater, R., Cornelissen, L., Fabrizi, L. et al. (2010) Oral sucrose as an analgesic drug for procedural pain in newborn infants: A randomised controlled trial. *Lancet* 376(9748), 1225–1232.

Stevens, B., Yamada, J., Beyene, J. et al. (2005) Consistent management of repeated procedural pain with sucrose in preterm neonates: Is it effective and safe for repeated use over time? *Clinical Journal of Pain* 21, 543–548.

Stevens, B., Yamada, J. and Ohlsson, A. (2010) Sucrose for analgesia in newborn infants undergoing painful procedures. *Cochrane Database of Systematic Reviews* issue 13.

Suresh, S., Wang, S., Porfyris, S., Kamanski-Sol, R. and Steinhorn, D. (2008) Massage therapy in outpatient pediatric chronic pain patients: Do they facilitate significant reductions in levels of distress, pain, tension, discomfort and mood alterations? *Pediatric Anesthesia* 18, 884–887.

Tanabe, P., Ferket, K., Thomas, R., Paice, J. and Marcantonio, R. (2002) The effect of standard care, ibuprofen, and distraction on pain relief and patient satisfaction in children with musculoskeletal trauma. *Journal of Emergency Medicine* 28(2), 118–125.

Tsao, J.C.I. (2007) Effectiveness of massage therapy for chronic, non-malignant pain: A review. *Evidence Based Complementary and Alternative Medicine* 4(2), 165–179.

Tsao, J.C.I., Evans, S., Meldrum, M., Altman, T. and Zeltzer, L.K. (2008) A review of CAM for procedural pain in infancy: Part II. Other interventions, *Evidence Based Complementary and Alternative Medicine*, 5(4), 399–407.

Uman, L.S., Chambers, C.T., McGrath, P.J. and Kisely, S. (2010) Psychological interventions for needle-related procedural pain and distress in children and adolescents. *Cochrane Database of Systematic Reviews* issue 11.

Uvnas-Moberg, K., Marchini, G. and Winberg, J. (1993) Plasma cholecystokinin concentrations after breast feeding in healthy 4-day-old infants. *Archives of Disease in Childhood* 68(spec no 1), 46–48.

van Tilburg, M.A., Chitkara, D.K., Palsson, O.S. et al. (2009) Audio-recorded guided imagery treatment reduces functional abdominal pain in children: A pilot study. *Pediatrics* 124(5), e890–897.

Walker, L.S., Williams, S.E., Smith, C.A., Garber, J., Van Slyke, D.A. and Lipani, T.A. (2006) Parent attention versus distraction: Impact on symptom complaints by children with and without chronic functional abdominal pain. *Pain* 122, 43–52.

Weydert, J.A., Shapiro, D.E., Acra, S.A., Monheim, C.J., Chambers, A.S. and Ball, T.M. (2006) Evaluation of guided imagery as treatment for recurrent abdominal pain in children: A randomised controlled trial. *BMC Pediatrics* 6(29), 1–10.

Wolitzky, K., Fivush, R., Zimand, E., Hodges, L. and Rothbaum, B.O. (2005) Effectiveness of virtual reality distraction during a painful medical procedure in pediatric oncology patients. *Psychology and Health* 20(6), 817–824.

Wu, S., Sapru, A., Stewart, M.A. et al. (2009) Using acupuncture for acute pain in hospitalized children. *Pediatric Critical Care Medicine* 10(3), 291–296.

Yu, H., Yongfeng, L., Shuzen, L. and Xianoming, M. (2009) Effects of music on anxiety and pain in children with cerebral palsy receiving acupuncture: A randomized controlled trial. *International Journal of Nursing Studies* 46, 1423–1430.

Zeltzer, L.K., Tsao, J.C.I., Stelling, C., Powers, M., Levy, S. and Waterhouse, M. (2002) A phase 1 study on the feasibility of an acupuncture/hypnotherapy intervention for chronic pediatric pain. *Journal of Pain and Symptom Management* 24, 437–446.

CHAPTER 6

Pain Assessment

Jennifer Stinson

Chronic Pain Programme, The Hospital for Sick Children;
Lawrence S. Bloomberg Faculty of Nursing, University of Toronto, Canada

Lindsay Jibb

Division of Haematology/Oncology, Department of Pediatrics,
The Hospital for Sick Children, Canada

Introduction

This chapter will provide an overview of the assessment of pain in children from neonates to adolescents. The difference between pain assessment and measurement will be highlighted, the key steps in pain assessment identified and the need to take a pain history discussed. Self-report, behavioural and physiological indicators of pain in children will be reviewed. The importance of clear documentation about pain assessment and frequency of pain assessment are also discussed. Information about commonly used pain tools will be provided and the factors to be considered when choosing a pain assessment tool will be outlined. Research relating to pain assessment practices is discussed in Chapter 1.

Healthcare Professionals' Role in Pain Assessment

Many healthcare professionals are involved, either directly or indirectly, in the assessment of children's pain. However, nurses have the most contact with children receiving health care. This places them in a unique position to identify children who are experiencing pain; to appropriately assess the pain and its impact on the child and family; to relieve pain using available resources; and to evaluate the effectiveness of those actions. This chapter will provide the theoretical knowledge required by nurses, and other healthcare professionals, to enable them to successfully assess pain in children.

Managing Pain in Children: A Clinical Guide for Nurses and Healthcare Professionals, Second Edition.
Edited by Alison Twycross, Stephanie Dowden, and Jennifer Stinson.
© 2014 John Wiley & Sons, Ltd. Published 2014 by John Wiley & Sons, Ltd.

Pain Measurement and Pain Assessment

Pain measurement generally describes the quantification of pain intensity. For example, we commonly ask 'How much does it hurt?' The emphasis is on the quantity, extent or degree of pain (Johnston, 1998).
Pain assessment is a broader concept than measurement and involves clinical judgement based on observation of the nature, significance and context of the child's pain experience (Johnston, 1998).

The majority of pain assessment tools focus on *measuring* pain intensity. However, a wider *assessment* provides information such as where the pain is and what it is like. This helps the healthcare professional to make decisions regarding the most likely cause of the pain and to choose the most appropriate intervention.

Pain assessment includes measurement (e.g. pain intensity) but the emphasis is on the multidimensional nature of pain. Pain assessment involves exploring the:

- intensity of the pain;
- location of the pain;
- duration of the pain;
- sensory qualities of the pain (e.g. word descriptors);
- cognitive aspects of the pain (e.g. perceived impact on activities of daily life);
- affective aspects of the pain experience (e.g. pain unpleasantness);
- contextual and situational factors that may influence the child's perception of pain (see Chapter 3).

Assessing Pain in Children

Pain assessment is the first step in the management of pain. To treat pain effectively, ongoing assessment of the presence and severity of pain and the child's response to treatment is essential (American Medical Association, 2007). Pain assessment poses many challenges in infants and children because of:

- the subjective and complex nature of pain;
- developmental and language limitations that preclude comprehension and self-report;
- dependence on others to infer pain from behavioural and physiological indicators;
- the social context of pain (i.e. differences in pain perception and expression depending on age, sex, race and ethnicity).

(Drendel et al. 2011)

When assessing pain in children there are three key steps (Box 6.1).

BOX 6.1

Key steps: Pain assessment

- Step 1: Record a pain history
- Step 2: Assess the child's pain using a developmentally appropriate pain assessment tool
- Step 3: Reassess pain having allowed time for pain-relieving interventions to work

Parents and significant family members know their child best and can recognise subtle changes in manner or behaviour. They have a particularly important role in pain assessment and should be involved at all three steps.

Step 1: Taking a pain history

Conducting a thorough history of the child's prior pain experiences and current pain complaints is the first step in pain assessment. Standardised pain history forms (Hester and Barcus 1986; Ball and Bindler 1995; Hester et al. 1998) have been developed for talking with children and parents about pain. For the child in acute pain, the questions outlined in Table 6.1 usually provide the clinician with sufficient pain history information.

For a child with chronic pain a more detailed pain history needs to be taken. This includes information about:

- the description of the pain;
- associated symptoms;
- temporal or seasonal variations;
- impact on activities of daily living (e.g. school, sport, play and self-care);
- pain-relieving measures used.

Further detail about questions to ask children and parents about chronic pain can be seen in Table 6.2 (see also Figure 6.1).

Table 6.1 Pain history for children with acute pain

Child's questions	Parent's questions
Tell me what pain is	What word(s) does your child use in regard to pain?
Tell me about the hurt you have had before	Describe the pain experiences your child has had before
Do you tell others when you hurt? If yes, who?	Does your child tell you or others when he or she is hurting?
What do you want to do for yourself when you are hurting?	How do you know when your child is in pain?
What do you want others to do for you when you are hurt?	How does your child usually react to pain?
What don't you want others to do for you when you hurt?	What do you do for your child when he or she is hurting?
What helps the most to take your hurt away?	What does your child do for him- or herself when he or she is hurting?
Is there anything special that you want me to know about when you hurt? (If yes, have child describe)	What works best to decrease or take away your child's pain?
	Is there anything special that you would like me to know about your child and pain? (If yes, describe)

Source: Hester and Barcus (1986); Hester et al. (1998)

Table 6.2 Pain history questions for children with chronic pain and their parents/carers

Description of pain	**Type of pain** – *Is the pain acute* (e.g. medical procedures, postoperative pain, accidental injury), *recurrent* (e.g. headaches) *or chronic* (e.g. juvenile idiopathic arthritis)? **Onset of pain** – *When did the pain begin? What were you doing before the pain began? Was there any initiating injury, trauma or stressors?* **Duration** – *How long has the pain been present?* (e.g. hours/days/weeks/months) **Frequency** – *How often is pain present? Is the pain always there or is it intermittent? Does it come and go?* **Location** *Where is the pain located? Can you point to the part of the body that hurts?* (Body outlines can be used to help children indicate where they hurt.) Children over 3 to 4 years of age can mark an 'X' on body maps to indicate painful areas, shade in with crayons areas of pain or choose different colours to represent varying degrees of pain intensity. An example of a body map for eliciting information about the location of pain from children and adolescents can be seen in Figure 6.1. *Does the pain go anywhere else?* (e.g. radiates up or down from the site that hurts). Pain radiation can also be indicated on body diagrams. **Intensity** *What is your pain intensity at rest? What is your pain intensity with activity?* (Use a developmentally appropriate intensity assessment tool.) *Over the past week what is the least pain you have had? What is the worst pain you have had? What is your usual level of pain?* **Unpleasantness** *How unpleasant/bothersome is the pain right now?* (Use a developmentally appropriate unpleasantness assessment tool.) *Over the past week what is the least unpleasant/bothersome your pain has been? What is most unpleasant/bothersome your pain has been? How unpleasant/bothersome is it usually?* **Quality of pain** School-age children can communicate about pain in more abstract terms. *Describe the quality of your pain* (e.g. word descriptors such as sharp, dull, achy, stabbing, burning, shooting or throbbing). Word descriptors can provide information on whether the pain is nociceptive or neuropathic in nature or a combination of both.
Associated symptoms	*Are there any other symptoms that go along with or occur just before or immediately after the pain* (e.g. nausea, vomiting, light-headedness, tiredness, diarrhoea, or difficulty walking)? *Are there any changes in the colour or temperature of the affected extremity or painful area?* (These changes most often occur in children with conditions such as complex regional pain syndromes.)
Temporal or seasonal variations	*Is the pain affected by changes in seasons or weather?* *Does the pain occur at certain times of the day* (e.g. after eating or going to the toilet)?

Continued

Table 6.2 Continued

Impact on daily living	*Has the pain led to changes in daily activities and/or behaviours* (e.g. sleep disturbances, change in appetite, decreased physical activity, change in mood, or a decrease in social interactions or school attendance)? *What level would the pain need to be so that you could do all your normal activities (e.g. tolerability)? What level would the pain need to be so that you won't be bothered by it?* (Rated on same developmentally appropriate scale as pain intensity.) *What brings on the pain or makes the pain worse* (e.g. movement, deep breathing and coughing, stress etc.)?
Pain relief measures	*What has helped to make the pain better? What medication have you taken to relieve your pain? If so, what was the medication and did it help? Were there any side effects?* It is important to also ask about the use of physical, psychological and complementary and alternative treatments, if tried, and how effective these methods are in relieving pain. The degree of pain relief (or change in pain intensity) after a pain-relieving treatment/intervention should be determined.

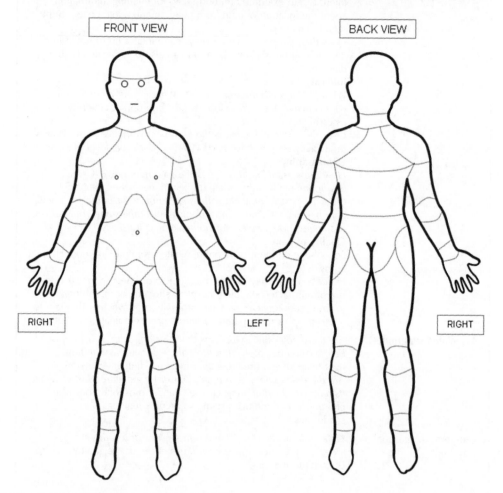

FRONT VIEW   BACK VIEW

RIGHT   LEFT   RIGHT

Figure 6.1 Body map from the Standardized Universal Pain Evaluation for pediatric rheumatology providers (SUPER-KIDZ) tool.
Source: BioMedCentral

Other factors that can affect an individual child's perception of pain should also be considered. These are discussed in Chapter 3.

Case study: Julie

The nurse asks Julie, an 8-year-old girl, if she is having pain. She denies being in pain, even though she is lying on her left side holding her abdomen with her knees flexed up to it.

- What might be some underlying factors leading Julie to deny her pain?
- How should the nurse assess Julie's pain?

Step 2: Assessing the child's pain using an developmentally appropriate pain assessment tool

The three approaches to measuring pain are:

- self-report (what the child says);
- behavioural indicators (how the child behaves);
- physiological indicators (how the child's body reacts).

These three approaches may be used separately but have also been combined in several pain assessment tools that are available for use in practice. Self-report tools should be used with children who are:

- old enough to understand and use self-report scale (e.g. older than 3 years);
- not overtly distressed;
- not cognitively impaired.

(Stinson et al. 2006a)

With infants, toddlers, and preverbal, cognitively impaired and sedated children, behavioural pain assessment tools should be used (von Baeyer and Spagrud 2007). If the child is overtly distressed (e.g. due to pain, anxiety or some other stressor), no meaningful self-report can be obtained at that time. Instead, the child's pain should be estimated using a behavioural pain assessment tool until the child is less distressed (e.g. following the administration of analgesic drugs).

Case study: Samir

Samir is a 14-year-old Iranian boy with a previous medical history of migraine headaches. He has come to the hospital with a 10-day history of headaches, joint pain, right leg pain and anorexia. He looks unwell and his vital signs are: heart rate 136, respiratory rate 32, blood pressure 124/70, oxygen saturation 98% and temperature 37.0°C orally. He lives at home with his mother, father and two brothers. He is a good student and enjoys school, playing football and listening to music. He has had blood testing in the past and is very fearful of needles. The emergency department nurse is carrying out an initial assessment of Samir.

- What would a thorough pain assessment with Samir include?
- How could the nurse involve Samir's family in the pain assessment? What questions should be asked?
- How would the assessment change if Samir was cognitively impaired?

Self-report tools

Several self-report pain assessment tools have been designed for use with school-aged children.

Verbal rating scales

- Verbal rating scales (VRS) consist of a list of simple word descriptors or phrases to indicate varying degrees or intensities of pain.
- Each word or phrase has an associated number on a VRS.
- Children are asked to select the word or phrase that best represents their level of pain intensity, and the score is the number associated with the chosen word.
- One example of a VRS is using word descriptors of *not at all* = 0, *a little bit* = 1, *quite a lot* = 2 and *most hurt possible* = 3 (Goodenough et al. 1997).

Faces pain scales

- Faces pain scales present the child with drawings or photographs of facial expressions representing different levels of pain intensity, in rank order (Figures 6.2 and 6.3).
- The child is asked to select the picture of a face that best represents their pain intensity, and their score is the number of the expression chosen.
- Faces scales have been well validated for use in children aged 5–17 years across several ethnic and cultural groups (Stinson et al. 2006a; Tomlinson et al. 2010; de Silva et al. 2011).
- There are two types of faces scales – line drawings (e.g. Faces Pain Scale–Revised, Figure 6.2) and photographs (e.g. Oucher, Figure 6.3).
- Faces pain scales with a happy and smiling *no pain* face or faces with tears for *most pain possible* have been found to affect the pain scores recorded. For example, the smiling lower anchor of the Wong-Baker FACES Pain Scale (accessible at: http://painconsortium.nih.gov/pain_scales/Wong-Baker_Faces.pdf) has been found to produce higher pain ratings than those with neutral faced anchors (Chambers and Craig 1998). Faces pain scales with neutral expressions for *no pain* such as that developed by Hicks et al. (2001) (Figure 6.2) are, therefore, generally recommended.
- Some of the more commonly used and well-validated faces pain scales are outlined in Table 6.3.

Numerical pain scales

- A numerical rating scale (NRS) consists of a range of numbers (e.g. 0–10 or 0–100) that can be represented in verbal or graphical format (Figure 6.4).
- Children are told that the lowest number represents *'no pain'* and the highest number represents *'the most pain possible'*. The child is instructed to circle, record or state the number that best represents their level of pain intensity.

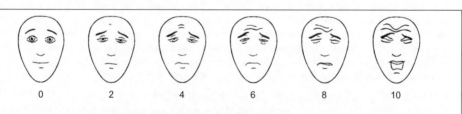

From Pain, 2001; 93:173-183. Used with permission from IASP. Numbers are for reference and are not shown to children. Scale and instructions in many languages are available online for clinical and research use at http://www.iasp-pain.org/Content/NavigationMenu/GeneralResourceLinks/FacesPainScaleRevised/default.htm

Figure 6.2   Faces Pain Scale–Revised.
Source: Hicks et al. 2001. This Faces Pain Scale-Revised has been reproduced with the permission of The International Association for the Study of Pain® (IASP®). This figure has been reproduced with permission of the International Association for the Study of Pain® (IASP). The figure may not be reproduced for any other purpose without permission.

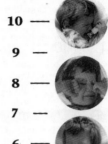

OUCHER!

10 —
9 —
8 —
7 —
6 —
5 —
4 —
3 —
2 —
1 —
0 —

http://www.oucher.org

Figure 6.3 Oucher.
Source: The Caucasian version of the Oucher was developed and copyrighted in 1983 by Judith E. Beyer, Ph.D., RN. (University of Missouri-Kansas City School of Nursing), USA. Reproduced with Permission from Dr. Judith Beyer.

No pain	0	1	2	3	4	5	6	7	8	9	10	Most pain

Figure 6.4 Numerical Rating Scale (NRS).

- Verbal NRS tend to be the most frequently used pain intensity tool with children over 8 years of age in clinical practice.
- They have the advantage that they can be verbally administered without a print copy and are easy to score. They do require numeracy skills and, therefore, should be used in older school-aged children and adolescents.
- While there is evidence of their reliability and validity in adults, before 2009 there was little testing of NRS in children. There is some early evidence that they are reliable and valid in older children (aged 8 years and over) and adolescents, for acute pain (von Baeyer et al. 2009; Bailey et al. 2010; Connelly and Neville 2010; Page et al. 2012).
- There is inconclusive evidence regarding the ability of NRS to detect changes in pain in response to medical treatments and procedures in children with chronic pain.
- Further research is needed on the lower age limit of children that can use the scale as well as standardised age-appropriate anchors and instructions for use (von Baeyer et al. 2009).

Table 6.3 Validated faces pain tools

Tool	Characteristics	Considerations
Faces Pain Scale–Revised (FPS-R) (Hicks et al. 2001)	• The Faces Pain Scale (FPS) (Bieri et al. 1990) was altered to ensure it was compatible in scoring with other self-rating and behavioural scales • Six gender-neutral faces (Figure 6.2) • Faces range from *no pain* to *as much pain as possible* • Scored 0–10	• Intended for use in children aged 5–12 years old but has been used in children aged 4–18 years • Well-established evidence of reliability, validity and ability to detect change (Stinson et al. 2006a; Tomlinson et al. 2010) • High clinical utility (quick and easy to use) • Translated into >35 languages • Disadvantages: limited evidence regarding interpretability of scores and mixed evidence about the acceptability of the scale to children
Oucher – photographic scale (Beyer et al 2009)	• Six photographs of ethnically/culturally specific faces presented vertically alongside Oucher numerical rating scale (Figure 6.3; instructions accessible at www.oucher.org) • Available as Caucasian, Hispanic, Afro-American and Asian scales • Scored 0–10	• Intended for use in children aged 3–7 years but has been used in children aged 3–18 years • Well-established evidence of reliability, validity and ability to detect change. Its use in younger children (3- to 4-year-olds) requires further testing (Stinson et al. 2006a; Tomlinson et al. 2010) • Moderate clinical utility • Mixed acceptability compared to other faces scales • Disadvantages: photos are not gender or ethnically neutral and are of children with acute rather than chronic pain, limiting the clinical contexts in which it can be used • Practical issues: cost to purchase scales and need to disinfect between patients
Wong-Baker FACES Pain Scale (Wong and Baker 1988)	• Six hand-drawn faces ranging from smiling to crying (accessible at: http://painconsortium.nih.gov/pain_scales/Wong-Baker_Faces.pdf) • Face 1 = 'no hurt', face 2 = 'hurts a little bit', face 3 = 'hurts little more', face 4 = 'hurts whole lot', face 5 = 'hurts worst' • Scored 0–5 or 0–10	• Intended for use in children aged 3–18 years • Well-established evidence of reliability, validity and ability to detect change (Stinson et al. 2006a; Tomlinson et al. 2010) • High clinical utility (quick and simple to use, requires minimal instruction) • High acceptability (well-liked by children and healthcare professionals) • Translated into more than 10 languages • Readily available (can be obtained free of charge) and easily reproduced by photocopying • Wearable badges are available for purchase • Disadvantages include: smiling *no pain* face results in higher reported pain scores compared to neutral face (Chambers and Craig 1998; Chambers et al. 2005), worst pain face has tears and not all children cry when in pain

- An example of a well-validated scale incorporating a graphic NRS is the Oucher (Beyer et al. 2009; Figure 6.3). The Oucher comprises two separate scales; the photographic faces scale and a 0–10 vertical NRS. Older school-aged children and adolescents normally use the NRS.

Graphic rating scales
- The most commonly used graphic rating scale is the *Pieces of Hurt Tool* (Hester 1979).
- This tool consists of four tokens (e.g. poker chips), representing *'a little hurt'* to *'the most hurt you could ever have'*.
- The child is asked to select the token that represents his/her pain intensity and the tool is scored from 0 to 4.
- The Pieces of Hurt Tool has been well-validated for acute procedural and hospital-based pain and is recommended for use in pre-school children (Stinson et al. 2006a).
- The Pieces of Hurt Tool is easy to use and score and the instructions have been translated into several languages including Arabic, Thai and Spanish and validated for use in Jordanian (Gharaibeh and Abu-Saad 2002) and Thai (Suraseranivongse et al. 2005) children.
- Drawbacks to its use include cleaning the chips after each patient and the potential to lose chips.

Visual analogue scales
- Visual analogue scales (VAS) require the child to select a point on a vertical or horizontal line where the ends of the line are defined as the extreme limits of pain intensity.
- The child is asked to make a mark along the line to indicate the intensity of their pain. There are many versions of VAS for use with children.
- In addition, creative strategies have been employed to improve the reliability and validity of VAS for use in children by using graphic or other methods to enhance the child's understanding of the tool (e.g. Colour Analogue Scale; McGrath et al. 1996, Figure 6.5).
- VAS have been extensively researched and have been recommended for most children aged 8 years and older (Stinson et al. 2006a).
- While VAS are easy to reproduce, photocopying may alter the line length and VAS pain assessment also requires the extra step of measuring the line, which increases the burden and likelihood for errors in assessment.

Multidimensional pain tools
Although pain intensity is the most commonly recorded measure of a painful episode, a more comprehensive pain assessment is often necessary, for example, for children with chronic pain. In this situation it is necessary to assess factors such as pain triggers, the types of sensation that are experienced and how the pain interferes with aspects of everyday life. Table 6.4 outlines three self-report pain tools that have been shown to be reliable and valid multidimensional pain measures.

Pain diaries are another way to track pain in children with recurrent or chronic pain. While paper-based diaries have been used in clinical and research practice for decades, they are prone to recall biases and poor compliance. More recently, real-time data collection methods using electronic hand-held devices have been developed for children with recurrent and chronic pain (Palermo et al. 2004; Stinson et al. 2006b, 2008; Lewandowski et al. 2009; Connelly et al. 2010; Jacobs et al. 2012).

Colored Analog Scale staff side (left) and child side (right)

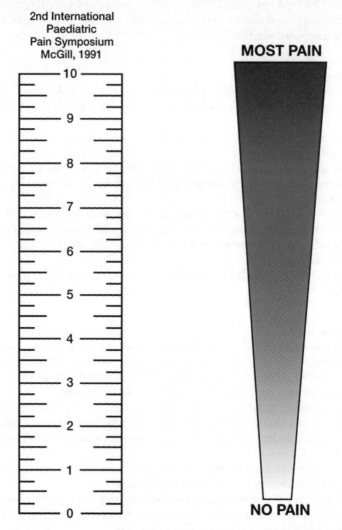

Figure 6.5 Coloured analogue scale.
Source: McGrath PA, Seifert CE, Speechley KN, Booth JC, Stitt L, and Gibson MC. A new analogue scale for assessing children's pain: an initial validation study. PAIN® 1996 March 64(3); 435–443. This figure has been reproduced with permission of the International Association for the Study of Pain® (IASP).

Additional information

For further information about self-report tools see:
Stinson, J.N., Yamada, J., Kavanagh, T., Gill, N. and Stevens, B. (2006) Systematic review of the psychometric properties and feasibility of self-report pain measures for use in clinical trials in children and adolescents. *Pain* **125**(1–2), 143–157.
Huguet, A., Stinson, J.N. and McGrath, P.J. (2010) Measurement of self-reported pain intensity in children and adolescents. *Journal of Psychosomatic Research* **68**(4), 329–336.
Tomlinson, D., von Baeyer, C.L., Stinson, J.N. and Sung, L. (2010) A systematic review of faces scales for the self-report of pain intensity in children. *Pediatrics* **26**(5), 1168–1198.

Table 6.4 Validated multidimensional self-report pain tools

Tool	Components	Considerations
Adolescent Pediatric Pain Tool (APPT) (Savedra et al. 1989)	Pain intensity measured using: • a 0–100 mm word graphic rating scale • body outline to describe location of pain • word descriptors	• Originally developed for children and adolescents with postoperative pain; has been used in children with acute and chronic disease-related pain (e.g. cancer, sickle cell disease, arthritis) • Intended for use in children aged 5–16 years; used in children from 4–18 years • Well-established evidence of reliability, validity and ability to detect change • Easy to use, well-liked, requires minimal training and takes 3–6 minutes to complete
Pediatric Pain Assessment Tool (PPAT) (Abu-Saad et al. 1990)	Pain intensity measured using: • 0–10 cm VAS • body outline (number of body areas marked) • 32 word descriptors	• Initially developed for acute medical and postoperative pain; has also been used with recurrent pain (headaches) and chronic pain (arthritis) • Intended for use in children aged 5–16 years; used in children up to 17 years • Well-established evidence of reliability and validity and some evidence of ability to detect change • Child, parent and healthcare professional forms • Easy to use and takes 5–10 minutes to complete
Pediatric Pain Questionnaire (PPQ) (Varni et al. 1987)	Pain intensity measured using: • 0–10 cm VAS anchored with happy and sad faces for present and worst pain • gender-neutral body outline to describe location of pain (number of body areas marked) • pain intensity (choosing four of eight coloured crayons to represent various levels of pain intensity from none, mild, moderate and severe) • 46 word descriptors to assess the sensory, affective and evaluative qualities of pain	• Originally developed for children and adolescents with recurrent and chronic pain (e.g. juvenile arthritis) • Intended for use in children aged 5–16 years; used in children 4–18 years • Child, adolescent and parent versions • Children younger than 7 years will usually need to be read the instructions to complete the VAS and body outline. Young children appear to be able to complete the tool without issue (Benestad et al. 1996) • Well-established evidence of reliability and validity and some evidence of ability to detect change • Minimal training and takes 10–15 minutes to complete • Website: www.pedsgl.org

Behavioural tools

The tools developed to assess pain in infants and young children generally use behavioural indicators of pain. A wide range of specific, expressive, behaviours have been identified in infants and young children that are indicative of pain. These are:

- individual behaviours (e.g. crying and facial expression);
- large body movements (e.g. withdrawal of the affected limb, touching the affected area, and the movement or tensing of limbs and torso);
- changes in social behaviour or appetite;
- changes in sleep/wake state or cognitive functions.

Case study: Baby Jessica

Jessica was born at 31 weeks gestational age. Now 15 days old, she is hospitalised in the neonatal intensive care unit for monitoring of prematurity. Her vital signs are: heart rate 179, respiratory rate 60, blood pressure 50/32, oxygen saturation 88% and temperature 38.0°C axillary. She is also mildly lethargic. Jessica's nurse suspects she is septic and requests that the attending physician further assess the baby. Following the physician's assessment, a septic workup is ordered. This includes intravenous blood test for a complete/full blood count, electrolyte levels and blood cultures and urine cultures. While the student nurse is preparing for the venepuncture and urinary catheter insertion the medical team arrives on the unit for medical rounds and generates a discussion as follows:

- Jessica's doctor asks the nursing student to tell the group about pain assessment for this baby and which validated tool should be used. How should the student answer?
- The doctor then asks the group, 'What will a baby in pain look like? Will a lethargic baby behave in the same way when in pain?' How should the group answer?

Behavioural tools are indicated for children who are:

- too young to understand and use self-report scales (e.g. less than 3 years old)
- too distressed to use self-report scales
- impaired in their cognitive or communication abilities
- very restricted by bandages, surgical tape, mechanical ventilation or paralysing or sedating drugs
- whose self-report ratings are considered to be exaggerated, minimised or unrealistic due to cognitive, emotional or situational factors

Source: von Baeyer and Spagrud (2007); von Baeyer et al. (2011)

A variety of behavioural pain tools have been developed and validated for use in infants and children (Table 6.5) (see also Figure 6.6).

Additional information

For further information about behavioural tools that can be used with children aged 3–18 years see: von Baeyer, C.L. and Spagrud, L.J. (2007) Systematic review of observational (behavioural) measures for children and adolescents aged 3 to 18 years. *Pain* **127**, 140–150.

Table 6.5 Validated behavioural tools

Tool	Indicators	Considerations
Children's Hospital of Eastern Ontario Pain Scale (CHEOPS) (McGrath et al. 1985)	Crying, facial expression, verbalisations, torso activity, whether and how child touches wound, leg position	• Intended for use in children aged 1–7 years but has been used in children 4 months to 17 years • Procedural and postoperative pain • Indicators are scored on a four-point scale (0, 1, 2, 3) with a total score from 4 to 13, but no indication of what mild, moderate or severe pain score ranges would be • Well-established evidence of reliability, validity and ability to detect change (von Baeyer and Spagrud, 2007) • Length of tool and confusing scoring system makes it complicated to use in everyday clinical practice (low/ medium clinical utility) • Cannot be used in intubated or paralysed patients
COMFORT Scale (Ambuel et al. 1992)	Alertness, calmness or agitation, respiratory response, blood pressure, heart rate, muscle tone, physical movement, facial tension. More recently modified to include crying for non-ventilated infants (van Dijk et al. 2000)	• Intended for use in children 0 to 17 years of age but has been used in children 0 to 18 years on ventilator or in critical care (only validated tool for this purpose) • Used to rate pain-related to heart surgery, child repositioning to improve oxygenation and mechanical ventilation (von Baeyer and Spagrud, 2007) • Well-established evidence of reliability and validity; however, inconsistent ability to detect change (von Baeyer and Spagrud, 2007) • Eight indicators scored from 1–5 with a total score from 8 to 40 • Administration time is about 3 minutes • 2 hours training to use tool needed
Revised FLACC (r-FLACC) (Malviya et al. 2006) (Table 6.6)	Facial expression, leg movement, activity, cry and consolability	• Initially developed as FLACC (Merkel et al. 1997) and intended for use in children aged 2 months to 8 years but has been used in children aged 0–18 years • Later amended to r-FLACC to include pain behaviours common to individuals with cognitive impairments • Used in cognitively impaired children aged 4–21 years (Malviya et al. 2006) • Validated for procedural and postoperative pain • Indicators are scored on a 0–2 scale, with a total score from 0 to 10 • Well-established evidence of reliability and validity; however, inconsistent ability to detect change demonstrated with FLACC (von Baeyer and Spagrud, 2007) • Simple to use, score and interpret. High clinical utility (von Baeyer and Spagrud 2007; Voepel-Lewis et al. 2008). • Cannot be used in paralysed patients. Some preliminary data suggests it may be useful with ventilated patients (Voepel-Lewis et al. 2010) • Important to note that consolability requires (a) an attempt to console and (b) a subjective rating of response to that intervention, which complicates the scoring

Categories	Scoring		
	0	**1**	**2**
Face	No particular expression or smile	Occasional grimace or frown, withdrawn, disinterested, *appears sad or worried*	Frequent to constant frown, clenched jaw, quivering chin, *distressed looking face, expression of fright or panic* *Individualised behaviour:*
Legs	Normal position or relaxed, *usual tone and motion to limbs*	Uneasy, restless, tense, *occasional tremors*	Kicking, or legs drawn up, *marked increase in spasticity, constant tremors or jerking* *Individualised behaviour:*
Activity	Lying quietly, normal position, moves easily, *regular rhythmic respirations*	Squirming, shifting back and forth, *tense or guarded movements, mildly agitated (e.g. head back and forth, aggression),shallow splinting respirations, intermittent sighs*	Arched, rigid, or jerking, *severe agitations, head banging, shivering (non-rigours), breath holding, gasping or sharp intakes of breath, severe splinting* *Individualised behaviour:*
Cry	No cry (awake or asleep)	Moans or whimpers, occasional complaint, *occasional verbal outburst or grunt*	Crying steadily, screams or sobs, frequent complaints, *repeated outbursts, constant grunting* *Individualised behaviour:*
Consolability	Content, relaxed	Reassured by occasional touching, hugging, or being talked to, distractible	Difficult to console or comfort, *pushing away caregiver, resisting care or comfort measures* *Individualised behaviour:*

Each of the five categories (F) face, (L) legs, (A) activity, (C) cry and (C) consolability is scored from 0 to 2, which results in a total score between 0 and 10. Revisions to original FLACC (Merkel et al. 1997) for children with cognitive impairments are indicated in italics.

Figure 6.6 Revised FLACC (r-FLACC) Behavioural Scale.
Source: © 2002, The Regents of the University of Michigan

Physiological indicators

Neonates and children display metabolic, hormonal, and physiological responses to pain. These physiological reactions all indicate the activation of the sympathetic nervous system, which is part of the autonomic nervous system, and is responsible for the *fight or flight* response associated with stress (Sweet and McGrath 1998). These physiological changes should be recognised as:

- usually reflecting stress reactions;
- being only loosely correlated with self-report of pain;
- occurring in response to other states such as exertion, fever and anxiety.

(von Baeyer and Spagrud 2007)

On their own, physiological indicators do not constitute a valid clinical pain measure for children. A multidimensional or composite tool that incorporates physiological and behavioural indicators, as well as self-report is, therefore, preferred whenever possible (von Baeyer and Spagrud 2007; Arif-Rahu et al. 2012).

Physiological parameters that can indicate that a child is in pain are outlined in Table 6.6.

Other physiological indicators of pain include sweating and dilated pupils.

Table 6.6 Physiological indicators used to assess pain

Observation	Change indicating pain
Heart rate	Increases when in pain (after an initial decrease)
Respiratory rate and pattern	There is conflicting evidence about whether this increases or decreases, but there is a significant shift from baseline. Breathing may become rapid and/or shallow
Blood pressure	Increases when a child is in acute pain
Oxygen saturation	Decreases when a child is in acute pain

Source: Sweet, S.D. & McGrath, P.J. (1998). This table has been reproduced with permission of the International Association for the Study of Pain® (IASP). The figure may not be reproduced for any other purpose without permission

Pain Assessment Tools for Neonates

There are several pain assessment tools that combine behavioural and physiological indicators as well as contextual factors (e.g. gestational age, sleep/wake state) for assessing pain in neonates. These tools have varying degrees of established reliability and validity (Table 6.7). The Premature Infant Pain Profile (PIPP) (Stevens et al. 1996) has been the most rigorously validated.

Facial activity has been the most comprehensively studied behavioural pain assessment indicator in neonates. It is the most reliable and consistent sign of pain across populations and types of pain (Craig 1998). The facial actions associated with acute pain in neonates are identified in Box 6.2 and are portrayed in Figure 6.7.

Table 6.7 Some validated pain assessment tools for neonates

Tool	Indicators	Considerations
CRIES (Crying, Requires O₂ for saturation above 95, Increased vital signs, Expression, and Sleeplessness) (Krechel and Bildner 1995)	Cry, O₂ saturation, heart rate/blood pressure, expression and sleeplessness	• Full-term neonates (32–60 weeks gestation) • Assesses postoperative pain • Indicators are scored on a three-point scale (0, 1, 2) with a total score from 0 to 10 • Evidence of reliability and validity (Duhn and Medves 2004) and some evidence of ability to detect change • Easy to remember and use (high clinical utility) • Uses oxygenation as a measure, which can be influenced by many other factors • BP measurements may upset neonates
Neonatal Infant Pain Scale (NIPS) (Lawrence et al. 1993)	Facial expression, cry, breathing patterns, arms, legs, state of arousal	• Preterm and term neonates • Assesses procedural pain • Operational definitions for indicators are provided • Indicators are scored on a two-point (0, 1) or three-point (0, 1, 2) scale at one-minute intervals, before, during, and following a procedure • Evidence of reliability and validity (Duhn and Medves 2004) • Hard to remember (limited clinical utility) • Cannot be used in intubated or paralysed neonates
Premature Infant Pain Profile (PIPP) (Stevens et al. 1996)	Gestational age, behavioural state, heart rate and oxygen saturation, brow bulge, eye squeeze, and nasolabial furrow	• Preterm and term neonates (e.g. 28–40 weeks gestation) • Initially developed for procedural pain, requires further evaluation with very low birthweight neonates and with non-acute and post-surgical pain populations • Includes contextual indicators (e.g. gestation and behavioural state) • Indicators are scored on a four-point scale (0, 1, 2, 3) for a total score of 0 to 21 based on the gestation of the neonate • Score of 6 or less generally indicates minimal or no pain, while scores greater than 12 indicate moderate to severe pain • Most rigorously evaluated tool; evidence of reliability, validity and ability to detect change (Stevens et al. 2010) • Further research required to establish feasibility and clinical utility (Stevens et al. 2010) • Pain assessments take 1 minute (early evidence of good clinical utility) • A revised version of the PIPP is currently undergoing testing that includes changes to scoring of individual items and total score

BOX 6.2

Facial actions associated with acute pain in neonates

- Bulging brow
- Eyes squeezed tightly shut
- Deepening of nasolabial furrow
- Open lips
- Mouth stretched vertically and horizontally
- Taut tongue

Source: Craig (1998)

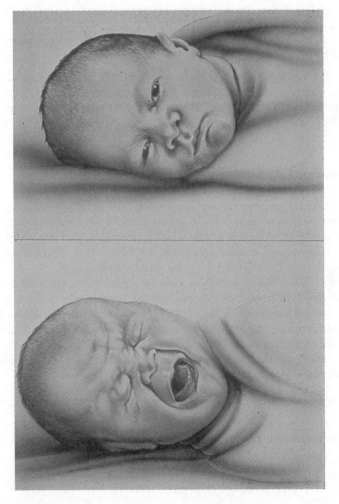

Figure 6.7 Neonatal Pain Facial Expression.
Source: Grunau RVE, Craig KD. Pain expression in neonates: facial action and cry. PAIN® 1987 March 28(3); 395–410. This figure has been reproduced with permission of the International Association for the Study of Pain® (IASP). The figure may not be reproduced for any other purpose without permission.

Pain Assessment in Ventilated Children

Assessing pain in ventilated infants and children remains a special challenge for clinicians (Ramelet et al. 2004; Boyle et al. 2006). Ventilated children may not be able to express their pain because:

- they are intubated;
- they are usually sedated (with or without pharmacological paralysis);
- they may have neurological impairment due to trauma, health condition or medications.

Other factors that add to the complexity of assessing pain in ventilated children include:

- difficulty differentiating pain from distress, anxiety and agitation;
- the child's age (e.g. limited range of pain behaviours in young infants; older children may be able to self-report);
- the severity of the child's illness may alter physiological and behavioural responses that would be seen in healthy children.

The COMFORT scale remains the only tool that has been well validated for pain assessment in ventilated children (Table 6.5). However, the major limitation of this tool is that it does not differentiate between pain and sedation (Ramelet et al. 2004). The COMFORT scale can be accessed at: http://painconsortium.nih.gov/pain_scales/index.html.

Pain Assessment in Cognitively Delayed Children

Infants and children with cognitive impairment or developmental delay who are unable to report pain may be at greater risk for under-treatment of pain. These include children with moderate or severe cerebral palsy, neurodevelopmental disorders, severe developmental delay and autism spectrum disorders. It is particularly difficult to accurately assess pain experienced by these children (Box 6.3).

While these children are generally unable to report pain, credible assessment can usually be obtained from the parent or another person who knows the child well (Breau et al. 2002; Hunt et al. 2004, 2007). However, proxy judgements have been shown to underestimate the pain experience of others (Kelly et al. 2002; Barakat et al., 2008; Rajasagaram et al. 2009).

Factors to consider in the assessment of pain in children with a significant cognitive impairment include:

BOX 6.3

Reasons for increased risk of under-treatment of pain

- Multiple medical problems may cause or be a source of pain
- Undergo multiple procedures that are often painful
- Idiosyncratic behaviours, such as moaning or laughing, may mask expression of pain or confuse observers
- Many pain behaviours, such as changes in facial expression and patterns of sleep or play, are already inconsistent and difficult to interpret because of physical problems
- Comfort of these children may be valued less by society

Source: McGrath (1998)

- underlying condition/process (e.g. impact on neurological or musculoskeletal system, progressive or stable);
- developmental level (e.g. cognition, communication, motor function);
- usual behaviour and health condition (e.g. baseline condition, pain experiences);
- usual means of communication (e.g. verbal, non-verbal, pain behaviours);
- caregiver's views;
- impact of concurrent illnesses (e.g. social, emotional, physical);
- differential diagnosis (e.g. all possible sources of distress and pain).

(Oberlander et al. 1999; Ely et al. 2012)

Behavioural cues used to identify pain in neurologically impaired children

- Facial expression
- Vocalisations (e.g. moaning)
- Changes in posture and movements
- Physiological changes (i.e. sweating, pallor or flushing)
- Alterations in sleeping and eating
- Change in mood and sociability

Source: McGrath et al. (1998); Fanurik et al. (1999)

Parents and caregivers may report a diversity of behavioural responses to pain but the categories outlined above are common to almost all children and can provide clues to caregivers and healthcare workers that the child might be experiencing pain. This underlines the importance of obtaining a thorough baseline history from caregivers of children with cognitive impairments.

While there are several pain assessment tools for this population, three tools have been found reliable and are well validated. These are the:

- Non-Communicating Children's Pain Checklist–Revised (NCCPC-R; Breau et al. 2002; Figure 6.8);
- Revised Faces, Legs, Activity, Cry, Consolability (r-FLACC; Malviya et al. 2006; Figure 6.6);
- Paediatric Pain Profile (PPP) (Hunt et al. 2004, 2007) (see www.ppprofile.org.uk/).

The NCCPC-R has been used to assess acute pain (e.g. resulting from a fall), chronic pain (e.g. due to a medical condition) and postoperative pain, in neurologically impaired children. Postoperative pain has also been assessed with the r-FLACC, and the PPP has been used to assess persistent daily pain in this group of children. Synthesised data from an evidence-based review, feedback from a family-based hospital advisory board and a quality improvement study with nurses and parents caring for children with cognitive impairments supported using the r-FLACC over the PPP in practice (Chen-Lim et al. 2012). The clinical utility of the r-FLACC has also been rated higher than other tools for neurologically impaired children, suggesting it may be more readily adopted into clinical practice (Voepel-Lewis et al. 2008).

Additional information

Further information about the assessment of pain in cognitively delayed children can be found in: Oberlander, T.E. and Symons, F. (2006) *Pain in children and adults with developmental disabilities*, Paul H. Brookes Publishing Company, Baltimore, MD.

Please indicate how often this person has shown the signs in *Subscales I to IV* in the <u>last 5 minutes</u>. For *Subscale VII*, please indicate how often this sign was observed <u>in the past 24 hours</u>. Please circle a number for each item. If an item does not apply to this person (for example, this person does not eat solid food or cannot reach with his/her hands), then indicate "not applicable" for that item.

0 = NOT AT ALL	1 = JUST A LITTLE	2 = FAIRLY OFTEN	3 = VERY OFTEN	NA = NOT APPLICABLE

I. Vocal

1. Moaning, whining, whimpering (fairly soft)...	0	1	2	3	NA
2. Crying (moderately loud)...	0	1	2	3	NA
3. Screaming/yelling (very loud)...	0	1	2	3	NA
4. A specific sound or word for pain (e.g. a word, cry or type of laugh).................	0	1	2	3	NA

II. Social

5. Not cooperating, cranky, irritable, unhappy...	0	1	2	3	NA
6. Less interaction with others, withdrawn...	0	1	2	3	NA
7. Seeking comfort or physical closeness	0	1	2	3	NA
8. Being difficult to distract, not able to satisfy or pacify.............................	0	1	2	3	NA

III. Facial

9. A furrowed brow..	0	1	2	3	NA
10. A change in eyes, including: squinching of eyes, eyes opened wide, eyes frowning	0	1	2	3	NA
11. Turning down of mouth, not smiling..	0	1	2	3	NA
12. Lips puckering up, tight, pouting, or quivering..	0	1	2	3	NA
13. Clenching or grinding teeth, chewing or thrusting tongue out	0	1	2	3	NA

IV. Activity

14. Not moving, less active, quiet..	0	1	2	3	NA
15. Jumping around, agitated, fidgety...	0	1	2	3	NA

V. Body and Limbs

16. Floppy	0	1	2	3	NA
17. Stiff, spastic, tense, rigid	0	1	2	3	NA
18. Gesturing to or touching part of the body that hurts	0	1	2	3	NA
19. Protecting, favoring or guarding part of the body that hurts	0	1	2	3	NA
20. Flinching or moving the body part away, being sensitive to touch.....................	0	1	2	3	NA
21. Moving the body in a specific way to show pain (e.g. head back, arms down, curls up, etc.)	0	1	2	3	NA

VI. Physiological

22. Shivering	0	1	2	3	NA
23. Change in color, pallor	0	1	2	3	NA
24. Sweating, perspiring	0	1	2	3	NA
25. Tears..	0	1	2	3	NA
26. Sharp intake of breath, gasping...	0	1	2	3	NA
27. Breath holding...	0	1	2	3	NA

VII. Eating/Sleeping

28. Eating less, not interested in food..	0	1	2	3	NA
29. Increase in sleep..	0	1	2	3	NA
30. Decrease in sleep..	0	1	2	3	NA

SCORE SUMMARY:

Category:	I	II	III	IV	V	VI	VII	TOTAL
Score:								

Figure 6.8 Non-Communicating Children's Pain Checklist–Revised (NCCPC-R).
Source: Reproduced with permission from Dr. Lynn Breau. Version 01.2004 © 2004 Lynn Breau, Patrick McGrath, Allen Finley, Carol Camfield.

Choosing the Right Pain Assessment Tool

There are an abundance of reliable, valid and clinically useful pain assessment tools for assessing pain in neonates, infants, children and adolescents (Duhn and Medves 2004; Stinson et al. 2006a; von Baeyer and Spagrud 2007). However, no easily administered, widely accepted, uniform technique exists for assessing pain for all children (Stinson et al. 2006a; von Baeyer and Spagrud 2007). Box 6.4 identifies some of the factors to be considered when selecting a pain tool for use in everyday practice.

BOX 6.4

Choosing a pain assessment tool for everyday use

The tool needs to be:
- *reliable* (e.g. consistent and trustworthy ratings regardless of time, setting or who is administering the tool)
- *valid* (e.g. unequivocally measures a specific dimension of pain)
- *responsive* (e.g. able to detect change in pain due to treatment)
- *feasible* to use (e.g. simple to use and not long, short training time, easy to administer and score)
- *practical* (e.g. for assessing different types of pain)

The tool should also be:
- developmentally and culturally appropriate for the client group
- easily and quickly understood by patients
- well-liked by patients, clinicians and researchers
- inexpensive and easy to obtain, reproduce, distribute and disinfect
- available in various languages or easily translatable

Source: Data from Hester et al. (1998); McCaffery and Pasero (1999); Twycross and Shields (2005); von Baeyer (2006); McGrath (2007)

BOX 6.5

Key points to consider when choosing a pain assessment tool for an individual child

- Selection of the right tool will depend on the child's condition, age, ethnic background and cognitive/developmental level
- Careful explanation and appropriate timing of administration are necessary
- It is helpful for children to have an opportunity to practice using the tool before pain is expected, for example in a surgical pre-admission programme
- Offer the child a chance to practise using the tool by having them rate hypothetical situations that would produce low (e.g. paper cut) and high levels of pain (e.g. stepping on a nail)

Source: Data from McCaffery and Pasero (1999); von Baeyer (2006)

Additional information

Within the hospital setting it will usually be necessary to have more than one pain assessment tool to cater for all patient groups.
Each pain assessment tool should, whenever possible, use a **common metric** – e.g. all rate pain from 0–10 or 0–5.
This means that a pain score of 5 will mean the same whichever pain assessment tool is used and will thus aid effective communication about children's pain.
For more information about why a common metric is important see: Hicks, C.L., von Baeyer, C.L., Spafford, P.A., van Korlaar, I. and Goodenough, B. (2001) The Faces Pain Scale–Revised: Toward a common metric in pediatric pain measurement. *Pain* **93**, 173–183.

The key points to consider when choosing a pain assessment tool for an individual child are outlined in Box 6.5. An example of an algorithm for assessing pain in hospitalised children can be seen in Figure 6.9 (Palozzi et al. 2010).

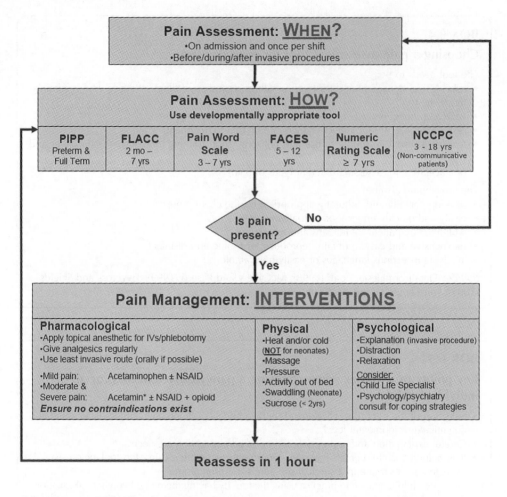

Figure 6.9 Example of an algorithm for assessing pain in hospitalised children. NB acetami-
nophen = paracetamol; child life specialist = play therapist.
Source: Reproduced with permission from Palozzi L, Campbell F and Hurdowar A. Palozzi, L.,
Campbell, F. & Hurdowar A. (2010). Pain Management Clinical Practice Guideline, Policies and
Procedures Database. The Hospital for Sick Children.

How Often Should Pain be Assessed?

Effective pain management depends on regular assessment of the presence and severity
of pain and the patient's response to pain management interventions. Every patient
should have their pain assessed:

- when they visit an emergency department or an ambulatory clinic;
- on admission to hospital;
- at least once per shift (while they are an inpatient);
- before, during and after an invasive procedure.

Pain should be assessed regularly following surgery and/or if the patient has a known
painful medical condition. In these cases, pain should be assessed hourly for the first
6 hours. After this, if the pain is well controlled, it can be assessed less frequently
(e.g. every 4 hours). If the pain is fluctuating, regular assessment should continue for

48–72 hours; after this the pain intensity will normally have peaked and be starting to subside. Chronic pain assessment may be more complex than acute pain assessment and should be detailed and multidimensional in nature. Chronic pain management is also likely to benefit from longitudinal pain assessment (i.e. frequent assessments over a period of days to weeks). (The management of acute pain is discussed in more detail in Chapter 7 and the management of chronic pain is discussed in Chapter 8.)

Documentation

Regular assessment and documentation of pain allows effective treatment and communication among members of the healthcare team and with the patient and family. Standardised forms and tools (e.g. admission assessment forms, vital signs chart) for the documentation of pain encourages initial assessment and ongoing reassessments. These forms can also be used for documenting efficacy of pain-relieving interventions. Including pain intensity ratings on the vital signs record reminds staff to consider pain as seriously as other vital signs they measure.

Summary

- Pain assessment is vital for effective pain management.
- The first step in assessing pain is recording a pain history.
- The second step in pain assessment is assessing the child's pain using a developmentally appropriate pain assessment tool.
- The third step is evaluating the effectiveness of the pain-relieving interventions used.
- Validated and reliable pain assessment tools are available for children of all ages.
- The child's self-report of pain is important and should be sought whenever possible.
- Children who are non-verbal or who have cognitive impairments are vulnerable to having their pain underestimated.
- Physiological, behavioural and self-report indicators can all be used to assess children's pain.
- Pain should be assessed regularly to detect the presence of pain and to evaluate the effectiveness of treatments.
- Documentation of pain facilitates regular reassessment of pain and follow-up.

Key to Case Studies

See Boxes 6.6, 6.7 and 6.8.

BOX 6.6

Julie

Julie may not want to say she has pain for fear of being given an injection or needle to deliver the pain medicine. There may also be cultural reasons for denying she has pain. It would be important to explore the reasons for her refusal.

Appropriate tools to assess her pain would be to use a self-report tool such as the FPS-R as well as a behavioural tool like the R-FLACC. By using both tools you can talk to Julie about the discordance between the two tools to try and discover why she is reluctant to talk about her pain.

BOX 6.7

Samir

A thorough assessment of Samir's pain involves taking a history of his prior pain experiences and current pain complaints. Standardised forms with questions such as those in Table 6.1 have been developed for talking to children and parents about pain and can help guide history taking. It would be important to assess the influence of culture on his pain beliefs. Current pain should be assessed with a valid age-appropriate pain assessment tool. For Samir, a self-report tool like an NRS or a multidimensional pain tool (e.g. APPT) would be good choices.

Samir's family members know him best and can recognise subtle changes in his manner or behaviour. They are, therefore, central to assessing his pain. The nurse should ask Samir's family if they have noticed any changes in his mood, physical activity level, engagement in schoolwork, social interactions or sleep patterns.

With cognitively impaired children it is important to obtain a detailed history from the parents about the behaviours they consider to indicate pain. You would then use a behavioural tool that has been validated in this population such as the NCCPC-R or the r-FLACC.

BOX 6.8

Jessica

Infants cannot express their pain verbally, so behavioural and physiological tools are used to assess pain. Physiological indicators include increased heart rate, decreased oxygen saturation and changes in respiratory pattern. Physiological indicators must be considered in the context of a multidimensional pain assessment, as they are not valid tools when used alone.

As Jessica is only 33 weeks, using the PIPP pain assessment tool is preferable as it has the greatest validity for babies born prematurely.

A baby in pain may display several pain behaviours. Facial activity (e.g. brow bulge, eye squeeze) has been the most comprehensively studied and is the most reliable and consistent pain behaviour. Sleeplessness and cry can also be indicators of infant pain. These responses may be less obvious in a lethargic infant, making consideration in this context (e.g. sepsis requiring painful procedures) important to Jessica's assessment.

Additional information

National Institutes of Health (NIH) Pain Consortium is a source of commonly used pain intensity assessment tools used in children, available from: http://painconsortium.nih.gov/pain_scales/index.html

Partners Against Pain provides printable PDFs of commonly used paediatric pain scales, available at: www.partnersagainstpain.com/hcp/pain-assessment/tools.aspx

Ped-IMMPACT: Recommendations for the design, execution and interpretation of paediatric pain clinical trials including PDFs of systematic reviews of self-report and behavioural pain tools for 3–18 years, available at: www.immpact.org/meetings.html

Royal College of Nursing provides information on RCN pain assessment guidelines and recommended pain assessment tools in children, available at: www.rcn.org.uk/development/practice/clinicalguidelines/pain

Acknowledgements

We would like to thank Ms Grace Lee and Dr Bonnie Stevens for preparing the case study and questions about Jessica.

References

Abu-Saad, H.H., Kroonen, E. and Halfens, R. (1990) On the development of a multidimensional Dutch pain assessment tool for children. *Pain* **43**(2), 249–256.

Ambuel, B., Hamlett, K.W., Marx, C.M. and Blumer, J.L. (1992) Assessing distress in pediatric intensive care environments: the COMFORT scale. *Journal of Pediatric Psychology* **17**, 95–109.

American Medical Association (2007) *Pain Management: Pediatric Pain Management*. American Medical Association. Available from: www.ama-cmeonline.com/pain_mgmt/printversion/ama_painmgmt_m6.pdf (accessed January 2013).

Arif-Rahu, M., Fisher, D. and Matsuda, Y. (2012) Biobehavioral measures for pain in the pediatric patient. *Pain Management Nursing* **13**(3), 157–168.

Bailey, B., Daoust, R., Doyon-Trottier, E., Dauphin-Pierre, S. and Gravel, J. (2010) Validation and properties of the verbal numeric scale in children with acute pain. *Pain* **149**(2), 216–221.

Ball, J. and Bindler, R. (1995) Pain assessment and management. In: *Pediatric Nursing: Caring for Children* (eds J. Ball and R. Bindler). Appleton & Lange, Norwalk, CT.

Barakat, L.P., Simon, K., Schwartz, L.A. and Radcliff, J. (2008) Correlates of pain-rating concordance for adolescents with sickle cell disease and their caregivers. *Clinical Journal of Pain* **24**(5), 438–446.

Benestad, B., Vinje, O., Veierod, B.M. and Vandvik, I.K. (1996) Quantitative and qualitative assessment of pain in children with juvenile chronic arthritis based on the Norwegian version of the Pediatric Pain Questionnaire. *Scandinavian Journal of Rheumatology* **25**(5), 293–299.

Beyer, J.E., Villarruel, A.M. and Denyes, M.J. (2009) *The Oucher: A User's Manual and Technical Report*. (www.oucher.org/downloads/2009_Users_Manual.pdf) (accessed: January 2013).

Bieri, D., Reeve, R.A., Champion, G.D. Addicoat, L and Ziegler, J.B. (1990) The Faces Pain Scale for the self-assessment of the severity of pain experienced by children: Development, initial validation and preliminary investigation for ratio scale properties. *Pain* **41**,139–150.

Boyle, E.M., Freer, Y., Wong, C.M., McIntosh, N. and Anand, K.J.S. (2006) Assessment of persistent pain or distress and adequacy of analgesia in preterm ventilated infants. *Pain* **124**, 87–91.

Breau, L.M., McGrath, P.J., Camfield, C. and Finley, G.A. (2002) Psychometric properties of the Non-communicating Children's Pain Checklist–Revised. *Pain* **99**, 349–357.

Chambers, C.T. and Craig, K.D. (1998) An intrusive impact of anchors in children's faces pain scales. *Pain* **78**(1), 27–37.

Chambers, C., Hardial, J., Craig, K., Court, C. and Montgomery, C. (2005) Faces scales for the measurement of postoperative pain intensity in children following minor surgery. *Clinical Journal of Pain* **21**(3), 277–285.

Chen-Lim, M.L., Zarnowsky, C., Green, R., Shaffer, S., Holtzer, B. and Ely, E. (2012) Optimizing the assessment of pain in children who are cognitively impaired through the quality improvement process. *Journal of Pediatric Nursing* **27**(6), 750–759.

Connelly, M. and Neville, K. (2010) Comparative prospective evaluation of the responsiveness of single-item pediatric pain-intensity self-report scales and their uniqueness from negative affect in a hospital setting. *Journal of Pain* **11**(12), 1451–1460.

Connelly, M., Anthony, K.K., Sarniak, R., Bromberg, M.K., Gil, K.M. and Schanberg, L.E. (2010) Parent pain responses as predictors of daily activities and mood in children with juvenile idiopathic arthritis: The utility of electronic diaries. *Journal of Pain and Symptom Management* **79**(3), 579–590.

Craig, K.D. (1998) The facial display of pain in infants and children. In: *Measures of pain in infants and children, Progress in Pain Research Management*, Vol. 10 (eds G.A. Finley and P.J. McGrath), pp. 103–121. IASP Press, Seattle.

de Silva, F.C., Santos Thuler, F.C. and de Leon-Casasola, O.A. (2011) Validity and reliability of two pain assessment tools in Brazilian children and adolescents. *Journal of Clinical Nursing* **20**(13–14), 1842–1848.

Drendel, A.L., Kelly, D.T. and Ali, S. (2011) Pain assessment in children: Overcoming challenges and optimizing care. *Pediatric Emergency Care* **27**(8), 773–781.

Duhn, L.J. and Medves, J.M. (2004) A systematic integrative review of infant pain assessment tools. *Advances in Neonatal care* **4**(3), 126–140.

Ely, E., Chen-Lim, M.L., Zarnowsky, C., Green, R., Shaffer, S. and Holtzer, B. (2012) Finding the evidence to change practice for assessing pain in children who are cognitively impaired. *Journal of Pediatric Nursing* **27**(4), 402–410.

Fanurik, D., Koh, J.L., Schmitz, M.L., Harrison, R.D. and Conrad, T.M. (1999) Children with cognitive impairment: Parent report of pain and coping. *Developmental and Behavioral Pediatrics* **20**(4), 228–234.

Gharaibeh, M. and Abu-Saad, H. (2002) Cultural validation of pediatric pain assessment tools: Jordanian perspective. *Journal of Transcultural Nursing* 13(1), 12–18.

Goodenough, B., Thomas, W., Champion, G. et al. (1997) Pain in 4- to 6-year-old children receiving intramuscular injections: A comparison of the faces pain scale with Oucher self-report and behavioural measures. *Clinical Journal of Pain* 13(1), 60–73.

Hester, N. (1979) The preoperational child's reaction to immunization. *Nursing Research* 28(4): 250–255.

Hester, N.O. and Barcus, C.S. (1986) Assessment and management of pain in children. *Pediatrics Nursing Update* 1(14), 1–8.

Hester, N.O., Foster, R.L., Jordan-Marsh, M. Ely, E., Vojir, C.P. and Miller, K.L. (1998) Putting pain measurement into clinical practice. In: *Measurement of Pain in Infants and Children, Progress in Pain Research Management*, Vol. 10 (eds G.A. Finley and P.J. McGrath), pp. 179–198. IASP Press, Seattle.

Hicks, C.L., von Baeyer, C.L., Spafford, P.A., van Korlaar, I. and Goodenough B. (2001) The Faces Pain Scale–Revised: Toward a common metric in pediatric pain measurement. *Pain* 93, 173–183.

Hunt, A., Goldman, A., Seers, K. et al. (2004) Clinical validation of the paediatric pain profile. *Developmental Medicine and Child Neurology* 46(1), 9–18.

Hunt, A., Wisbeach, A., Seers, K. et al. (2007) Development of the paediatric pain profile: Role of video analysis and saliva cortisol in validating a tool to assess pain in children with severe neurological disability. *Journal of Pain and Symptom Management* 33(3), 276–289.

Jacobs, E., Stinson J., Duran, J. et al. (2012) Usability testing of a smartphone for accessing a web-based e-diary for self-monitoring of pain and symptoms in sickle cell disease. *Journal of Pediatric Hematology/Oncology* 34(5), 326–335.

Johnston, C. (1998) Psychometric issues in the measurement of pain. In: *Measurement of Pain in Infants and Children, Progress in Pain Research Management*, Vol. 10 (eds G.A. Finley and P.J. McGrath), pp. 5–20. IASP Press, Seattle.

Kelly, A.M., Powell, C.V. and Williams, A. (2002) Parent visual analogue scale ratings of children's pain do not reliably reflect pain reported by child. *Pediatric Emergency Care* 18(3), 159–162.

Krechel, S.W. and Bildner, J. (1995) CRIES: A new neonatal postoperative pain measurement score. Initial testing of validity and reliability. *Pediatric Anesthesia* 5, 53–61.

Lawrence, J., Alcock, D., McGrath, P., Kay, J., MacMurray, S.B. and Dulberg, C. (1993) The development of a tool to assess neonatal pain. *Neonatal Network* 12, 59–66.

Lewandowski, A.S., Palermo, T.M., Kirchner, H.L. and Drotar, D. (2009) Comparing diary and retrospective reports of pain and activity restriction in children and adolescents with chronic pain conditions. *Clinical Journal of Pain* 25(4), 299–306.

Malviya, S., Voepel-Lewis, T., Burke, C., Merkel, S. and Tait, A.R. (2006) The revised FLACC observational pain tool: Improved reliability and validity for pain assessment in children with cognitive impairment. *Pediatric Anethesia* 16, 258–265.

McCaffery, M. and Pasero, C. (1999) *Pain: Clinical Manual*, 2nd edition. Mosby, St. Louis.

McGrath, P., Seifert, C., Speechley, K., Booth, J., Stitt, L. and Gibson, M. (1996) A new analogue scale for assessing children's pain: An initial validation study. *Pain* 64, 435–443.

McGrath, P.A. (2007) Pain assessment in children. In: *Encyclopedia of Pain* (eds R.F. Schmidt and W.D. Willis), pp. 645–1648. Springer-Verlag, Berlin and Heidelberg.

McGrath, P.J. (1998) Behavioral measures of pain. In: *Measurement of Pain in Infants and Children, Progress in Pain Research Management*, Vol. 10 (eds G.A. Finley and P.J. McGrath), pp. 83–102. IASP Press, Seattle.

McGrath, P.J., Johnson, G., Goodman, J.T., Schillinger, J., Dunn, J. and Chapman, J. (1985) CHEOPS: A behavioral scale for rating postoperative pain in children. In: *Proceedings of the Fourth World Congress on Pain. Advances in Pain Research and Therapy*, Vol. 9 (eds H.L. Fields, R. Dubner and F. Cervero), pp.395–401. Raven Press.

McGrath, P.J., Rosmus, C., Campbell, M.A. and Hennigar, A. (1998) Behaviours caregivers use to determine pain in non-verbal, cognitively impaired individuals. *Developmental Medicine and Child Neurology* 40, 340–343.

Merkel, S.I., Voepel-Lewis, T., Shayevitz, J.R. and Malviya, S. (1997) The FLACC: A behavioral scale for scoring postoperative pain in young children. *Pediatric Nursing* 23(3), 292–297.

Oberlander, T.F, O'Donnell, M.E. and Montgomery, C.J. (1999) Pain in children with significant neurological impairment. *Developmental and Behavioral Pediatrics* 20(4), 235–243.

Page, M.G., Katz, J., Stinson, J., Isaac, L., Martin-Pichora, A.L., and Campbell, F. (2012) Validation of the numerical rating scale for pain intensity and unpleasantness in pediatric acute postoperative pain: Sensitivity to change over time. *Journal of Pain* 4, 359–369.

Palermo, T., Valenzuela, D. and Stork, P. (2004) A randomized trial of electronic versus paper pain diaries in children: Impact on compliance, accuracy, and acceptability. *Pain* 107, 213–219.

Palozzi, L., Campbell, F. and Hurdowar A. (2010) *Pain Management Clinical Practice Guideline, Policies and Procedures Database*. Hospital for Sick Children, Toronto.

Rajasagaram, U., Taylor, D.M., Braitberg, G., Pearsell, J.P. and Capp, B.A. (2009) Paediatric pain assessment: Differences between triage nurse, child and parent. *Journal of Paediatrics and Child Health* 45(4), 199–203.

Ramelet, A, Abu-Saad, H.H., Rees, N. and McDonald, S. (2004) The challenges of pain measurement in critically ill young children: A comprehensive review. *Australian Critical Care* 17(1), 33–45.

Savedra, M.C., Tesler, M.D., Holzemer, W.L. and Ward, J.A. (1989) *Adolescent Pediatric Pain Tool (APPT): Preliminary User's Manual*. University of California, San Francisco, School of Nursing.

Stevens, B., Johnston, C., Petryshen, P. and Taddio, A. (1996) Premature Infant Pain Profile: Development and initial validation. *Clinical Journal of Pain* 12, 13–22.

Stevens, B., Johnston, C., Taddio, A., Gibbins, S. and Yamada, J. (2010) The Premature Infant Pain Profile: Evaluation 13 years after development. *Clinical Journal of Pain* 26(9), 813–830.

Stinson, J., Yamada, J., Kavanagh, T., Gill, N. and Stevens, B. (2006a) Systematic review of the psychometric properties and feasibility of self-report pain measures for use in clinical trials in children and adolescents. *Pain* 125(1–2), 143–157.

Stinson, J., Petroz, G., Tait, G., Feldman, B., Streiner, D., McGrath, P. and Stevens, B. (2006b) E-Ouch: Usability testing of an electronic chronic pain diary for adolescents with arthritis. *Clinical Journal of Pain* 22(3), 295–305.

Stinson, J., Stevens, J., Feldman, B. et al. (2008) Construct validity of a multidimensional electronic pain diary for adolescents with arthritis. *Pain* 136(3), 281–292.

Stinson, J., Connelly, M., Jibb, L.A. et al. (2012) Developing a standardized approach to the assessment of pain in children and youth presenting to pediatric rheumatology providers: A Delphi survey and consensus conference process followed by feasibility testing. *Pediatric Rheumatology* 10(7), 1–10.

Suraseranivongse, S., Montapaneewat, T., Monon, J., Chainhop, P., Petcharatana, S. and Kraiprasit, K. (2005) Cross-validation of a self-report scale for postoperative pain in school-aged children. *Journal of the Medical Association of Thailand* 88(3), 412–418.

Sweet, S.D. and McGrath, P.J. (1998) Physiological measures of pain. *Measurement of Pain in Infants and Children, Progress in Pain Research Management, Vol. 10* (eds G.A. Finley and P.J. McGrath), pp. 59–81. IASP Press, Seattle.

Tomlinson D., von Baeyer, C.L., Stinson, J.N. and Sung, L. (2010) A systematic review of faces scales for the self-report of pain intensity in children. *Pediatrics* 26(5), 1168–1198.

Twycross, A. and Shields, L. (2005) Reliability and validity in practice: Assessment tools. *Paediatric Nursing* 17(9), 43.

van Dijk, N., de Boer, J.B., Koot, H.M., Tibboel, D., Passchier, J. and Duivenvoorden, H.J. (2000) The reliability and validity of the COMFORT scale as a postoperative pain instrument in 0 to 3-year-old infants. *Pain* 84, 367–377.

Varni, J.W., Thompson, K.L. and Hanson, V. (1987) The Varni/Thompson Pediatric Pain Questionnaire: I. Chronic musculoskeletal pain in juvenile rheumatoid arthritis. *Pain* 28, 27–38.

Voepel-Lewis, T., Malviya, S., Tait, A.R. et al. (2008) A comparison of the clinical utility of pain assessment tools for children with cognitive impairment. *Anesthesia and Analgesia* 106(1), 71–78.

Voepel-Lewis, T., Zanotti, J., Dammeyer, J.A. and Merkel, S. (2010) Reliablity and validity of the Face, Legs, Activity, Cry, Consolability behavioral tool in assessing acute pain in critically ill patients. *American Journal of Critical Care* 19(1), 55–61.

von Baeyer, C.L. (2006) Children's self-reports of pain intensity: Scale selection, limitations and interpretation. *Pain Research and Management* 11(3), 157–162.

von Baeyer, C.L. and Spagrud, L.J. (2007) Systematic review of observational (behavioral) measures for children and adolescents aged 3 to 18 years. *Pain* 127, 140–150.

von Baeyer, C.L., Spagrud, L.J., McCormick, J.C., Choo, E., Neville, K. and Connelly, M.A. (2009) Three new datasets supporting use of the Numerical Rating Scale (NRS-11) for children's self-reports of pain intensity. *Pain* 143(3), 223–227.

von Baeyer, C.L., Uman, L.S., Chambers, C.T., and Gouthro, A. (2011) Can we screen young children for their ability to provide accurate self-reports of pain? *Pain* 152, 1327–1333.

Wong, D.L. and Baker, C.M. (1988) Pain in children: Comparison of assessment scales. *Pediatric Nursing* 14(1), 9–17.

CHAPTER 7

Managing Acute Pain in Children

Sueann Penrose

Children's Pain Management Service, Royal Children's Hospital, Australia

Lori Palozzi

Department of Anesthesia and Pain Medicine, The Hospital for Sick Children, Canada

Stephanie Dowden

Paediatric Palliative Care, Princess Margaret Hospital for Children, Australia

Introduction

This chapter will review the causes of acute pain in childhood. Strategies for managing acute pain in both hospital and community settings will be provided, with an emphasis on pharmacological management. Best-practice management of specialist analgesic modalities such as intravenous (IV) infusions, patient-controlled analgesia (PCA) and regional anaesthesia (RA) will be discussed in detail. Information about the different analgesic drugs is outlined in Chapter 4, the use of different physical and psychological pain-relieving interventions in Chapter 5 and procedural pain management in Chapter 10.

What is Acute Pain?

Acute pain is short-lived (lasting days to weeks). It usually has a single obvious cause (e.g. tissue damage due to surgery or injury) and has a protective purpose. Acute pain is proportionate to the severity of tissue damage, is generally easy to treat with single modalities (pharmacological or physical) and is expected to resolve as healing takes place (Goldman 2002). Pain lasting over 3 months is classified as chronic or persistent. However, it is likely that acute pain and chronic pain are on a continuum, rather

Managing Pain in Children: A Clinical Guide for Nurses and Healthcare Professionals, Second Edition. Edited by Alison Twycross, Stephanie Dowden, and Jennifer Stinson.
© 2014 John Wiley & Sons, Ltd. Published 2014 by John Wiley & Sons, Ltd.

Table 7.1 Causes of acute pain

Cause	Examples
Injury	Musculoskeletal injuries, lacerations, contusions, burns
Childhood illnesses	Earache (otalgia), pharyngitis, headache, abdominal pain, musculoskeletal pain, dental caries, immunisation pain
Medical procedures	Venepuncture, IV cannulation, wound care, fracture reduction, immunisations, lumbar puncture, bone marrow aspiration
Surgery	Postoperative pain and surgical devices
Medical conditions	Cancer, sickle cell disease, haemophilia, arthritis, pancreatitis, inflammatory bowel disease, osteogenesis imperfecta, migraine

Source: Data from Schechter (2006, 2008)

than being separate entities (Macintyre et al. 2010). (See Chapter 2 for further information about the physiology of pain and Chapter 8 for a discussion about chronic pain.)

Causes of Acute Pain in Childhood

Injury, childhood illnesses, medical procedures, surgery and medical conditions are causes of acute pain in childhood (Acworth et al. 2009). These causes are identified in Table 7.1 and discussed further below.

Injury

Unintentional injuries from falls, collisions, burns and cuts are the most common cause of acute pain in childhood and contribute to one-third of Emergency Department (ED) attendances (Acworth et al. 2009; Mickalide and Carr 2012). Within the ED setting musculoskeletal pain in children is persistently undertreated despite high levels of pain being identified (Ali et al. 2010; Dong et al. 2012). Injuries to preschool children generally happen in the home (Bayreuther et al. 2009), while school-aged children's injuries occur at school, during sport and through road traffic accidents (both as passengers and pedestrians) (Mickalide and Carr 2012).

Childhood illnesses

Childhood illnesses frequently cause acute pain. Acute otitis media and pharyngitis are the most frequent diagnoses in children attending community-based health services (Schechter 2006). Pain from tooth decay is prevalent in children of low socio-economic backgrounds with limited access to dental care (Goes et al. 2008; Moura-Leite et al. 2008).

Surgery/medical investigations

A substantial number of children still experience moderate to severe pain while in hospital, despite improvement in pain management practices (Kozlowski et al. 2012;

Stevens et al. 2012; Twycross and Collis 2012; Twycross et al. 2013). Intravenous cannulation, venepuncture, surgery and medical investigations are the most likely reasons for this pain.

Medical conditions

Sickle cell disease (SCD) is an important medical cause of acute pain in childhood. SCD pain is described as worse than surgical pain and equivalent to terminal cancer pain (Zempsky 2010). Vaso-occlusive episodes cause very severe pain requiring presentation to hospital for management (Meier and Miller 2012). Despite the need for hospital presentations the majority (90%) of SCD pain episodes are managed at home (Zempsky 2010).

Other medical conditions such as arthritis, cancer, systemic lupus erythematosus, haemophilia, inflammatory bowel disease and epidermolysis bullosa have combined acute and chronic pain components due to the disease process, treatment or medical investigations (McClain 2006; Riley et al. 2011; WHO 2012). Acute pain associated with these conditions can cause considerable suffering, may be poorly recognised, and under-treatment may be compounded by the negative attitudes of clinicians (Zempsky 2010; Riley et al. 2011).

Developmental disabilities

Children with developmental disabilities (e.g. Down's syndrome, cerebral palsy and autism) are another group with very high prevalence of pain (75–85%) (Oberlander and Symons 2006). They experience acute pain from multiple sources (Table 7.2) as well as chronic pain from their underlying condition. Due to cognitive and communication impairments, pain in these children is difficult to identify and consequentially is often under-treated (Breau and Burkitt 2009; Temple et al. 2012).

Table 7.2 Causes of pain in children with developmental disabilities

Cause	Example
Assistive devices	Pressure areas or rubbing from orthotics, splints, prostheses
Surgery	Scoliosis surgery, femoral osteotomy, tendon transfers, release of contractures
Oral health	Periodontal disease, dental caries, temporomandibular pain
Drug toxicity	Adverse effects of drugs, especially anti-epilepsy drugs (e.g. pancreatitis, mucositis, gingivitis, neuropathies)
Gastrointestinal disorders	Gastro-oesophageal reflux, gastritis, oesophagitis, constipation, gastric feeding tube problems
Musculoskeletal	Hip dislocation, spasticity, muscle spasm, positioning difficulties, immobility, joint problems
Childhood illnesses	Late recognition/presentation of childhood illnesses with consequential increased pain, illness severity and complications

Source: Data from Oberlander and Symons (2006)

Pain Assessment

The assessment of pain is detailed in Chapter 6. A thorough assessment is an essential first step for determining the pain-relieving interventions required. Acute medical pain may include exacerbation of the underlying disease, for example, acute abdominal pain with Crohn's disease or a joint bleed with haemophilia. Acute pain from injury or surgery is primarily due to tissue damage and inflammation. *All* possible sources of pain and discomfort should be considered including haemorrhage or haematoma, compartment syndrome, urinary retention, bladder spasms, muscle spasms, vomiting, nausea and itching.

Physical and Psychological Interventions

Many of the physical and psychological interventions discussed in Chapter 5 are suitable for acute pain. In the pre-hospital and ED setting, use of the RICE method (Rest, Ice, Compression/splinting and Elevation) for soft-tissue and musculoskeletal injuries and haemophilia bleeds is effective (Riley et al. 2011; Gourde and Damian, 2012). For SCD pain, heat is beneficial but *ice* should not be used (Meier and Miller 2012). For *all* children, strategies that diminish the emotional aspects of pain are beneficial (American Society of Anaesthesiologists [ASA] 2012).

Pharmacological Interventions

Current research about the use of analgesics for acute pain in children is summarised below.

Non-opioids

- Combining paracetamol (acetaminophen) and nonsteroidal anti-inflammatory drugs (NSAIDs) has been shown to be opioid-sparing following myringotomy (Tay and Tan 2002), minor orthopaedic surgery (Hiller et al. 2006), inguinal surgery (Hong et al. 2010) and multiple dental extractions (Gazal and Mackie 2007).
- Early use of non-opioids reduces the odds of serious postoperative adverse events in children (Voepel-Lewis et al. 2013).
- Ibuprofen alone provides equivalent analgesia to paracetamol and codeine for children with extremity injuries (Friday et al. 2009).
- A meta-analysis of 27 randomised controlled trials (RCTs) found that peri-operative NSAIDs decreased opioid requirements and postoperative nausea and vomiting (PONV) during the first 24 hours after surgery (Michelet et al. 2012).
- Patients who received peri-operative IV propacetamol/paracetamol required 30% less opioid immediately postoperatively than those receiving a placebo (Tzortzopoulou et al. 2011).
- Infants undergoing major (non-cardiac) surgery receiving IV paracetamol had significantly reduced morphine requirements in the first 48 hours postoperatively (Ceelie et al. 2013).
- Ketamine used preoperatively for tonsillectomy and adenotonsillectomy decreased postoperative analgesic requirements (Aydin et al. 2007).

Opioids

- Opioids are the mainstay for treating severe SCD pain. PCA with background infusion provides optimal analgesia in this population (Jacob et al. 2008; Zempsky 2010).
- Intranasal fentanyl provides equivalent analgesia to oral morphine for burns dressings (Borland et al. 2005).
- Intranasal fentanyl is equivalent to IV morphine for acute pain in the paediatric ED setting and improves time to analgesia by up to 50% (Borland et al. 2007, 2009).
- An RCT explored the use of morphine and hydromorphone PCA for postoperative pain in children. Comparable pain control was demonstrated with similar rates of opioid-related adverse effects for both drugs (Karl et al. 2012).
- Postoperative IV tramadol provides similar analgesia to IV paracetamol after adenotonsillectomy in children (Uysal et al. 2011).

Local anaesthetics

- Local anaesthetic (LA) block of the dorsal penile nerve was the most effective intervention for neonatal circumcision (Brady-Fryer et al. 2009).
- LA infiltration prior to tonsillectomy was found to reduce pain and analgesic requirement postoperatively in children (Naja et al. 2005).
- Intra-operative LA reduces postoperative pain following dental extractions (APA 2012).

Regional anaesthesia

- Dobereiner et al. (2010) examined 17 RCTs to determine the best drug for paediatric caudal epidural. Levobupivacaine, bupivacaine and ropivacaine were equivalent in efficacy, but bupivacaine produced a longer-acting motor block.
- Addition of clonidine or ketamine to paediatric caudal epidural improved analgesia compared to using LA alone (Schnabel et al. 2011a, 2011b).
- The addition of opioids to epidural or caudal provided equivalent or improved analgesia to LA alone but increased side-effects, particularly itch, respiratory depression and PONV (Cho et al. 2009; Shukla et al. 2011; Singh et al. 2011).

Pain Management Guidelines

A list of pain management guidelines is provided in Chapter 1. Guidelines specific to acute pain management are outlined in Box 7.1.

Aims of Pain Management

As pain is a biopsychosocial phenomenon (see Chapter 3), a combined approach should include pharmacological, physical and psychological strategies. The aims of managing acute pain in children are to:

- rapidly identify pain;
- prevent pain if possible;
- control pain by administering analgesia according to age, weight, pain severity and underlying medical condition;
- reduce surgical stress response;
- use multimodal analgesia;
- monitor to prevent adverse events;

- address emotional components of pain;
- continue pain control after discharge from hospital.

(Association of Paediatric Anaesthetists [APA] 2012; ASA 2012)

BOX 7.1

Acute pain management guidelines

American Society of Anesthesiologists (2012) *Practice guidelines for acute pain management in the perioperative setting: An updated report by the American Society of Anesthesiologists Task Force on Acute Pain Management.* Available from: http://journals.lww.com/anesthesiology/fulltext/2012/02000/practice_guidelines_for_acute_pain_management_in.11.aspx

Association of Paediatric Anaesthetists of Great Britain and Ireland (2012) *Good Practice in Postoperative and Procedural Pain*, 2nd edition. Available from: http://onlinelibrary.wiley.com/doi/10.1111/j.1460-9592.2012.03838.x/pdf

Macintyre, P.E., Schug, S.A., Scott, D.A., Visser, E.J., Walker, S.M.; APM:SE Working Group of the Australian and New Zealand College of Anaesthetists and Faculty of Pain Medicine (2010) *Acute Pain Management: Scientific Evidence*, 3rd edition. ANZCA & FPM, Melbourne. Available from: http://sydney.edu.au/medicine/pmri/pdf/Acute-pain-management-scientific-evidence-third-edition.pdf.

Guidelines relating to sickle cell disease pain

Updated sickle cell guidelines are due to be published by the US National Heart Lung and Blood Institute (National Institute of Health in 2013: www.nhlbi.nih.gov/guidelines/scd/index.htm

The National Institute of Health and Care Excellence (NICE) (2012): www.nice.org.uk/nicemedia/live/13772/59765/59765.pdf

---

Surgical stress response

Acute pain induces effects ranging from tissue injury and inflammation to activation of metabolic, immune and hormone systems. These cause a stress response involving changes in systemic blood flow, blood pressure, heart rate and pulmonary function leading to complications and negative health outcomes. The magnitude is related to the size and site of injury (enhanced in abdominal and thoracic regions).

Different analgesic modalities have varied effects on both pain-relief and reducing the body's stress response with simple analgesics being less effective than opioids that are in turn less effective than regional anaesthesia.

Source: Wolf (2012)

Practice point

Poorly managed postoperative pain may result in:

- increased morbidity;
- slowed recovery time;
- prolonged hospital stay;
- delayed return to normal activities;
- decreased patient and family satisfaction;
- increased risk of chronic pain.

The consequences of unrelieved pain are discussed further in Chapter 1.

BOX 7.2

Two-step strategy for pain management

Step 1 (mild pain)

Paracetamol (acetaminophen) and/or ibuprofen

Step 2 (moderate to severe pain)

Strong opioid (morphine is recommended as first-line)
Adjuvant analgesics may be added at either step to enhance pain relief.

Source: WHO (2012)

Table 7.3 Treatment of pain at home

Type of pain	Treatment
Otalgia	Ibuprofen or paracetamol appear to be equally as effective in managing pain associated with otitis media (Perrott et al. 2004; Macintyre et al. 2010) Topical local anaesthesia to the ear canal is effective for managing pain from acute otitis media (Bolt et al. 2008; Wood et al. 2012)
Acute pharyngitis	Although glucocorticoid use has been associated with faster reduction of pain when compared to placebo (Korb et al. 2010) they offer no significant benefit over simple analgesics (paracetamol and NSAIDs) in children (Drutz 2012) Medicated topical therapies (sprays or lozenges) offer no advantage over saltwater gargling or sucking hard candy (Drutz 2012)
Dental pain	NSAIDs alone provide adequate analgesia following dental extractions (APA 2012)

World Health Organization (WHO) analgesic ladder

The WHO analgesic ladder (WHO 2012), discussed in Chapter 4, offers a two-step strategy for treating pain, recommending that analgesics are given according to pain severity (Box 7.2). Acute pain is short-lived, and once controlled, a step-down rather than a step-up approach should be used, as the pain is expected to diminish over hours or days. Analgesia should be given regularly in the initial phase, then as needed for comfort (APA 2012). If the pain does not lessen as expected, this may indicate complications or an alternative diagnosis.

Pain management in the community setting

Most mild childhood pain is managed by parents at home using physical and psychological strategies and (if required) Step 1 analgesics (Table 7.3). Moderate pain can be controlled with Step 1 analgesics and low doses of Step 2 analgesics with the addition of LA in the majority of situations. Severe acute pain is initially managed by parents, community health professionals or emergency responders before referral to hospital for intensive management.

Pain management in the hospital setting

Pain experienced in hospital can vary in intensity, and both steps of the WHO analgesic ladder may be required. Infants and children have widely variable analgesia requirements; clinicians must take this into consideration. An algorithm to support decision-making can be seen in Figure 7.1. For analgesic regimes for specific types of surgery, refer to the APA (2012) guidelines.

Suggested Pain Management Regimes for Acute Pain

Non-opioid analgesia

Non-opioid analgesics are important in acute pain management, and for mild pain may be all that is required. For moderate to severe pain, they are key components of multimodal analgesia and are opioid sparing. Intravenous preparations of paracetamol and some NSAIDs are now widely available and are used intra-operatively, when patients are allowed nothing by mouth or when rapid onset of analgesia is required. (Information about dosing for non-opioid analgesics can be found in Chapter 4.)

Practice point

Multimodal analgesia is the combination (by the same or different routes) of two or more analgesic drugs with different mechanisms of action to provide analgesia, which:

- improves pain scores and provides greater pain relief;
- allows for lower drug doses, thus minimises adverse effects;
- allows analgesia to be individualised to the patient or patient group;
- targets pain at different points of the pain pathway (see Chapter 2).

Multimodal analgesia is particularly useful for peri-operative pain, and patients with severe acute pain from sickle cell crisis, pancreatitis or acute cancer pain also benefit from this approach.

Source: Yaster (2010); ASA (2012); Young and Buvanendran (2012)

Opioid analgesia

Opioids are safe and effective for children of all ages (Macintyre et al. 2010). Pethidine (meperidine) is *NOT* routinely used in children due to the problem of norpethidine toxicity (see Chapter 4). Instead, morphine, diamorphine (in the UK), oxycodone, hydromorphone or fentanyl is used.

Oral opioids

Oral opioids are used for moderate to severe pain in conjunction with non-opioid analgesics. If the child can take medications by mouth, oral opioids may be given in place of parenteral opioids or after infusions have ceased. A small number of children require oral opioids for an extended time. The use of long-acting (sustained-release) and short-acting (normal-release) opioids has been shown to be safe and effective after major surgery in children (Czarnecki et al. 2004). (The use of oral opioids is detailed in Chapters 4 and 9.)

Analgesia decision algorithm

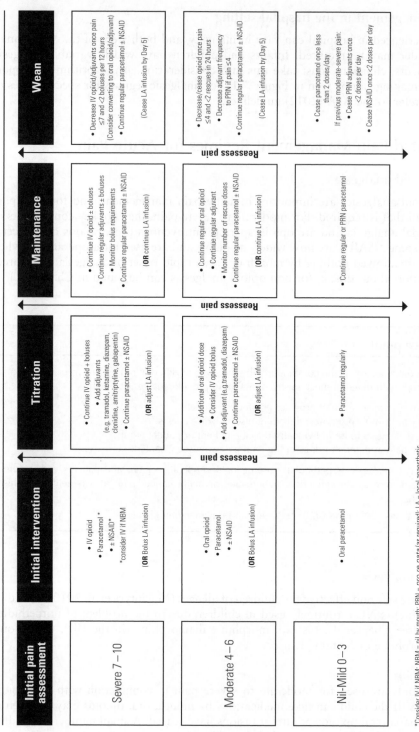

Figure 7.1 Analgesia decision algorithm.
Source: Developed by Dowden SJ, Penrose S and Palmer GM, Department of Anaesthesia & Pain Management, The Royal Children's Hospital, Melbourne. Adapted from The Sherbrooke Algorithm for Acute Pain, Falanga et al. 2006.

Practice point

Oral opioids should be for short-term use (ideally weeks).
If the pain is extended (i.e. lasting over 4–6 weeks) the patient should be referred to a pain specialist or chronic pain service for review.

Intranasal opioids

- Intranasal fentanyl provides safe and effective needle-free analgesia in a variety of clinical settings and is acceptable to children (Borland et al. 2009; Finn and Harris 2010; Mudd 2011).
- Intranasal diamorphine is widely used in the UK for acute pain and procedural pain in children (Finn and Harris 2010; Hadley et al. 2010).

Parenteral opioids

Intramuscular injections are disliked by children and are less effective than other methods of opioid delivery (Macintyre et al. 2010). Methods such as subcutaneous or intravenous bolus or infusion and PCA are preferred.

Intravenous and subcutaneous routes

- The same dose of morphine can be given via intravenous or subcutaneous route (by bolus, PCA or infusion) with no difference in efficacy (Macintyre et al. 2010).
- If more than two or three intermittent opioid bolus doses are required in a 24-hour period, a continuous infusion or PCA may be more appropriate.

Intermittent opioid boluses

Intermittent opioid boluses are used to manage short-term moderate to severe pain episodes (e.g. fracture reduction or following minor surgery). They are helpful in achieving rapid pain control prior to starting an infusion or PCA (e.g. with postoperative pain) or as a *rescue* for severe pain exacerbation. Tables 7.4, 7.5 and 7.6 contain suggested opioid bolus dosing guidelines.

Continuous opioid infusions

Continuous opioid infusions are used for moderate to severe pain that is expected to last for more than 24 hours where intermittent bolus dosing provides inadequate analgesia, and PCA or oral analgesia are not suitable (due to medical condition, age,

Table 7.4 Suggested intravenous or subcutaneous opioid bolus dosing guidelines for children (<50 kg)

Drug	Bolus	Frequency
Morphine	50–100 µg/kg	2- to 3-hourly
Fentanyl	0.5–1 µg/kg	1- to 2-hourly
Hydromorphone	10–20 µg/kg	2- to 4-hourly

Source: Data from Kraemer and Rose (2009); APA (2012)
Note: dosing guidelines vary between organisations and countries. The authors have described doses or dose ranges based on the best available evidence at time of publication. Readers are advised to follow their own institution's guidelines.

Table 7.5 Suggested intravenous morphine bolus dosing guidelines for full-term neonates/infants (1–3 months)

Drug	Bolus	Frequency
Morphine	25–50 µg/kg	3- to 4-hourly

Source: Data from Kraemer and Rose (2009); APA (2012)
Note: dosing guidelines vary between organisations and countries. The authors have described doses or dose ranges based on the best available evidence at time of publication. Readers are advised to follow their own institution's guidelines.

Table 7.6 Suggested intranasal opioid bolus dosing guidelines for children (over 3 years (<50 kg))

Drug	Bolus	Frequency
Diamorphine	0.1 mg/kg	Single dose
Fentanyl	1–2 µg/kg	Single dose

Source: Data from Kraemer and Rose (2009); APA (2012)
Note: dosing guidelines vary between organisations and countries. The authors have described doses or dose ranges based on the best available evidence at time of publication. Readers are advised to follow their own institution's guidelines.

Table 7.7 Suggested intravenous opioid infusion dosing guidelines for children (<50 kg)

Drug	Loading dose	Start rate	Infusion range	Bolus dose
Morphine	50–100 µg/kg	20 µg/kg/h	5–40 µg/kg/h	10–20 µg/kg each 10 min as required
Morphine*	50–100 µg/kg	20 µg/kg/h	0–20 µg/kg/h	10–20 µg/kg bolus each 20–30 min as required
Hydromorphone	10–20 µg/kg	2 µg/kg/h	2–8 µg/kg/h	2–4 µg/kg each 10 min as required
Fentanyl	0.6–1 µg/kg	0.5 µg/kg/h	0.5–2.5 µg/kg/h	0.3 µg/kg each 5–10 min as required

*Nurse-controlled infusion
Source: Data from Kraemer and Rose (2009); Macintyre et al. (2010); APA (2012)
Note: dosing guidelines vary between organisations and countries. The authors have described doses or dose ranges based on the best available evidence at time of publication. Readers are advised to follow their own institution's guidelines.

cognitive function or physical limitations). Continuous infusion allows for constant pain relief and decreases staff workload compared to intermittent opioid boluses (Macintyre et al. 2010).

- Initial infusion rates vary according to age and weight and should be titrated to the child's response (Macintyre et al. 2010).
- Bolus doses may be prescribed for breakthrough pain.

Tables 7.7, 7.8 and 7.9 contain suggested opioid infusion dosing guidelines.

Table 7.8 Suggested intravenous morphine infusion dosing guidelines for infants (1–3 months)

Drug	Loading dose	Start rate	Infusion range	Bolus dose
Morphine	25–50 µg/kg	10 µg/kg/h	5–20 µg/kg/h	10 µg/kg each 30 min

Source: Data from Kraemer and Rose (2009); Macintyre et al. (2010); APA (2012)
Note: dosing guidelines vary between organisations and countries. The authors have described doses or dose ranges based on the best available evidence at time of publication. Readers are advised to follow their own institution's guidelines.

Table 7.9 Suggested intravenous morphine infusion dosing guidelines for term neonates

Drug	Loading dose	Start rate	Infusion range	Bolus dose
Morphine	10–25 µg/kg	5 µg/kg/h	5–10 µg/kg/h	5–10 µg/kg each 60 min

Source: Data from De Lima and Browning (2010); Macintyre et al. (2010); APA (2012)
Note: dosing guidelines vary between organisations and countries. The authors have described doses or dose ranges based on the best available evidence at time of publication. Readers are advised to follow their own institution's guidelines.

Case study: Billy

Billy is a 6-year-old boy who underwent surgery 6 hours ago to remove a perforated appendix via laparotomy. He has a nasogastric tube in situ (on free drainage) and is allowed nothing by mouth. He has a morphine PCA with no background infusion. He has not used the PCA since surgery. He is complaining of 'a sore tummy' and is lying very still and reluctant to move. He has a respiratory rate of 30 and shallow respirations. His parents are with him.

- What is significant about Billy's behaviour?
- What education would you give Billy and his parents regarding the PCA?
- What are the consequences of inadequate pain relief following abdominal surgery?

Patient-controlled analgesia

PCA uses a programmable infusion pump to allow patients to self-administer analgesia. The aim is optimal pain relief and improved patient and parent satisfaction. The use of small, frequent boluses allow the patient to titrate the analgesia to their pain, thus receiving only what they need (Grass 2005; APA 2012).

- PCA has become the gold standard for acute pain management since its introduction into paediatric medicine in the early 1990s (Grass 2005; Kraemer and Rose 2009).
- PCA is used for the management of moderate to severe pain in children over 5 or 6 years (Kraemer and Rose 2009).
- PCA is commonly used for postoperative pain (APA 2012), pain related to trauma and burns (Gandhi et al. 2010), SCD (van Beers et al. 2007; Jacob et al. 2008), and pain from cancer and during palliative care (Anghelescu et al. 2012).
- PCA is safe, effective and viewed as a highly satisfactory method of analgesia delivery by staff, patient and families. Adverse effects are rare and can be reduced by

the addition of opioid-sparing analgesics and close monitoring (Grass 2005; Kraemer and Rose 2009; Macintyre et al. 2010).

- Other advantages of PCA include improved analgesia during sleep-wake cycles and movement as well as increased autonomy for the child (Kraemer and Rose 2009; Franson 2010).

When using PCA:

- It is important that the child's parents understand the concept of PCA, so they can support their child in its use.
- Unless allowed by an institutional protocol the PCA should *ONLY* be used by the patient, to reduce the risk of opioid-induced adverse effects (Wuhrman et al. 2007).
- Children who are unwilling or unable to use PCA should have an opioid infusion or PCA-by-proxy instead (see below).

A useful resource for parents relating to PCA can be found at: www.aboutkidshealth.ca/En/ HealthAZ/TestsAndTreatments/PainReliefSedationAnaesthesia/Pages/PCA-Patient-Controlled-Analgesia.aspx

---

Practice point

To use PCA the child must:

- have the cognitive ability to associate pressing the PCA button with receiving pain relief;
- be physically able and willing to press the button to control their pain.

The terminology used for PCA administration is outlined in Box 7.3. Table 7.10 details suggested PCA dosing guidelines.

BOX 7.3
PCA terminology*

Bolus dose: When the patient presses the remote button, the PCA delivers the programmed bolus dose of analgesia.

Lockout time: The PCA will not deliver a dose during lockout time, even if the button is pressed. This allows each bolus to reach peak effect before another bolus, thus reducing the risk of overdose. The lockout time is usually set at 5–10 minutes.

Good try/bad try: A *good try* is when the PCA delivers a dose of analgesia. A *bad try* is when the patient presses the button during the lockout time and no bolus dose is delivered.

Dose duration: This ranges from 30 to 90 seconds, depending on the PCA pump. The dose duration can be increased to prevent problems such as light-headedness or nausea associated with a rapid peak of onset of analgesia.

Background: A *continuous* infusion that may be added to improve analgesia. Generally a background infusion is only used for patients with high opioid requirements. Adding a background infusion increases the likelihood of opioid-induced adverse effects.

4-hour limit: This setting may be used to limit the amount of medication the patient may request in a 4-hour period.

*Terminology varies slightly in different countries and with different PCA pumps
Source: Data from Grass (2005); San Diego Patient Safety Council (2009)

Table 7.10 Suggested PCA dosing guidelines for children (<50 kg)

Drug	Loading dose	Bolus dose	Lockout time	Background infusion rate	4-hour limit
Morphine	40–100 µg/kg	20 µg/kg	5–10 min	Nil *or* 4–10 µg/kg/h	Nil *or* 400 µg/kg
Hydromorphone	10 µg/kg	2–4 µg/kg	5–10 min	Nil *or* 0.5–2 µg/kg/h	Nil *or* 60 µg/kg
Fentanyl	0.5–1 µg/kg	0.3–0.5 µg/kg	5 min	Nil *or* 0.2–0.4 µg/kg/h	Nil *or* 10 µg/kg

Source: Data from Kraemer and Rose (2009); Macintyre et al. (2010); APA (2012)

Note: dosing guidelines vary between organisations and countries. The authors have described doses or dose ranges based on the best available evidence at time of publication. Readers are advised to follow their own institution's guidelines.

PCA-by-proxy

PCA-by-proxy is the delivery of medication from a PCA device by someone other than the patient, typically either a parent or nurse. It is sometimes called *parent-controlled* or *nurse-controlled* analgesia. PCA-by-proxy is used when the child is too young, physically unable, or cognitively impaired, or during end-of-life care (Franson 2010). When the designated proxy is carefully chosen and educated, PCA-by-proxy is safe and effective (Wuhrman et al. 2007; Krane 2008; Howard et al. 2010; Anghelescu et al. 2012).

A position paper on PCA-by-proxy by the American Society for Pain Management Nursing (ASPMN) can be found at: www.aspmn.org/Organization/documents/PCAbyProxy-final-EW_004 .pdf

---

Practice point

When commencing an opioid infusion or PCA, or if the rate is to be increased:

- a loading dose may be required to ensure therapeutic plasma levels are reached quickly;
- it takes approximately four half-lives (approximately 8 hours for morphine/hydromorphone; approximately 1.5 hours for fentanyl) for opioids to reach steady-state plasma concentration.

Source: Trescot et al. (2008)

Other analgesic infusions

Other analgesic drugs, such as tramadol or ketamine, are used for acute pain when opioids are contraindicated or adjunct analgesia is required (Bozkurt 2005; Dahmani et al. 2011; APA 2012). These are usually prescribed by a pain service or anaesthetist, and may be administered via PCA or IV infusion. There is variable evidence for their efficacy in children:

- The addition of ketamine to morphine PCA or infusion improved analgesic efficacy in children with mucositis pain with no increase in side effects (James et al. 2010).
- In a review of 35 RCTs administration of ketamine was associated with decreased pain intensity and non-opioid analgesic requirement in the immediate postoperative period but did not show a postoperative opioid-sparing effect (Dahmani et al. 2011).

Further guidance about ketamine infusions can be found at: www.rch.org.au/anaes/pain _management/Ketamine_Infusion/

Optimising the Safety of Analgesic Drugs

Safe administration of analgesic drugs requires education of all involved and careful attention to the organisational aspects in delivering pain-relief (Macintyre et al. 2010; APA 2012). Strategies for optimising the safety of analgesic drugs are outlined in Box 7.4. Suggested observations for infants and children receiving opioid infusion or PCA are outlined in Table 7.11 (see also Box 7.5).

Practice point

If a patient on opioids is receiving other medication that can cause sedation (e.g. antihistamines, benzodiazepines or anti-epilepsy drugs) there is an increased risk of sedation and respiratory depression.

BOX 7.4

Optimising the safety of analgesic drugs

- Appropriate patient selection considering medical condition, comorbidities, age, surgery/procedure, emotional state and concurrent medications
- Staff adequately trained and supported, with sufficient staff numbers to safely monitor patients
- Education about all aspects of analgesics to clinicians, children and families
- Clear guidelines and expectation they will be followed
- Risk minimisation: labelling, standard drug concentrations, smart pump technology, specific charts, double-checking of pump programming and prescriptions, documentation, and appropriate patient monitoring
- Avoiding co-administration of sedatives or opioids by different routes
- Regular review of efficacy and adverse effects of analgesia
- Reportable safety limits individualised to patient type or age groups
- Emergency protocols to manage adverse events
- Pain service or pain link nurses to guide/direct staff
- Regular audit of pain management

Source: Data from Macintyre et al. (2010); Morton and Errera (2010); APA (2012)

Table 7.11 Suggested observations for infants and children receiving opioid infusion or PCA

Parameter	Suggested frequency	Comments
Sedation score	1-hourly for the duration of the opioid infusion/PCA	Use a validated paediatric sedation scale (e.g. University of Michigan Sedation Scale, Box 7.6)
Respiratory rate and heart rate	1-hourly for the duration of the opioid infusion/PCA	
Pain score	1-hourly while awake	Use a developmentally appropriate pain assessment scale (see Chapter 6)
Nausea/vomiting assessment	1-hourly for the first 12 hours, then 4-hourly as indicated	
Pulse oximetry	As indicated (Box 7.5)	

Source: RCH (2012a, 2012b). Used with permission.
Note: observation requirements vary between organisations and countries. Readers are advised to follow their own institution's guidelines.

BOX 7.5

Indications for pulse oximetry

Pulse oximetry **MUST BE** used **continuously** in high-risk patients with:
- University of Michigan Sedation Scale (UMSS) sedation score >2
- age under 6 months
- significant cardiorespiratory impairment
- sleep apnoea, snoring or airway obstruction
- spot oximetry less than 94% SaO_2

Or in patients receiving:
- supplementary oxygen
- concurrent sedative agents

Clinical indicators for **'spot'** pulse oximetry are:
- tachypnoea or bradypnoea
- respiratory distress
- pallor or cyanosis or impaired oxygenation
- confusion or agitation
- hypotension
- nurse concern

Source: Department of Anaesthesia and Pain Management, The Royal Children's Hospital, Melbourne 2011. Used with permission.
Note: observation requirements vary between organisations and countries. Readers are advised to follow their own institution's guidelines.

Practice point

Any adverse effects relating to specialist analgesia techniques should be reported urgently to the pain service or anaesthetist.
Any observations outside reportable limits or outside normal values for age should be reported.
The effectiveness of the analgesia should be documented in the child's healthcare record.

Managing Adverse Effects of Opioids

The incidence of complications related to opioid analgesics in children is 1:2,000 for serious complications and 1:10,000 for persisting sequelae at 12 months (Morton and Errera 2010). Opioids cause a number of adverse effects (sedation, nausea, vomiting, urinary retention, pruritus and constipation) but it is important to consider *all* possible causes and not assume that the opioid alone is responsible (Macintyre et al. 2010; APA 2012). Adverse effects will be discussed in order of clinical significance (see also Chapter 4).

Sedation/respiratory depression

Assessing sedation is the key to early identification and treatment of opioid-induced respiratory depression (Pasero 2009). A lower dose of opioid is required to induce sedation than respiratory depression, for this reason monitoring of sedation provides effective early detection (Jarzyna et al. 2011).

Practice point

Respiratory depression from opioids is caused by:

- decreased responses to hypercapnia and hypoxia;
- depression of the cough reflex;
- decreased tidal volume (by decreased respiratory rate).

The best clinical indicator is increasing sedation.
Decreased rate of breathing and decreased oxygen saturation are *LATE* signs.

Source: Pasero (2009); APA (2012)

Sedation should be assessed using a validated sedation scale to ensure consistency between clinicians (Box 7.6 outlines a sedation tool). If required, an opioid antagonist (most commonly, naloxone) should be administered. All patients receiving opioids should have standing orders for naloxone to minimise delays. Box 7.7 suggests a protocol to manage opioid-induced respiratory depression.

BOX 7.6

University of Michigan Sedation Scale (UMSS)

0	Awake and alert
1	Minimally sedated: may appear tired/sleepy, responds to verbal conversation and/or sound
2	Moderately sedated: somnolent/sleeping, easily aroused with light tactile stimulation or simple verbal command
3	Deep sedation: deep sleep, arousable only with deep or significant physical simulation
4	Unarousable
S	Patient is sleeping

Source: Data from Malviya et al. (2002, 2006)

BOX 7.7

Protocol to manage opioid-induced respiratory depression in children

If opioid-induced respiratory depression is suspected:
- Cease the opioid
- Stimulate the patient (shake gently, call by name, ask to breathe)
- Administer oxygen
- Administer naloxone if indicated

Indications for naloxone

If patient is *significantly sedated* (University of Michigan Sedation Scale 3):
- Administer naloxone 2 µg/kg via IV push and repeat **every 1–2 min** as required (maximum 5 doses)

If patient *cannot be roused and/or is apnoeic* (University of Michigan Sedation Scale 4):
- Manage airway/resuscitate
- Administer naloxone **10 µg/kg** via IV push and repeat **every 1–2 min** as required (maximum 5 doses)

Suggested dilution: 0.4 mg naloxone in 20 mL normal saline = 20 µg/mL

Continue to monitor the patient closely. Naloxone has a shorter duration of action than most opioids, thus repeated doses may be required. In some situations a naloxone infusion will be necessary.

Source: Adapted from Pasero (2009); RCH (2012c). Used with permission.

Additional management of sedation
- If the child is receiving PCA or opioid infusion, consider reducing or ceasing the background infusion or reducing the bolus size.
- Optimise doses of non-opioid analgesics, including adjuvant analgesics.
- Check for other contributing factors (e.g. sedatives, dose error, hypoxia, sepsis, hypovolaemia, renal impairment or electrolyte imbalance).

(Kraemer and Rose 2009)

Nausea and vomiting

Nausea and vomiting is caused by complex mechanical and chemical interactions between the brain (vomiting centre, chemoreceptor trigger zone [CTZ] and vestibular apparatus in the middle ear) and the gastrointestinal tract. Postoperative nausea and vomiting (PONV) in children is *multifactorial* (i.e. due to type of surgery, anaesthesia, prolonged fasting, opioids, antibiotics, other drugs, ileus, pain, psychological distress, electrolyte imbalance, renal dysfunction), although opioids are generally considered to be the primary cause (Kovac 2007).

When deciding how best to treat PONV *all* possible causes should be considered, as this may influence antiemetic selection. The following need to be taken into account:

- Children have a significantly higher PONV rate than adults, which can be compounded in children with a prior history of PONV or motion sickness (Kovac 2007).
- The 2006 Consensus Guidelines for Managing PONV (Gan et al. 2007) suggest identifying children at high-risk for PONV, treating aggressively with prophylactic

Table 7.12 Antiemetic drugs for prevention and management of postoperative nausea and vomiting in children (<50 kg)

Antiemetic class	Drug doses
Serotonin antagonists	Ondansetron: 0.1–0.15 mg/kg IV/oral 8-hourly as required (maximum dose 8 mg) Granisetron: 40 µg/kg IV DAILY as required (maximum dose 0.6 mg) Tropisetron: 0.1 mg/kg IV DAILY as required (maximum dose 2 mg)
Corticosteroid	Dexamethasone: 0.15 mg/kg IV SINGLE DAILY DOSE (maximum of 3 days)
Dopamine antagonist	Metoclopramide*: Loading dose 0.5 mg/kg IV (maximum dose 20–30 mg); maintenance dose 0.2 mg/kg IV/oral 6–8-hourly as required (maximum dose 20 mg)
Dopamine antagonist	Droperidol: 10–15 µg/kg IV 8-hourly as required (maximum dose 1.25 mg)
Antihistamine	Promethazine: 0.5 mg/kg IV 8-hourly as required (maximum dose 25 mg) Dimenhydrinate: 0.5–2 mg/kg IV 8-hourly as required (maximum dose 25 mg) Diphenhydramine: 0.5–1 mg/kg IV 6-hourly (maximum dose 50 mg) Cyclizine: 1 mg/kg IV/oral 8-hourly as required (maximum dose 50 mg)

*In addition to being a dopamine antagonist, metoclopramide has prokinetic actions on the gastrointestinal tract: enhancing gastric emptying and gut motility

Serotinin, histamine, dopamine and acetylcholine are all neurotransmitters involved in the process of nausea and vomiting

Source: Data from Gan et al. (2007); Kovac (2007); Friedrichsdorf et al. (2011)

Note: dosing guidelines vary between organisations and countries. The authors have described doses or dose ranges based on the best available evidence at time of publication. Readers are advised to follow their own institution's guidelines.

antiemetic therapy and using a combination of different antiemetic agents from different classes for best results (Table 7.12):

○ Moderate to high risk for PONV = prophylaxis with *two antiemetics* (different classes);

○ High risk PONV or failed prophylaxis = combination therapy with *two or three antiemetics* (different classes).

Practice point

Non-operative nausea and vomiting related to pain or analgesics will usually only require single antiemetic therapy, using drugs acting on the CTZ (e.g. serotonin antagonists), but some children require rotation to another opioid or low-dose naloxone infusion.

Source: Friedrichsdorf et al. (2011)

An algorithm for managing PONV can be found at: www.rch.org.au/anaes/pain_management/Postoperative_Nausea_Vomiting_PONV/

Urinary retention

Urinary retention following surgery is also multi-factorial (i.e. due to opioids, pain, bladder spasm, constipation, dehydration, neuraxial blockade or anxiety about using a bedpan or bottle). Even if one cause seems likely, others such as pre-existing neurological deficits or bladder dysfunction may be significant (Macintyre et al. 2010).

Consider:

- conservative management (e.g. observation, reassurance, manual expression of bladder);
- encouragement strategies (e.g. increase privacy, commode by the bed, encourage male patients to stand up if possible, or running water);
- intermittent catheterisation or indwelling urinary catheter may be required.

(Rosen and Dower 2011)

If the retention is likely to be opioid-induced, consider:

- reducing the opioid dose;
- administering low dose opioid antagonist.

(Monitto et al. 2011)

Pruritus (itch)

- Pruritus is caused by opioid-induced histamine release and usually settles within two or three days of commencing opioids.
- Despite the tendency for clinicians to prescribe antihistamines for this problem, they are not very effective and cause sedation, constipation and urinary retention.
- Low-dose opioid antagonist is effective.

(Monitto et al. 2011; Rosen and Dower 2011)

Constipation

- Constipation is an expected side-effect of opioids, caused by delayed gastric emptying and decreased peristaltic activity of the bowel.
- Unlike almost all other adverse opioid effects it does not resolve after a few days and needs management for the duration of the opioid therapy.
- Preventive measures should be implemented *early* following commencement of opioids. Ideally a combination of stool softener and a stimulant laxative should be used.
- Ensuring adequate fluids and a high-fibre diet will assist in constipation management.
- Peripherally acting opioid antagonists may offer alternative management (see Chapter 4).

(Kraemer and Rose 2009; Rosen and Dower 2011)

Low-dose opioid antagonist

For opioid-induced adverse effects such as itch, urinary retention or antiemetic-resistant PONV, low-dose opioid antagonist (naloxone) can be administered as:
Intermittent IV bolus dose (e.g. naloxone 0.5–1 µg/kg each 2–4 hours)
or IV infusion (e.g. naloxone 0.25–1 µg/kg/h)

Source: Kraemer and Rose (2009); Monitto et al. (2011)

Case study: Jack

Jack is a 10-year-old boy who has had bilateral femoral osteotomies. He has an epidural infusion (inserted at T12 dermatome level) for pain management. He has a urinary catheter in situ. He returned to the ward from the operating theatre at 1600. At 2300 Jack is unable to move his legs. You assess his sensory block with ice. It is covering T12 to S1 dermatomes bilaterally. He says he has no pain.

- What is the Bromage score and what score would you give Jack?
- Why is ice used to assess the sensory block?
- Why is it important to know the amount of sensory and motor block?

Regional Anaesthesia

Regional anaesthesia (RA) or *neuraxial analgesia* is the administration of local anaesthetic (LA) into the epidural space (caudal or epidural), around a peripheral nerve plexus or into the intrathecal space (spinal) to block pain transmission (Chapters 2 and 4). RA provides excellent analgesia, reduces surgical stress response and can significantly diminish the need for opioids and other analgesics (Macintyre et al. 2010; APA 2012; Walker and Yaksh 2012). RA is used in infants and children of all ages. It needs to be managed by suitably trained staff to minimise complications (Llewellyn and Moriarty 2007; Macintyre et al. 2010).

Central blocks

- The most frequently used central RA technique in children is the caudal block, which is used for surgical procedures below the umbilical region. It is usually a single-dose technique (Patel 2006).
- Epidurals are used for major surgery of the spine, chest and abdomen (thoracic epidural) or lower limbs (lumbar epidural). They are delivered by patient-controlled epidural anaesthesia (PCEA) or continuous infusion. It can be the sole technique or used in conjunction with general anaesthesia (Patel 2006; Saudan et al. 2008; Moriarty 2012).
- In neonates, epidurals are inserted into the caudal epidural space, then threaded to the lumbar or thoracic levels as required (Macintyre et al. 2010; APA 2012).
- Intrathecal analgesia is administered as a single dose or by infusion and provides an alternative to general anaesthesia (Walker and Yaksh 2012).

Peripheral blocks

- The use of peripheral nerve (*perineural*) blocks are increasing and in some case replacing central RA techniques as the analgesia is comparable with fewer adverse effects. They are most useful for site-specific analgesia (e.g. limb surgery) and are administered as a single dose or by infusion (Dadure and Capdevila 2012; Suresh et al. 2012).
- Continuous peripheral nerve blocks (CPNB) enable prolonged analgesia and can be delivered via a portable pump, allowing early discharge from hospital (Ivani and Mossetti 2010; Dadure and Capdevila 2012).

Table 7.13 Local anaesthetic solutions and additives for regional anaesthesia in children (<50 kg)

Local anaesthetic	Dose	Infusion rate	Neonate/Infant dose	Comments
Bupivacaine Levobupivacaine Ropivacaine	0.0625%–0.25%	0.1–0.4 mL/kg/h	Lower concentration and infusion rate	0.125% is generally used
Additive	**Dose**	**Neonate/Infant dose**	**Comments**	
Morphine	10–50 µg/kg	Lower dose	Preservative free	
Fentanyl	0.5–1 µg/kg	Lower dose		
Clonidine	0.5–2 µg/kg	May cause apnoea		
Ketamine or S-ketamine	0.25–5 mg/kg	Minimal data	Preservative free	

Source: Data from Macintyre et al. (2010); APA (2012); Walker and Yaksh (2012)
Note: dosing guidelines vary between organisations and countries. The authors have described doses or dose ranges based on the best available evidence at time of publication. Readers are advised to follow their own institution's guidelines.

- Depending on the LA used, analgesia can last for 6 to 24 hours with a single-dose technique or longer with infusion. Bupivacaine, levobupivacaine and ropivacaine are the LA drugs most often used. Opioids, clonidine or ketamine may be added to the LA solution (APA 2012) (see Table 7.13).

Optimising the Safety of Regional Anaesthesia

The practices to optimise safety suggested in Box 7.4 also apply to RA techniques. Suggested observations required for children receiving RA infusions are outlined in Table 7.14.

Practice point

Any adverse events or concerns relating to the regional anaesthesia should be reported urgently e.g. to the pain service or anaesthetist.
Any observations outside reportable limits or outside normal values for age should be reported.
The effectiveness of the analgesia should be documented in the child's healthcare record.

Best practice management for regional analgesia

Sensory and motor block
Assessment of sensory and motor block enables early detection of complications and ensures analgesia can be optimised. The method for assessment of sensory block is outlined in Box 7.8. Figure 7.2 demonstrates the dermatome distribution in children.

Table 7.14 Suggested observations for children receiving regional anaesthesia

Parameter	Suggested frequency	Comments
Sedation score	1-hourly for the duration of the epidural infusion	Use a validated paediatric sedation scale (See Box 7.6)
Respiratory rate and heart rate	1-hourly for the duration of the epidural infusion	
Temperature and blood pressure	1-hourly for *the first 4 hours* then 4-hourly until epidural ceased	
Pain score	1-hourly while awake	Use developmentally appropriate pain assessment scale (see Chapter 6)
Nausea/vomiting score	1-hourly for the first 12 hours, then 4-hourly as indicated	
Pulse oximetry	As indicated (see Box 7.5)	
Sensory and motor assessment	4-hourly	See Box 7.8 and 7.9

Source: RCH (2011, 2012d). Used with permission.
Note: observation requirements vary between organisations and countries. Readers are advised to follow their own institution's guidelines.

BOX 7.8

Assessment of sensory block

Rationale

Sensory nerve fibres respond to pain, temperature, touch and pressure. As pain and temperature nerve fibres are similarly affected by local anaesthetic drugs, changes in temperature perception indicate the anaesthetised area.

At each vertebra, nerve roots exit from the spinal cord bilaterally. Dermatomes are areas of skin that are primarily innervated by a single spinal nerve.

It is important to assess sensory block:

- to ensure effective pain relief;
- to ensure the block is not too extensive, which may increase the risk of complications.

Procedure

1. Explain procedure to patient/parent.
2. Wrap an ice cube in tissue/paper towel leaving part exposed.
3. Place ice on an area well away from the affected dermatomes (e.g. face) and ask the patient to tell you how cold it feels to them.
4. Apply the ice to an area likely to be numb on the same side of the body and ask the patient 'Does this feel the same cold as your face/arm or different?' Patients may report the ice feeling colder, warmer or the same.
5. Apply the ice to areas above and below this point until you can determine the upper and lower margins of the block.
6. Repeat the procedure on the opposite side of the body. (Blocks may be uneven or unilateral.)
7. Document the blocked dermatomes on the observation chart. Record both the upper and lower margins of the block, e.g. T7–L1, L = R **or** R: T7–L1, L: T10–L2.
8. It is possible to assess dermatome levels on infants or non-verbal/cognitively impaired children by observing flinching and facial expression in response to ice on presumed blocked and unblocked dermatomes. Another way is by observing the patient's response to movement and response to very gentle palpation of the operative site.

Source: RCH (2010a). Used with permission.

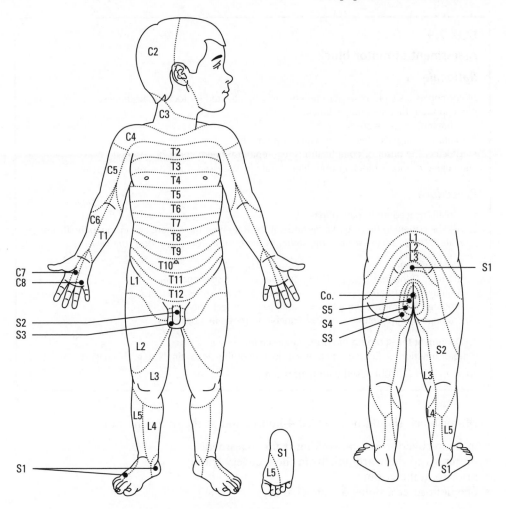

Figure 7.2 The distribution of dermatomes in children.
Source: Royal Children's Hospital, Melbourne.

Sensory block should be assessed **4-hourly** and at the following times:

- in the recovery room on waking from anaesthetic;
- on return to the ward/unit from the recovery room;
- if the patient complains of pain;
- one hour after a bolus or rate change.

The patient should be reviewed by the pain service or anaesthetist *if:*

- the block is higher than T3 dermatome;
- there is no block;
- the block is insufficient to relieve pain.

The method for assessment of motor block is outlined in Box 7.9. Figure 7.3 demonstrates the Bromage scale to assess motor function in children.

BOX 7.9

Assessment of motor block

Rationale

Motor nerves (as well as sensory nerves) may be affected by local anaesthetics. It is important to assess motor block:

- to prevent pressure areas
- to ensure the patient is safe to walk (if permitted)
- to detect the onset of complications (e.g. epidural haematoma or abscess)

The degree of motor block in both legs should be assessed using the Bromage scale.

Procedure

1. Explain procedure to patient/parent
2. Ask the patient to flex their knees and ankles. Rate their movement according to the Bromage scale. *(The Bromage scale is the standard method of assessing motor function.)*

   Bromage score:
   Bromage 0 (none)   = full flexion of knees and feet
   Bromage 1 (partial)   = just able to move knees and feet
   Bromage 2 (almost complete)   = able to move feet only
   Bromage 3 (complete)   = unable to move feet or knees

3. Document the score on the observation chart.

If motor function is different in each leg document this accordingly, e.g. Bromage L) 2, R) 0

Source: RCH (2010b). Used with permission.

Motor block should be assessed **4-hourly** and at the following times:

- in the recovery room on waking from anaesthetic;
- on return to the ward/unit from the recovery room;
- prior to ambulation;
- one hour after a bolus or rate change.

The patient should be reviewed by the pain service or anaesthetist *if there is:*

- any major change in motor function (particularly any *sudden* change);
- almost complete or complete motor block in legs (Bromage score 2–3);
- reduced motor function in hands or fingers with thoracic epidural.

Practice point

Assessing sensory and motor block can assist in ensuring optimal efficacy of continuous peripheral nerve blocks. As the nerve block affects a single limb, a modified assessment is required. The type and frequency of assessment should be guided by the region being blocked and specific institutional protocols.

Catheter position and insertion site

- The catheter insertion site should be inspected at least 8-hourly for redness, tenderness, leaking and dressing integrity.

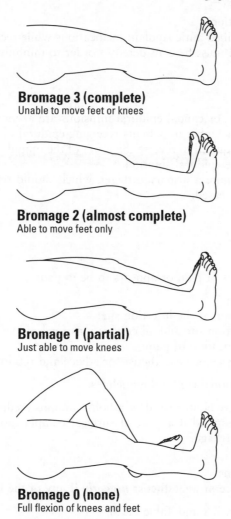

Bromage 3 (complete)
Unable to move feet or knees

Bromage 2 (almost complete)
Able to move feet only

Bromage 1 (partial)
Just able to move knees

Bromage 0 (none)
Full flexion of knees and feet

Figure 7.3 The Bromage scale to assess motor function in children.
Source: Royal Children's Hospital, Melbourne

- The catheter markings should be checked to ensure that the catheter has not migrated (moved).

Pressure area care
- The decreased sensation and motor blockade produced by epidural and perineural analgesia can cause pressure sores and nerve compression.
- Usually the heels, medial and lateral malleoli and sacrum are involved but *all* pressure points are at risk.
- Superficial nerves (e.g. common peroneal nerve) are vulnerable to damage from unrecognised pressure due to decreased sensation.
- The use of pressure-relief devices (e.g. air mattresses, pressure pads) and meticulous nursing care minimises the risk (Llewellyn and Moriarty 2007).

Anticoagulant medication

- If a patient is prescribed anticoagulant medications while receiving RA, the timing for catheter removal must be considered in order to minimise bleeding risk (Macintyre et al. 2010).

Urinary retention

- Patients with lumbar or caudal epidural infusions are at increased risk of urinary retention. The risk is higher in patients receiving epidural opioids.
- Naloxone may be required to reverse the effect of the opioid and/or the opioid may be removed from the epidural solution.
- The patient may require a urinary catheter, which should remain in situ until the epidural infusion is ceased.

Problem solving

Inadequate analgesia

If the patient complains of pain or appears to be in pain:

- assess sensory block;
- check catheter position at the insertion site;
- check catheter, insertion site and all connections for leaking/dislodgement;
- assess severity and location of pain;
- contact the pain service or anaesthetist for advice and report findings.

Manage as per institutional epidural guidelines:

- The infusion rate may be increased or a bolus administered;
- A review may be required if at risk of surgical complications, e.g. compartment syndrome or haemorrhage.

Reportable observations

Contact the pain service or anaesthetist *urgently* if any of the following occur:

- high block >T3 (Box 7.8 and Table 7.15);
- back pain (Table 7.15);
- dense motor block: Bromage score 2–3 (Box 7.9 and Table 7.15);
- UMSS sedation score ≥3 +/– respiratory depression (Boxes 7.6 and 7.7);
- fever >38.5°C;
- hypotension;
- signs of local anaesthetic toxicity (Table 7.16);
- signs of infection at the catheter entry site (Table 7.17);
- oedema or swelling at catheter entry site.

Complications of Regional Anaesthesia

The incidence of RA complications is 1:2,000 for serious complications and 1:10,000 for persisting complications (Llewellyn and Moriarty 2007; Sethna et al. 2010; Polaner et al. 2012). The following tables outline RA complications and suggested treatment. Epidural insertion-related problems (Table 7.15) are outlined first, followed by drug-related problems (Table 7.16) and catheter-related problems (Table 7.17). Tables 7.16 and 7.17 apply to both epidural and perineural techniques.

Table 7.15 Complications related to insertion of epidural catheter

Problem	Comments	Treatment
Headache	May be due to dural tap (incidence 1–2%) May not present until patient mobilises	1. Analgesia 2. Bed rest 3. Fluids 4. Epidural blood patch if prolonged, typical postural headache
Back pain	Usually at insertion site Mild back pain is common and usually transient Moderate or severe back pain must be thoroughly investigated	1. Simple analgesics and reassurance for mild back pain with regular checkups until resolved 2. If moderate-severe pain and/or fever needs *urgent* review to rule out epidural abscess or haematoma (see below)
Sympathetic blockade	May cause hypotension (usually in children >8 years)	1. Posture (lie flat, NOT head down) 2. IV fluid bolus
High blockade (see Box 7.8)	Dermatome block higher than T3: Numbness or tingling in fingers or arms Horner's syndrome: miosis, ptosis, dry/warm skin on face (unilateral) Respiratory distress (*intercostal block*) Bradycardia (*high thoracic block*) Unconsciousness (*total spinal block*)	1. Resuscitation 2. Cease epidural infusion 3. The infusion might be recommenced at a lower rate if epidural position is confirmed
Dense motor block (see Box 7.9)	Usual immediately after surgery due to higher concentrations of solution used intra-operatively Prolonged dense motor block >6 hours after surgery must be investigated to rule out epidural abscess or haematoma	1. Regularly assess amount of motor block (using Bromage scale) 2. Report Bromage score 2–3 3. Investigate if indicated
Nerve damage	Very rare May present with weakness or numbness that is usually transient	1. Neurology referral 2. Investigate if indicated
Epidural abscess	Very rare Presents with moderate to severe back pain, fever, sensory or motor deficits, malaise	1. Urgent investigation: Full blood examination, inflammatory markers, blood culture, MRI 2. Urgent neurology or neurosurgical review
Epidural haematoma	Very rare Presents with moderate to severe back pain, sensory or motor deficits	1. Urgent investigation: Full blood examination, coagulation studies, MRI 2. Urgent neurology or neurosurgical review

Source: Data from Ragg (1997); Patel (2006); RCH (2011, 2012d); Moriarty (2012)

Table 7.16 Drug-related problems with regional anaesthesia

Problem	Comments	Treatment
Local anaesthetic drugs		
Overdose/ Toxicity	Signs of LA toxicity: dizziness, blurred vision, decreased hearing, restlessness, tremor, hypotension, bradycardia, arrythmia, seizures, sudden loss of consciousness	1. Resuscitation 2. Management of cardiac, neurological and respiratory side-effects 3. Cease RA infusion
Allergy	Extremely rare Signs of anaphylaxis or allergic reaction may be present	1. Resuscitation with IV fluids, adrenaline, antihistamines and steroids 2. Cease RA infusion
Opioids		
Respiratory depression (see Box 7.7)	Early or delayed	1. Resuscitation 2. Administer naloxone 3. Cease infusion 4. Opioid dose decreased or removed from LA solution
Nausea and vomiting	More frequent with morphine vs. fentanyl or hydromorphone	1. Give antiemetic(s) 2. Opioid dose decreased or removed from LA solution
Pruritus	More frequent with morphine vs. fentanyl or hydromorphone	1. Low dose naloxone 2. Opioid dose decreased or removed from LA solution
Urinary retention		1. Try simple measures 2. Low dose naloxone 3. Urinary catheter 4. Opioid dose decreased or removed from LA solution
Sedation	UMSS score >3 (see Box 7.6)	1. Cease epidural 2. Urgent assessment 3. Opioid dose decreased or removed from LA solution
Clonidine		
Sedation	Clonidine increases sedation	1. May need clonidine dose decreased or removed from LA solution
Hypotension/ bradycardia	Clonidine increases hypotension	1. Consider IV fluid bolus 2. Monitor urine output and BP 3. May need clonidine dose decreased or removed from LA solution

Source: Data from Ragg (1997); RCH (2011, 2012d); Lonnqvist (2012); Moriarty (2012); Suresh et al. (2012)

Pain Problem-Solving

An important component of pain management is problem-solving why analgesia is inadequate or why the child is not responding as expected. It is useful to consider all possibilities. Sometimes distress may not be due to pain; for example, an infant crying can be due to hunger, parental separation or being in an unfamiliar place. Sometimes the prescribed analgesia is inadequate for activity and the patient is only comfortable when they stay still.

Table 7.17 Catheter-related problems with regional anaesthesia

Problem	Comments	Treatment
Leakage	Common Often unrelated to effectiveness of infusion	1. Reinforce dressing with gauze pad taped under pressure 2. Use occlusive dressing with high fluid permeability 3. Monitor leakage 4. Seek advice if in pain
Occlusion or kinking	Catheters easily occlude or kink Kinking may be subcutaneous or on the skin where the catheter or filter is secured	1. Check catheter tubing, filter and the infusion giving set 2. Check all adhesive taping 3. Try a bolus 4. Increase the pump infusion pressure 5. Change the infusion rate
Dislodgement	Preventable with meticulous securing of catheter at time of insertion and regular checks of all taping	1. Partial dislodgement may not adversely affect the block 2. Full dislodgement may require alternative analgesia
Disconnection	Preventable with meticulous securing of catheter and filter and regular checks of all connections	1. Disconnection is often at the filter 2. The catheter may need to be removed if disconnection occurs and alternate analgesia ordered

Source: Data from Ragg (1997); RCH (2011, 2012d); Dadure and Capdevila (2012)

Practice point

When assessing for efficacy of analgesia, ensure it is sufficient:

- for rest and sleep;
- for movement and turning;
- for deep breathing and coughing;
- for physiotherapy and nursing care;
- to enable mobilising.

Source: Kraemer and Rose (2009)

Asking yourself questions such as 'If this were me or my child, what could the problem be? Would this situation be painful?' can stimulate thinking. However, it is also useful to consider that if it looks like pain and sounds like pain it probably is pain! Involve the parents. Although they may not be able to pinpoint the cause, parents may be able to identify causative factors. Further suggestions for problem-solving are outlined in Table 7.18.

Practice point

Most surgical pain peaks 24–48 hours following surgery, then decreases rapidly. If there is worsening pain more than 48 hours after surgery, or at any time the pain appears *disproportional* to the surgery or underlying medical condition, reasons for this should always be considered and thoroughly investigated *in addition* to administering analgesics.

Table 7.18 Pain problem-solving

Problem	Possible cause/Considerations	Management
Pain escalation	What analgesia has been given and why is it inadequate?	Check the doses are correct Ensure ALL prescribed analgesics are given in a timely manner If required administer additional analgesia (titrate to comfort)
	Have Step 1 analgesics been given in addition to other analgesics?	
	Has the analgesia been given as prescribed? Are the doses appropriate for the child's weight, age or condition?	
	Are the infusion pumps functioning correctly? Is there a problem with drug delivery?	Check the infusion delivery device(s) and ensure it is functioning correctly
	Is the IV cannula or RA catheter in place and functioning normally?	Check the device is not leaking, blocked or dislodged
	Is the pain due to a medical or surgical complication (e.g. tight plaster, compartment syndrome, haemorrhage, haematoma, blocked wound drain, ileus)?	Request a medical or surgical review if complications are present or possible Address the underlying cause of the pain (e.g. split the plaster, adjust the drain(s), insert nasogastric tube)
	Has a *single dose* RA or perineural block regressed, requiring additional analgesia?	Administer additional analgesia
	Is the RA infusion providing adequate analgesia?	Review rate, consider a bolus Consider other analgesics
	Is the opioid infusion providing adequate analgesia?	Check rate, consider a bolus Consider other analgesics
Multiple *bad tries* or complaints of pain with PCA	Does the child understand how to use the PCA?	Re-educate if necessary
	Is the bolus dose adequate? Is the lockout time appropriate? Is a background infusion required? Is the analgesia adequate for the pain severity	Consider addition of background infusion or increase bolus size Consider other analgesics
	Consider other causes: anxiety, confusion, inappropriate use	Address and manage non-pain issues

Transition to Oral Analgesics

The transition from specialist analgesia techniques can be problematic if not planned carefully (Kraemer and Rose 2009). As the child's pain decreases and condition improves, oral medications are generally tolerated, which allows the specialist techniques to be weaned or ceased. If the child needs to remain fasting for extended period of time some Step 1 analgesic drugs can be given via the intravenous route.

It is important not to wean (decrease) analgesia too rapidly as this will slow recovery if the child becomes reluctant to mobilise or cough due to pain. Instead, encourage mobilisation while continuing specialist techniques, rather than ceasing them because it is the *expected day* the technique should finish. Ensuring additional rescue doses of analgesic drugs also relieves child and parental anxiety.

Weaning PCA

Most children self-wean from PCA, using it less as the pain improves, thus making a natural progression to simple analgesics. If the child is reluctant to cease using the PCA it may be helpful to negotiate an extended period of demand-only use on the PCA (Kraemer and Rose 2009). This is particularly useful for children after major surgery as it allows the clinician to leave the PCA for additional analgesia *rescues* while deciding if the prescribed oral analgesia is sufficient.

Practice point

Children who have required high doses or prolonged periods on opioids risk developing opioid abstinence syndrome (*withdrawal*) if opioids are decreased too rapidly. Instead a careful weaning regime should be implemented (see Chapter 4).

Weaning regional anaesthesia infusions

To minimise adverse effects, RA infusions are usually limited to 3 or 4 days (Moriarty 2012). Oral analgesia should be administered as soon as the RA infusion is ceased rather than waiting until sensation has returned. If the patient cannot receive oral analgesia, PCA or IV will be required. Analgesia needs to be given regularly for 12–24 hours with doses available for pain escalation. After this period, analgesia should be given on a PRN basis, depending on the surgery and expected pain.

Pain medications at home

Once the child is ready for discharge from hospital it is important that parents are given clear instructions about pain management and analgesics, the weaning plan and what to do if the pain is not well controlled (Kraemer and Rose 2009). Children needing to stay on Step 2 analgesic drugs for an extended period following discharge from hospital may require telephone follow-up or outpatient review to assist weaning and monitoring for chronic pain. An analgesia decision algorithm for weaning can be seen in Figure 7.1, and Figure 7.4 outlines a five-point plan for managing acute pain in children.

Summary

- Acute pain is a common childhood experience. It is generally of short duration and usually resolves completely.
- There are multiple causes of acute pain including childhood illnesses, injury, surgery or pre-existing medical conditions.
- Children with developmental disabilities experience significant pain in their daily life.
- Opioids are the mainstay for the management of severe acute pain but should be combined with simple analgesics as these have an opioid-sparing effect.
- Multimodal analgesia allows for optimal pain management, while minimising adverse effects by using combinations of analgesics at lower doses.

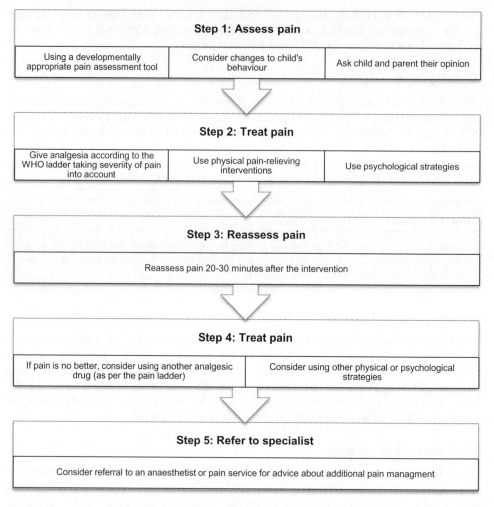

Figure 7.4   Five-step approach to acute pain management in children.

- Regional anaesthesia offers superior pain relief compared with most other analgesic techniques, as it can completely block pain.
- Close monitoring is key to prevention of serious adverse events related to opioid and regional analgesia techniques.
- Problem-solving can assist clinicians to improve the pain management of their patients.
- Any pain disproportional to the surgery or condition should always be investigated as it may indicate medical or surgical complications.
- Transition to oral analgesia following specialist analgesia techniques requires planning to ensure optimal pain management.
- Parents should be given clear instructions about managing pain at home following their child's discharge from hospital.

Key to Case Studies

See Box 7.10 and Box 7.11.

BOX 7.10

Billy

Billy is demonstrating signs of pain: immobility, pain complaints and elevated vital signs.

To establish Billy's understanding, ask him to tell you about the 'pain button' and how to use it. His parents are able assist by prompts to press the PCA button prior to movement or with complaints of pain. It may be appropriate to use PCA-by-proxy if Billy is not able to manage the PCA and the hospital protocols allow this.

Consequences of poorly managed abdominal pain include reduced chest expansion and atelectasis, reluctance to cough, immobility, prolonged hospitalisation and emotional distress.

BOX 7.11

Jack

The Bromage scale assesses motor function. Jack's Bromage score is 3.

Using an ice cube to determine altered temperature sensation indicates the area where the epidural is working.

Assessing the sensory block is important to ensure the epidural analgesia is sufficient for pain control. Assessing the motor block detects neurological deficits due to the LA or a complication.

Your main concern about a Bromage score of 3 should be an epidural haematoma. Although this is a rare complication it is an urgent reportable observation at any time. The anaesthetist or pain service should be immediately contacted and Jack should be examined. The epidural may need to be ceased until motor function returns. In addition, all bony areas such as heels, sacrum and malleoli are vulnerable to pressure, particularly with a dense motor block.

Additional information

Department of Anaesthesia and Pain Management, Royal Children's Hospital, Melbourne, Pain Clinical Practice Guidelines: www.rch.org.au/clinicalguide/guideline_index/Pain_Acute_Pain _Management_Link/

Great Ormond Street Hospital for Children, NHS Trust, Clinical Practice Guideline, Epidural Analgesia: www.gosh.nhs.uk/health-professionals/clinical-guidelines/epidural-analgesia/?locale=en

The New York School of Regional Anesthesia – Pediatric Epidural and Caudal Analgesia and Anesthesia in Children: www.nysora.com/regional_anesthesia/sub-specialties/pediatric_anesthesia/ index.1.html

---

References

Acworth, J., Babl, F., Borland, M. et al. (2009) Patterns of presentation to the Australian and New Zealand Paediatric Emergency Research Network. *Emergency Medicine Australasia* **21**(1), 59–66.

Ali, S., Drendel, A.L., Kircher, J. and Beno, S. (2010) Pain management of musculoskeletal injuries in children: Current state and future directions. *Pediatric Emergency Care* **26**(7), 518–524.

American Society for Pain Management Nursing (ASPMN) (2006) Authorized and Unauthorized ('PCA by Proxy') Dosing of Analgesic Infusion Pumps, Position Statement, American Society for Pain Management Nursing, available at: www.aspmn.org (accessed December 2012).

American Society of Anesthesiologists Task Force on Acute Pain Management (2012) Practice guidelines for acute pain management in the perioperative setting: An updated report by the American Society of Anesthesiologists Task Force on Acute Pain Management. *Anesthesiology* **116**(2), 248–273.

Anghelescu, D.L., Faughnan, L.G., Oaks, L. L., Windsor, K. Pei, D. and Burgoyne, L. (2012) Parent-controlled PCA for pain management in pediatic oncology: Is it safe? *Journal of Pediatric Hematology/Oncology* **34**(6), 416–420.

Association of Paediatric Anaesthetists of Great Britain and Ireland (APA) (2012) *Good Practice in Postoperative and Procedural Pain*, 2nd edition. Available from: http://onlinelibrary.wiley.com/doi/10.1111/j.1460-9592.2012.03838.x/pdf (accessed December 2012).

Aydin, O.N., Ugur, B., Ozgun, S., Eyigor, H. and Copcu, O. (2007) Pain prevention with intraoperative ketamine in outpatient children undergoing tonsillectomy or tonsillectomy and adenotomy. *Journal of Clinical Anesthesia* **19**, 115–119.

Bayreuther, J., Wagener, S., Woodford, M. et al. (2009) Paediatric trauma: injury pattern and mortality in the UK. *Archives of Disease in Childhood: Education and Practice Edition* **94**, 37–41.

Bolt, P., Barnett, P., Babl, F.E. and Sharwood, L.N. (2008) Topical lignocaine for pain relief in acute otitis media: Results of a double blind placebo-controlled randomized trial. *Archives of Disease in Childhood* **93**(1), 40–44.

Borland, M.L., Bergesio, R., Pascoe, E.M., Turner, S. and Woodger, S. (2005) Intranasal fentanyl is an equivalent analgesic to oral morphine in paediatric burns patients for dressing changes: A randomised double blind crossover study. *Burns* **31**(7), 831–837.

Borland, M., Jacobs, I., King, B. and O'Brien, D. (2007) A randomized controlled trial comparing intranasal fentanyl to intravenous morphine for managing acute pain in children in the emergency department. *Annals of Emergency Medicine* **49**, 335–340.

Borland, M.L., Clark, L.J. and Esson, A. (2009) Comparative review of the clinical use of intranasal fentanyl versus morphine in a paediatric emergency department. *Emergency Medicine Australasia* **20**, 515–520.

Bozkurt, P. (2005) Use of tramadol in children. *Pediatric Anesthesia* **15**, 1041–1047.

Brady-Fryer, B., Wiebe, N. and Lander, J.A. (2009) Pain relief for neonatal circumcision, *Cochrane Database Systematic Review* **issue 1**.

Breau, L.M. and Burkitt, C. (2009) Assessing pain in children with intellectual disabilities. *Pain Research and Management* **14**, 116–120.

Ceelie, I., de Wildt, S.N., van Dijk, M. et al. (2013) Effect of intravenous paracetamol on postoperative morphine requirements in neonates and infants undergoing major noncardiac surgery: A randomized controlled trial. *Journal of the American Medical Association* **309**(2), 149–154.

Cho, J.E., Kim, J.Y., Hong, J.Y. and Kil, H.K. (2009) The addition of fentanyl to 1.5 mg/ml ropivacaine has no advantage for paediatric epidural analgesia. *Acta Anaesthesiologica Scandinavica* **53**(8), 1084–1087.

Czarnecki, M.L., Jandrisevits, M.D., Theiler, S.C., Huth, M.M. and Weisman, S.J. (2004) Controlled-release oxycodone for the management of pediatric postoperative pain. *Journal of Pain Symptom Management* **27**(4), 379–386.

Dadure, C. and Capdevila, X. (2012) Peripheral catheter techniques. *Paediatric Anaesthesia* **22**(1), 93–101.

Dahmani, S., Michelet, D., Abback, P. et al. (2011) Ketamine for perioperative pain management in children: A meta-analysis of published studies. *Pediatric Anesthesia* **21**, 636–652.

De Lima, J. and Browning Carmo, K. (2010) Practical pain management in the neonate. *Best Practice and Research Clinical Anaesthesiology* **24**, 291–307.

Dobereiner, E.F, Cox, R.G., Ewen, A. and Lardner, D.R. (2010) Evidence-based clinical update: Which local anesthetic drug for pediatric caudal block provides optimal efficacy with the fewest side effects? *Canadian Journal of Anesthesia* **57**(12), 1102–1110.

Dong, L., Donaldson, A., Metzger, R. and Keenan, H. (2012) Analgesic administration in the emergency department for children requiring hospitalization for long-bone fracture. *Pediatric Emergency Care* **28**(2), 109–114.

Drutz, J.E. (2012) Symptomatic relief of sore throat in children and adolescents. In T.K. Duryea (ed.) *UpToDate*. www.uptodate.com (Accessed 21/12/12).

Falanga, I.J., Lafrenaye, S., Mayer, S.K. and Tetrault, J-P. (2006) Management of acute pain in children: Safety and efficacy of a nurse-controlled algorithm for pain relief. *Acute Pain* **8**(2), 45–54.

Finn, M. and Harris, D. (2010) Intranasal fentanyl for analgesia in the paediatric emergency department. *Emergency Medicine Journal* **27**(4), 300–301.

Franson, H. (2010) Postoperative patient-controlled analgesia in the pediatric population: A literature review. *American Association of Nurse Anesthetists Journal* **78**(5), 374–378.

Friday, J.H., Kanegaye, J.T., McCaslin, I., Zheng, A. and Harley, J.R. (2009) Ibuprofen provides analgesia equivalent to acetaminophen-codeine in the treatment of acute pain in children with extremity injuries: A randomized clinical trial. *Academic Emergency Medicine* **16**(8), 711–716.

Friedrichsdorf, S., Drake, R. and Webster, M.L. (2011) Gastrointestinal symptoms In: *Textbook of Interdisciplinary Pediatric Palliative Care* (eds J. Wolfe, P.S. Hind and, B.M. Sourkes), pp. 311–334. Elsevier Saunders, Philadelphia.

Gan, T.J., Meyer, T., Apfel C.C. et al. (2007) Society for Ambulatory Anesthesia Guidelines for the management of postoperative nausea and vomiting. *Ambulatory Anesthesiology* **105** (6), 1615–1628.

Gandhi, M., Thomson, C., Lord, D. and Enoch, S. (2010) Management of pain in children with burns. *International Journal of Pediatrics* **2010**, 1–10.

Gazal, G. and Mackie, I.C. (2007). A comparison of paracetamol, ibuprofen or their combination for pain relief following extractions in children under general anaesthesia: A randomized controlled trial. *International Journal of Pediatric Dentistry* **17**(3), 169–177.

Goes, P., Watt, R., Hardy, R. and Sheiham, A. (2008) Impacts of dental pain on daily activities of adolescents aged 14–15 years and their families. *Informal Healthcare* **66**(1), 7–12.

Goldman, B. (2002) Acute pain. In *Managing Pain: The Canadian Healthcare Professional's Reference* (ed. R.D. Jovey), pp 87–102. Healthcare and Financial Publishing, Toronto.

Gourde, J. and Damian, F.J. (2012) ED fracture pain management in children. *Journal of Emergency Nursing* **38**(1), 91–97.

Grass, J.A. (2005) Patient-controlled analgesia. *Anesthesia and Analgesia* **101**(5 Suppl): S44–S61.

Hadley, G., Maconochie, I. and Jackson, A. (2010) A survey of intranasal medication use in the paediatric emergency setting in England and Wales. *Emergency Medical Journal* **27**(7), 553–554.

Hiller, A., Meretoja, O.A., Korpela, R., Piiparinen, S. and Taivainen, T. (2006) The analgesic efficacy of acetaminophen, ketoprofen, or their combination for pediatric surgical patients having soft tissue or orthopedic procedures. *Anesthesia and Analgesia* **102**(5), 1365–1371.

Hong, J.Y., Won Han, S., Kim, W.O. and Kil, H.K. (2010) Fentanyl sparing effects of combined ketorolac and acetaminophen for outpatient inguinal hernia repair in children. *Journal of Urology* **183**(4): 1551–1555.

Howard, R.E., Lloyd-Thomas, A., Thomas, M. et al. (2010) Nurse-controlled analgesia (NCA) following major surgery in 10,000 patients in a children's hospital. *Paediatric Anaesthesia* **20**(2), 126–134.

Ivani, G. and Mossetti, V. (2010) Continuous central and perineural infusions for postoperative pain control in children. *Current Opinion in Anaesthesiology* **23**(5), 637–642.

Jacob, E., Hockenberry, M., Mueller, B.U., Coates, T.D. and Zeltzer, L. (2008). Analgesic response to morphine in children with sickle cell disease: A pilot study. *Journal of Pain Management* **2**(1), 179–190.

James, P.J., Howard, R.F. and Williams, D.G. (2010) The addition of ketamine to a morphine nurse-or patient-controlled analgesia infusion (PCA/NCA) increases analgesic efficacy in children with mucositis pain. *Paediatric Anaesthesia* **20**(9), 805–811.

Jarzyna, D., Jungquist, C., Pasero, C. et al. (2011) American Society for Pain Management Nursing Guidelines on monitoring for opioid-induced sedation and respiratory depression. *Pain Management Nursing* **12**(3), 118–145.

Karl, H.W., Tyler, D.C. and Miser, A.W. (2012) Controlled trial of morphine vs hydromorphone for patient-controlled analgesia in children with postoperative pain. *Pain Medicine* **13**(12), 1658–1659.

Korb, K., Scherer, M., and Chenot, J.F., (2010) Steroids as adjuvant therapy for acute pharyngitis in ambulatory patients: A systematic review. *Annals of Family Medicine* **8**(1), 58–63.

Kovac, A.L. (2007) Management of postoperative nausea and vomiting in children. *Pediatric Drugs* **9**(1), 47–69.

Kozlowski, L.J., Kost-Byerly, S., Colantuoni, E. et al. (2012) Pain prevalence, intensity, assessment and management in a hospitalized pediatric population. *Pain Management Nursing*, online early.

Kraemer, F.W. and Rose, J.B. (2009) Pharmacologic management of acute pediatric pain. *Anesthesiology Clinics* **27**, 241–268.

Krane, E.J. (2008) Patient-controlled analgesia? *International Anaesthesia Research Society* **107**, 15–17.

Llewellyn, N. and Moriarty, A. (2007) The national pediatric epidural audit. *Pediatric Anesthesia* **17**, 520–533.

Lonnqvist, P.A. (2012) Toxicity of local anaesthetic drugs: A pediatric perspective. *Pediatric Anaesthesia* **22**, 39–43.

Macintyre, P.E., Schug, S.A., Scott, D.A., Visser, E.J., Walker, S.M.; APM:SE Working Group of the Australian and New Zealand College of Anaesthetists and Faculty of Pain Medicine (2010) *Acute Pain Management: Scientific Evidence*, 3rd edition. ANZCA & FPM, Melbourne.

Malviya, S., Voepel-Lewis, T., Tait, A.R., Merkel, S., Tremper, K. and Naughton, N. (2002) Depth of sedation in children undergoing computed tomography: Validity and reliability of the University of Michigan Sedation Scale (UMSS). *British Journal of Anaesthesia* **88**(2), 241–245.

Malviya, S., Voepel-Lewis, T. and Tait, A. (2006) A comparison of observational and objective measures to differentiate depth of sedation in children from birth to 18 years of age. *Anaesthesia and Analgesia* **102**, 389–394.

McClain, B.C. (2006) Pediatric hospital-based pain care. In: *Bringing Pain Relief to Children: Treatment Approaches* (eds G.A. Finley, P.J. McGrath and C.T. Chambers), pp 1–30. Totowa, Humana Press.

Meier, E.R. and Miller, J.L. (2012) Sickle cell disease in children. *Drugs* **72**(7), 895–906.

Michelet, D., Andreu-Gallien, J., Bensalah, T. et al. (2012) A meta-analysis of the use of nonsteroidal antiinflammatory drugs for pediatric postoperative pain. *Anesthesia and Analgesia* **114**(2), 393–406.

Mickalide, A. and Carr, K. (2012) Safe kids worldwide: Preventing unintentional childhood injuries across the globe. *Pediatric Clinics of North America* **59**(6), 1367–1380.

Monitto, C.L., Kost-Byerly, S., White, E. et al. (2011) The optimal dose of prophylactic intravenous naloxone in ameliorating opioid-induced side effects in children receiving intravenous patient-controlled analgesia morphine for moderate to severe pain: A dose finding study. *Anesthesia and Analgesia* **113**(4), 834–842.

Moriarty, A. (2012) Pediatric epidural analgesia (PEA). *Paediatric Anaesthesia* **22**(1), 51–55.

Morton, N. and Errera, A. (2010) APA National audit of pediatric opioid infusions. *Pediatric Anesthesia* **20**, 119–125

Moura-Leite, F.R., Ramos-Jorge, M.L., Bonanato, K., Paiva, S.M., Vale, M.P. and Pordeus, I.A. (2008) Prevalence, intensity and impact of dental pain in 5-year-old preschool children. *Oral Health and Preventative Dentistry* **6**(4), 295–301.

Mudd, S. (2011) Intranasal fentanyl for pain management in children: A systematic review of the literature. *Journal of Pediatric Health Care* **25**(5), 316–322.

Naja, M.Z., El-Rajab, M., Kabalan, W., Ziade, M.F., and Al-Tannir, M.A. (2005) Pre-incisional infiltration for pediatric tonsillectomy: A randomized double-blind clinical trial. *International Journal of Pediatric Otorhinolaryngology* **69**(10), 1333–1341.

Oberlander, T.F. and Symons, F.L. (2006) *Pain in Children and Adults with Developmental Disabilities*. Paul Brookes Publishing Co., Baltimore, MD.

Pasero, C. (2009) Assessment of sedation during opioid administration for pain management. *Journal of PeriAnesthesia Nursing* **24**(3), 186–190.

Patel, D. (2006) Epidural analgesia for children. *Continuing Education in Anaesthesia, Critical Care and Pain* **6**(2), 63–66.

Perrott, D.A., Piira, T., Goodenough, B. and Champion, D. (2004) Efficacy and safety of acetaminophen vs ibuprofen for treating children's pain or fever. *Archives of Pediatric and Adolescent Medicine* **158**, 551–556.

Polaner, D.M., Taenzer, A.H., Walker, B.J. et al. (2012) Pediatric Regional Anesthesia Network (PRAN): A multi-institutional study of the use and incidence of complications of pediatric regional anesthesia. *Anesthesia and Analgesia* **115**(6), 1353–1364.

Ragg, P. (1997) Epidural analgesia in children In: *Manual of Acute Pain Management in Children* (I.M. McKenzie, P.B. Gaukroger, P.G. Ragg and T.C.K. Brown), pp. 47–61. Churchill Livingstone, New York.

Riley, R.R., Witkop, M. Hellman, E. and Akins, S. (2011) Assessment and management of pain in haemophilia patients. *Hemophilia* **17**(6), 839–846.

Rosen, D.A. and Dower, J. (2011) Pediatric pain management. *Pediatric Annals* **40**(5), 243–252.

Royal Children's Hospital (RCH), Melbourne (2010a) Assessment of sensory block. Available at: www.rch.org.au/anaes/pain_management/Assessment_of_sensory_block/ (accessed February 2013).

Royal Children's Hospital (RCH), Melbourne (2010b) Assessment of motor block. Available at: www.rch.org.au/anaes/pain_management/Assessment_of_motor_block/ (accessed February 2013).

Royal Children's Hospital (RCH), Melbourne (2011) Epidural infusions. Available at: www.rch.org.au/anaes/pain_management/Epidural_Infusion/ (accessed March 2013).

Royal Children's Hospital (RCH), Melbourne (2012a) Opioid infusion: Observations. Available at: www.rch.org.au/anaes/pain_management/Opioid_Infusion/ – Observations (accessed February 2013).

Royal Children's Hospital (RCH), Melbourne (2012b) Patient Controlled Analgesia: Observations. Available at: www.rch.org.au/anaes/pain_management/Patient_Controlled_Analgesia_PCA/ – Observations (accessed February 2013).

Royal Children's Hospital (RCH), Melbourne (2012c) Opioid infusion: Complications. Available at: www.rch.org.au/anaes/pain_management/Opioid_Infusion/ – Complications (accessed February 2013).

Royal Children's Hospital (RCH), Melbourne (2012d) Regional anaesthetics. Available at: www.rch.org.au/anaes/pain_management/Regional_Anaesthetic_Infusion_Blocks/ (accessed March 2013).

San Diego Patient Safety Council (2009) Tool Kit: Patient Controlled Analgesia (PCA) Guidelines of Care. Available from: www.patientsafetycouncil.org/Publications.html (accessed January 2013).

Saudan, S., Habre, W., Ceroni, D. et al. (2008) Safety and efficacy of patient controlled epidural analgesia following pediatric spinal surgery. *Paediatric Anaesthesia* 18(2), 132–139.

Schechter, N.L. (2006) Treatment of acute and chronic pain in the outpatient setting. In: *Bringing Pain Relief to Children: Treatment Approaches* (eds G.A. Finley, P.J. McGrath and C.T. Chambers), pp. 31–58. Totowa, Humana Press.

Schnabel, A., Poepping, D.M., Kranke, P., Zahn, P.K. and Pogatzki-Zahn, E.M. (2011a) Efficacy and adverse effects of ketamine as an additive for paediatric caudal anaesthesia: A quantitative systematic review of randomized controlled trials. *British Journal of Anaesthesia* 107(4), 601–611.

Schnabel, A., Poepping, D.M., Pogatzki-Zahn, E.M. and Zahn, P.K. (2011b) Efficacy and safety of clonidine as additive for caudal regional anesthesia: A quantitative systematic review of randomized controlled trials. *Paediatric Anaesthesia* 21(12), 1219–1230.

Sethna, N.F., Clendenin, D., Athiraman, U., Solodiuk, J., Rodriguez, D.P. and Zurakowski, D. (2010) Incidence of epidural catheter-associated infections after continuous epidural analgesia in children. *Anesthesiology* 113(1), 224–232.

Shukla, U., Prabhakar, T. and Malhotra, K. (2011) Postoperative analgesia in children when using clonidine or fentanyl with ropivacaine given caudally. *Journal of Anaesthesiology and Clinical Pharmacology* 27(2), 205–210.

Singh, R., Kumar, N. and Singh, P. (2011) Randomized controlled trial comparing morphine or clonidine with bupivacaine for caudal analgesia in children undergoing upper abdominal surgery. *British Journal of Anaesthesia* 106(1), 96–100.

Stevens, B.J., Harrison, D., Rashotte, J. et al. and CIHR Team in Children's Pain (2012) Pain assessment and intensity in hospitalized children in Canada. *Journal of Pain* 13(9), 857–865.

Suresh, S., Birmingham, P.K. and Kozlowski. R.J. (2012) Pediatric pain management. *Anesthesiology Clinics* 30(1), 101–117.

Tay, C.L. and Tan, S. (2002) Diclofenac or paracetamol for analgesia in paediatric myringotomy outpatients. *Anaesthesia and Intensive Care* 30(1), 55–59.

Temple, B., Dube, C., McMillan, D. et al. (2012) Pain in people with developmental disabilities: A scoping review. *Journal on Developmental Disabilities* 18(1), 73–86.

Trescot, A.M., Datta, S., Lee, M. and Hansen, H. (2008) Opioid pharmacology. *Pain Physician* 11, S135–S153.

Twycross, A. and Collis, S. (2012). How well is acute pain in children managed? A snapshot in one English hospital. *Pain Management Nursing*, online early.

Twycross, A., Finley, G.A., Latimer, M. (2013) Pediatric nurses' postoperative pain management practices: An observational study. *Journal for Specialists in Pediatric Nursing.* 18(3), 189–201.

Tzortzopoulou, A., McNicol, E.D., Cepeda, M.S., Francia, M.B., Farhat, T. and Schumann, R. (2011) Single dose intravenous propacetamol or intravenous paracetamol for postoperative pain. *Cochrane Database Systematic Review* issue 10.

Uysal, H.Y., Takmaz, S.A., Yaman, F., Baltaci, B. and Başar, H. (2011) The efficacy of intravenous paracetamol versus tramadol for postoperative analgesia after adenotonsillectomy in children. *Journal of Clinical Anesthesia* 23(1), 53–57.

van Beers, E., van Tuijn, C., Nieuwkerk, Friderich, P., Vranken, J. and Biemond, B. (2007) Patient Controlled analgesia versus continuous infusion of morphine during vaso-occlusive crisis in sickle cell disease, a randomized controlled trial. *American Journal of Haematology* 82(11), 955–960.

Voepel-Lewis, T., Wagner, D., Burke, C. et al. (2013) Early adjuvant used of non-opioids associated with reduced odds of serious postoperative opioid adverse events and need for rescue in children. *Pediatric Anesthesia* 23(2), 162–169.

Walker, S.M. and Yaksh, T.L. (2012) Neuraxial analgesia in neonates and infants: A review of clinical and preclinical strategies for the development of safety and efficacy data. *Anesthesia and Analgesia* **115**(3), 638–662.

Wolf, A.R. (2012) Effects of regional analgesia on stress responses to pediatric surgery. *Paediatric Anaesthesia* **22**(1), 19–24.

Wood, D.N., Nakas, N. and Gregory, C.W. (2012) Clinical trials assessing ototopical agents in the treatment of pain associated with acute otitis media in children. *International Journal of Pediatric Otorhinolaryngology* **76**(9), 1229–1235.

World Health Organization (2012) *WHO guidelines on the pharmacological treatment of persisting pain in children with medical illnesses.* World Health Organization, Geneva.

Wuhrman, E., Cooney, M.F., Dunwoody, C.J., Eksterowicz, N., Merkel, S. and Oaks, L.L. American Society for Pain Management Nursing (2007) Authorized and unauthorized ('PCA by proxy') dosing of analgesic infusion pumps: Position statement with clinical practice recommendations. *Pain Management Nursing* **8**(1), 4–11.

Yaster, M. (2010) Multimodal analgesia in children. *European Journal of Anaesthesiology* **27**(10), 851–857.

Young, A. and Buvanendran, A. (2012) Recent advances in multimodal analgesia. *Anesthesiology Clinics* **30**, 91–100.

Zempsky, W.T. (2010) Evaluation and treatment of sickle cell pain in the Emergency Department: Paths to a better future. *Clinical Pediatric Emergency Medicine* **11**(4), 265–273.

CHAPTER 8

Chronic Pain in Children

Jennifer Stinson

Chronic Pain Programme, The Hospital for Sick Children;
Lawrence S. Bloomberg Faculty of Nursing, University of Toronto, Canada

Kathy Reid

Paediatric Chronic Pain Program, Stollery Children's Hospital, Canada

Introduction

This chapter provides an overview of chronic pain in children. It defines and describes the main types of chronic pain experienced by children and adolescents and considers the impact on the child and family. Key factors that have been found to influence the development and maintenance of chronic pain are discussed. The principles of treatment are outlined and the role of the multidisciplinary team in the management of children's chronic pain is described.

What is Chronic Pain?

Chronic pain is a term used to describe persistent or recurrent pain. Chronic pain in children and adolescents is commonly defined as any prolonged pain that lasts longer than the expected healing time (arbitrarily defined as more than 3 to 6 months), or any recurrent pain that occurs at least three times throughout a period of 3 months (Van Den Kerkhof and van Dijk 2006; American Pain Society 2012).

The Pediatric Chronic Pain Task Force, which is part of the American Pain Society (APS), has provided a description of chronic pain in children:

> Chronic pain in children is the result of a dynamic integration of biological processes, psychological factors, and socio-cultural context, considered within a developmental trajectory. This category of pain includes persistent (ongoing) and recurrent (episodic) pain in children with chronic health conditions (e.g. arthritis or sickle cell disease) and pain that is a disorder itself (e.g. migraines, functional abdominal pain, complex regional pain syndrome) (/www.ampainsoc.org/advocacy/downloads/aps12-pcp.pdf).

Managing Pain in Children: A Clinical Guide for Nurses and Healthcare Professionals, Second Edition.
Edited by Alison Twycross, Stephanie Dowden, and Jennifer Stinson.
© 2014 John Wiley & Sons, Ltd. Published 2014 by John Wiley & Sons, Ltd.

Table 8.1 Differences between acute and chronic pain (adapted from Goldman 2002)

Characteristic	Acute pain	Chronic pain
Cause	Usually single obvious cause (e.g. tissue damage due to surgery)	Usually multiple causative or triggering factors Neuronal or CNS abnormality (plasticity, sensitisation)
Type	Nociceptive and/or neuropathic	Nociceptive, neuropathic or mixed
Purpose	Protective; activation of sympathetic nervous system	No protective function; rarely accompanied by signs of activation of sympathetic nervous system
Duration	Short-lived (days to weeks)	Long-lasting (>3 months) or recurring beyond time of normal healing May be associated with chronic disease
Pain intensity	Usually proportionate to severity of injury	Often out of proportion to objective physical findings
Treatment	Usually easy to treat with single modalities (pharmacological or physical)	More difficult to treat, requiring multidisciplinary, multimodal treatment approach
Outcome	Expected to resolve with healing	Pain persists in significant proportion (30–62%) (Perquin et al. 2003; El-Metwally et al. 2005; Martin et al. 2007); with smaller proportion developing pain-related disability (Huguet and Miró 2008)

Chronic pain in children is a serious health problem due to its complex nature, and can result in significant disability (Gauntlett-Gilbert and Eccleston 2007; Martin et al. 2007; Huguet and Miró 2008; Zernikow et al. 2012a). Table 8.1 outlines the main differences between acute and chronic pain.

Unlike acute pain, which usually has an identifiable cause, most chronic pain conditions in children are idiopathic (unexplained) in nature. This often results in patients and families continuing their search for an underlying cause for the pain, which leads to multiple medical investigations (in a vicious cycle of doctor-shopping) to find a diagnosis and cure. During this process the child often receives little, if any, appropriate pain management. This cycle elevates the child's fear and the parents' stress and anxiety, which may further contribute to pain symptoms and disability (Eccleston et al. 2003).

Practice point

Acute and chronic pain may occur concurrently. For example, children with arthritis might experience an acute flare in their pain while living with persistent chronic arthritic pain. Acute pain that is not properly treated may become chronic.

Children with chronic pain respond differently to those with acute pain and may not seem to be in pain. They may appear withdrawn and unresponsive, or have a seemingly exaggerated response to a usually non-painful stimulus such as a light touch (Eccleston et al. 2006).

Table 8.2 Prevalence of chronic pain in children

Pain sites	Prevalence (range)	Age differences	Gender differences
Headache	8–82.9%	Older > younger	Girls > boys
Abdominal pain	3.8–53.4%	Younger > older	Girls > boys
Back pain	13.5–24%	Older > younger	Girls > boys
Musculoskeletal/limb pain	3.9–40%	Older > younger	Girls > boys
Multiple pains	3.6–48.8%	Unclear	Girls > boys
Other/general pain	5–88%	Unclear – possible age and gender interaction	Girls > boys

Source: King et al. (2011)

How Common is Chronic Pain in Children?

There is growing evidence about the epidemiology of chronic pain in children (Van Den Kerkhof and van Dijk 2006; King et al. 2011). However, there are inconsistent findings on prevalence, with rates varying considerably across studies. Table 8.2 provides information regarding the nature and aggregated prevalence of chronic pain in children from 41 studies carried out between 1999 and 2009 (King et al. 2011). Prevalence estimates (median) range from 11% to 38%. These findings indicate that chronic pain is common in children and adolescents and that prevalence rates and or the recognition of it have increased over the past decade (Van Den Kerkhof and van Dijk 2006; King et al. 2011). Although no definition of chronic pain exists for infants, indicators for chronic pain in this age group do exist, including inability to settle, social withdrawal, sleep disturbances and poor feeding (Pillai Riddell et al. 2009).

The most common chronic pain conditions are headaches, abdominal pain, back pain and musculoskeletal pain. Children often report pain in multiple locations, with headache reported as most disabling (van Gessel et al. 2011). It is estimated that 5–8% of children with recurrent and persistent pain will develop significant pain-related disability that increases with age (Martin et al. 2007; Huguet and Miró 2008). Pain prevalence rates tend to increase with age, with the exception of abdominal pain (which is more prevalent in younger children), and girls generally report more pain than boys (Huguet and Miró 2008; Zernikow et al. 2012a). Psychosocial variables impacting pain prevalence include anxiety, depression, low self-esteem, other chronic health conditions and low socio-economic status (King et al. 2011).

Practice point

Despite the relatively high prevalence of chronic pain in children and its significant physical, psychological, social and economic impact on children and their families, it is often under-recognised and under-treated by clinicians.

The lack of objective signs (no sympathetic nervous system arousal, no overt distress) often leads the inexperienced clinician to diagnose the pain as functional or psychosomatic.

Viewing pain as either organic or non-organic is harmful because it leads to over-medicalisation (inappropriate investigations, procedures and interventions) or insufficient acknowledgement of the child's multidimensional experience and underlying neurophysiology.

Source: Kozlowska et al. (2008)

Table 8.3 Types of chronic pain in children

Category/Aetiology	Examples
Disease-related pain	Sickle cell disease Haemophilia Epidermolysis bullosa Osteogenesis imperfecta Rheumatological conditions Neuromuscular conditions (e.g. spasticity, dystonia) Post-viral infection (e.g. herpes) Cancer and treatment (e.g. chemotherapy, radiotherapy)
Injury-related pain	Burns Sprains, fractures Post-surgery (e.g. phantom limb pain, scar tissue, nerve damage) Complex regional pain syndrome (e.g. post-fracture or sprain)
Nonspecific (unexplained/ chronic benign pain)	Headache Recurrent abdominal pain Complex regional pain syndrome Low back pain Widespread chronic pain Chronic fatigue syndrome
Somatoform disorders	Pain disorder Conversion disorder

Aetiology or Causes of Chronic Pain

Chronic pain may be part of an ongoing/long-term medical condition, may develop following surgery, illness or injury, or may have no obvious cause (idiopathic) (Table 8.3). Chronic pain conditions can be nociceptive, neuropathic, or mixed (combination of nociceptive and neuropathic) in nature and/or associated with psychological factors. (For definitions of nociceptive and neuropathic pain see Chapter 2.)

- Musculoskeletal (e.g. bone, joint and muscle) pain is common (experienced by 10–35% of children) and is often associated with rheumatological conditions such as juvenile idiopathic arthritis and systemic lupus erythematosus (El-Metwally et al. 2004; O'Sullivan et al. 2011).
- One-fifth of preteens and early adolescents experienced new-onset weekly musculoskeletal pain over a one-year period (El-Metwally et al. 2007).
- Children with cancer can experience multiple sources of pain due to the cancer, its treatment (side-effects of chemotherapy and radiation) or secondary effects (e.g. infections) (Collins et al. 2008).
- In a longitudinal study of pain in children with advanced cancer, pain was consistently reported across all children with various types of cancer. Children most frequently reported head pain (31%), followed by abdomen, lower back, leg and feet pain (20% to 30%) (Van Cleve et al. 2012).
- The outcomes of childhood cancer-related pain extend into the adult life of cancer survivors. A recent questionnaire-based descriptive study of over 10,000 childhood cancer survivors and over 3,000 of their sibling controls revealed that adult survivors had an increased risk of reporting pain compared to siblings (Lu et al. 2011).

- Children with cognitive, motor and communication impairments are at particular risk of experiencing chronic pain due to their underlying condition and limited ability to self-report pain. For example, Ramstad et al. (2011) found that 62% of children and adolescents with cerebral palsy experienced moderate levels of recurrent musculoskeletal pain.
- Children with cognitive impairment may suffer from chronic pain related to headaches or self-injurious behaviours (Breau et al. 2006).
- Chronic pain is also common in children with neuromuscular disease (NMD) (Engel et al. 2009). In that study 55% (23/42) of adolescents with NMD reported chronic pain and the leg was the most common location of pain.

Pain disorders associated with psychological factors were previously referred to as psychogenic pain (i.e. real pain caused by psychological problems). They are now referred to as *somatoform disorders* (American Psychiatric Association 2000).

> Somatisation is the communication of emotional distress, troubled relationships and personal predicaments through bodily symptoms in the absence of clear physical pathology (Taylor and Garralda 2003).

Psychological factors are judged to play a major role in the onset, severity, exacerbation or maintenance of certain somatoform disorders. Pain is common in children with somatoform disorders (Mullick 2002). Pain that is solely psychological in nature is rare (<2%) (Taylor and Garralda 2003). The explanation of pain as psychogenic is often considered unhelpful, partly due to the misconceptions attached to such a diagnosis, and because all pain has psychological, social and biological components (Kozlowska et al. 2008).

Common Chronic Pain Conditions in Children and Adolescents

Headache

Headaches are distinguished and defined largely on the basis of their clinical features.

> Headaches have been classified by the International Headache Society (http://ihs-classification.org/en/).
> Classifications include primary and secondary headache. Primary headaches include migraine (with and without aura), tension-type headaches and new daily persistent headache.
> The term chronic headache is loosely defined as a headache for 15 or more days per month for 3 consecutive months or longer. The most common types in children are migraine with and without aura (Table 8.4) and chronic tension-type headaches. Tension-type headaches may progress to chronic headaches (Shashi 2012).
> New daily persistent headache (NDPH) is a relatively new term to categorise those individuals where the headache is daily and unremitting from very soon after onset (within 3 days at the most). The pain is typically bilateral, pressing or throbbing in quality and of mild to moderate intensity. There may be photophobia, phonophobia or mild nausea.

Headaches are the most commonly reported chronic pain in children (Zernikow et al. 2012a). For the common types of headaches in children, the actual causes are

Table 8.4 Types of paediatric migraines

Paediatric migraine without aura (65–85%)	Paediatric migraine with aura (15–30%)
At least 5 distinct attacks	Fulfils criteria for migraine without aura
Headache attack lasting 1–72 hours	Characterised by focal disturbances before or as the headache begins, such as visual, motor, or aphasia Gradual onset, lasting several minutes up to an hour
Headache has at least two of the following: • Bilateral location (frontal/temporal) or unilateral location • Pulsating quality • Moderate to severe intensity • Aggravated by routine physical activity	Two distinct types: Basilar migraine: Two or more symptoms of: • Dizziness, vertigo, tinnitus, visual disturbances, decreased hearing or ataxia as the aura Familial hemiplegic: • 'Stroke-like' qualities, with some degree of hemiparesis 30–60 minutes prior to the headache • At least one relative experienced similar attack
During headache, at least one of the following: • Nausea and/or vomiting • Photophobia and/or phonophobia (abnormal sensitivity to noise)	Headache begins during the aura or within 60 minutes
Not attributed to another disorder	Not attributed to another disorder

Source: Lewis (2009)

not known. Children may also develop secondary headaches. These are headaches that occur with another illness, condition or problem such as:

• trauma;
• strokes or other vascular disorders;
• intracranial disorders such as tumours or epilepsy;
• substances such as medication overuse;
• infections;
• disorders of the facial or cranial structures;
• psychiatric disorders.

(IHS Classification ICHD-II 2012)

Practice point

It is imperative to rule out serious neurological or neurosurgical causes for the headaches (for example, cerebral haemorrhage, shunt malfunction) prior to implementing chronic pain management strategies. A referral to a neurologist or additional investigations might be warranted.

Chronic abdominal pain

Case study: Suzie

Suzie, aged 13 years, presents with a 9-month history of cramping, peri-umbilical pain and nausea. She has seen her GP several times over the past 6 months for pain and has had three visits to the Emergency Room for pain. Her blood work (complete blood count, differential, erythrocyte sedimentation rate) is normal, her coeliac screen is negative and her abdominal x-ray shows faecal loading. She is on regular doses of laxatives. Suzie reports that she can't go to school as she feels she can't make it to the bathroom in time and that she is not sleeping very well at night.

- What additional assessments would you make to help with diagnosis and treatment?
- What pharmacological, physical and psychological therapies might help Suzie?

Chronic abdominal pain (CAP) is defined as three or more episodes of abdominal pain and associated gastrointestinal (GI) symptoms over a period of at least 3 months that are severe enough to interfere with normal activities (American Academy of Pediatrics 2005). Epidemiological studies suggest 8–25% of school children are affected by CAP (Huguet and Miró 2008). Pain in children with CAP is thought to be due to distension, muscle contractions and hypersensitivity of the mechanoreceptors which detect stretch. Children with CAP and irritable bowel syndrome (IBS) experience pain at lower levels of distention than healthy controls (Wood 2008).

Other research in this area has shown that:

- females appear to be affected by CAP slightly more than males (van Gessel et al. 2011);
- the majority of children with CAP have no obvious underlying cause for their pain and therefore are classified as having functional abdominal pain (Jones and Walker 2006).

Functional abdominal pain (FAP) is defined as abdominal pain without obvious pathology and includes functional dyspepsia (indigestion), irritable bowel syndrome, abdominal migraine and functional abdominal pain syndrome (Subcommittee on Chronic Abdominal Pain, 2005). Table 8.5 outlines diagnosis criteria and estimated incidence (percentage) within the four subgroups of FAP. Until recently the term recurrent abdominal pain (RAP) was used to describe this condition, but is now considered outdated. Up to 35% of children with FAP continue to report symptoms as adults and report symptoms consistent with diagnostic criteria for migraine and/or tension headaches (Walker et al. 2010).

The lack of an obvious cause for abdominal pain can result in considerable distress for the child and family, and it is essential that children are not subjected to unnecessary tests. The signs and symptoms that may indicate underlying pathology or 'red flags' and thus prompt further investigation include:

- pain away from the umbilicus;
- unexplained fever;
- weight loss, deceleration of linear growth (no longer following their line on growth chart);
- significant vomiting;
- blood in stool or urine;

Table 8.5 Types of functional abdominal pain

Diagnosis	Criteria
Irritable bowel syndrome (44.9%)	1. Abdominal discomfort or pain with two of three features: • Relieved with defecation • Onset associated with change in stool frequency • Onset associated with change in stool form/appearance 2. No structural or metabolic abnormalities to explain symptoms
Functional dyspepsia (15.9%)	1. Persistent or recurrent pain or discomfort centred in the upper abdomen 2. No evidence that organic disease is likely to explain symptoms 3. No evidence that dyspepsia is relieved by defecation or associated with change in stool frequency/form 4. May be characterised by abdominal fullness, bloating, nausea, early satiety
Functional abdominal pain syndrome (7.5%)	1. Continuous or nearly continuous abdominal pain in school-age children or adolescent 2. None or only occasional relation of pain to physiological events (e.g. eating). 3. Some loss of daily functioning 4. The pain is not malingering or feigned 5. Insufficient criteria for other functional GI disorders that would explain pain 6. No structural, inflammatory or metabolic abnormalities to explain symptoms
Abdominal migraine (4.7%)	1. Three or more episodes, in preceding 12 months, of midline abdominal pain lasting several hours to days, paroxysmal in nature 2. No evidence of metabolic, structural or central nervous system disease 3. Two of the following features: • headaches during episodes • photophobia during episodes • family history of migraines • headache confined to one side of head • sensory, visual or motor aura preceding episodes

Source: Jones and Walker (2006). With kind permission from Springer Science + Business Medi

- pain that awakens the child;
- jaundice;
- abdominal mass or organomegaly.
  (AAP Subcommittee and NASPGHAN Committee on Chronic Abdominal Pain 2005; Scholl and Allen 2007)

For children who do not have any of the above *red flags*, unnecessary testing not only increases healthcare costs (Dhroove et al. 2010), it rarely changes diagnosis or prognosis (Gieteling et al. 2008). Continued testing also increases the ongoing anxiety that 'something has been missed' or that there is a clearly identifiable cause. Mothers who received the message that abdominal pain was functional rather than organic using a biopsychosocial framework were more satisfied with the doctor's explanation and reported less anxiety than mothers who were provided with a biomedical explanation that ruled out disease and did not address multiple factors (Williams et al. 2009).

Musculoskeletal pain

Musculoskeletal pains are common in children. The most common musculoskeletal chronic pain conditions include complex regional pain syndrome (described under neuropathic pain), juvenile primary fibromyalgia, idiopathic chronic limb pain (growing pains) and back pain conditions (El-Metwally et al. 2005; Connelly and Schanberg 2006).

Chronic widespread pain is a term used to describe musculoskeletal pain in adults that is all over their body. However, in children and adolescents it is referred to as fibromyalgia syndrome (previously called juvenile fibromyalgia) (Zernikow et al. 2012b). It thought to affect between 1% and 15% of children and adolescents and is more common in females. Symptoms of fibromyalgia syndrome include musculoskeletal pain, tension headaches, sleep disturbances, fatigue and emotional distress. Parents of these children show increased anxiety and they often suffer from chronic pain themselves (Zernikow et al. 2012b). There also seems to be a high prevalence of anxiety disorders in children with fibromyalgia syndrome, and the presence of anxiety disorder is associated with poorer physician-rated physical functioning (Kashikar-Zuck et al. 2008a).

Idiopathic chronic limb pain in children is often referred to as *growing pains*. Growing pains typically present as recurrent bilateral non-articular pain in the lower extremities that occurs late in the day or at night. In severe cases, persistent pain can occur daily and have a significant impact on the child and family functioning (Pavone et al. 2011).

Chronic low back pain (LBP) was thought to be relatively uncommon in children. However, epidemiological evidence suggests that it is an important and increasing problem in school-age children and adolescents and has a marked impact on daily activities (Watson et al. 2002; Bejia et al. 2005). Psychosocial factors (Kopek and Sayre 2005; Diepenmaat et al. 2006), as well as physical activity and body positioning (e.g. guarding) during repeated activities (Bejia et al. 2005; Kopek and Sayre 2005; Diepenmaat et al. 2006; Jones and Macfarlane 2009) have been shown to increase the risk of LBP. Jones and Macfarlane (2009) found that predictors of pain persistence in children with LBP were peer relationship problems, being of smaller stature, prior report of widespread body pain, long duration of LBP episodes, and radiating leg pain. Of children with none of these factors at baseline, <5% went on to report persistent LBP. In contrast, of children with four or five factors, nearly 80% experienced persistent symptoms for up to 4 years.

Neuropathic pain

What is neuropathic pain?

Neuropathic pain is often described as burning, stabbing or shooting and may be spontaneous or *evoked* (i.e. having a trigger factor such as touch or change in temperature).

Neuropathic pain conditions may also be characterised by sensory disturbances such as *allodynia, dysaesthesia, hyperalgesia, hyperpathia* and *paraesthesia* (Box 8.1).

There may also be motor abnormalities such as tremor, spasms, atrophy, dystonia and weakness and autonomic disturbances such as cyanosis, erythema, mottling, increased sweating, swelling and poor capillary refill (Berde et al. 2003; Johnson 2004; Walco et al. 2010).

BOX 8.1

Terms associated with neuropathic pain

Allodynia: Severe pain triggered by innocuous (non-harmful) stimuli such as stroking, the touch of clothing on the affected area, or changes in temperature

Dysesthesia: An unpleasant abnormal sensation (e.g. shooting, tingling sensations), which may be spontaneous or evoked

Hyperalgesia: A reduced threshold to pain

Hyperpathia: Increased pain from stimuli that are normally painful (e.g. increased sharpness from a pin prick)

Paresthesia: An abnormal sensation (e.g. pins and needles), which may be spontaneous or evoked

---

Further information about the anatomy and physiology of neuropathic pain can be found in Chapter 2.

Examples of neuropathic pain in children include complex regional pain syndrome (CRPS) and phantom limb pain, which is pain that is felt in the area of a limb that has been amputated. Children with cancer also experience neuropathic pain, which may be due to the cancer treatment (e.g. chemotherapy or radiotherapy) or the underlying cancer itself (e.g. due to the tumour impinging on a spinal nerve root).

Common Types of Neuropathic Pain Conditions

Case study: Amanda

Amanda, aged 15 years, twisted her right ankle while dancing. She instantly felt pain but continued her lesson and over the next day noticed bruising and swelling. Her ankle was x-rayed and no fracture was found; however, as her ankle remained swollen and she complained of significant pain she was prescribed a support brace and the family purchased crutches to assist her with mobilisation.

Over the next few weeks, she was noted to have increased pain in her ankle, and stated 'my toes are blue'. She reported her foot and lower leg hurt to touch and she could not wear her shoes due to pain.

On examination her right foot appears blue compared to her left, with strong equal pulses bilaterally. Temperature differences are noted to touch between the limbs with the right leg feeling cooler that the left. Amanda describes her foot and lower leg as like 'feeling like it is on fire' and rates her pain severity at 8/10. She is afraid to go to school in case her foot gets bumped. Her mother is very concerned that 'something is very wrong'.

- What questions would you like to ask Amanda about her pain to help with diagnosis and treatment?
- What additional assessments would you make to help with diagnosis and treatment of Amanda's pain?
- What pharmacological, physical and psychological therapies might help Amanda?

Complex regional pain syndrome

What is complex regional pain syndrome?

Complex regional pain syndrome (CRPS) is a multifactorial syndrome of neuropathic pain. Both central and peripheral mechanisms are involved, including sensitisation of both the central and peripheral nervous systems, inflammation, and altered somatosensory representation in the brain. It is thought to possibly have a genetic factor (Bruehl 2010).

CRPS is further classified into two types: type 1 manifests following injury without a definable nerve lesion and type 2 occurs following damage to an identifiable nerve. CRPS type 2 is rarely seen in children. The clinical criteria for CRPS are outlined in Box 8.2.

CRPS in children differs from the presentation in adults in the following ways:

- It most commonly affects lower limbs, and skin temperature changes are often evident in that the limb is cooler.
- Sympathetic and neurological symptoms are less obvious.
- Children with CRPS have a better prognosis than adults.
- Most children will have complete resolution of symptoms with non-invasive treatment; a small proportion (20%) will continue to have pain or relapse.
- Early recognition and treatment are associated with the best chance of good outcomes.

(Berde et al. 2003; Low et al. 2007; Tan et al. 2008)

BOX 8.2

Clinical diagnostic criteria for CRPS

CRPS is a clinical diagnosis based on the following:

1. Continuing pain disproportionate to the inciting event
2. Must report at least one symptom in *three of the four* following categories:
   (a) Sensory: hyperesthesia or allodynia
   (b) Vasomotor: temperature asymmetry, and/or skin colour changes, and/or skin colour asymmetry
   (c) Sudomotor/oedema; oedema and/or sweating changes and/or sweating asymmetry
   (d) Motor/trophic; decreased range of motion and/or motor dysfunction (such as weakness, tremor) and/or changes to hair, skin or nails
3. Must display at least one sign *at the time of evaluation* in *two or more* of the following categories:
   (a) Sensory: evidence of hyperalgesia (to pin prick) and/or allodynia (to light touch and/or temperature sensation and/or deep somatic pressure and/or joint movement
   (b) Vasomotor: evidence of temperature asymmetry (>1°C) and/or skin colour changes and/or asymmetry
   (c) Sudomotor/Oedema evidence of oedema and/or sweating changes and/or sweating asymmetry
   (d) Motor/trophic: evidence of decreased range of motion and/or motor dysfunction (weakness, tremor) and/or trophic changes (hair, skin, nails)
4. There is no other diagnosis that better explains the signs and symptoms.

Source: Harden et al. (2007)

Phantom limb pain

Congenital or traumatic (accidental or surgical) loss of a limb can result in sensations in the missing limb. These sensations can be classified as sensations which are non-painful, called phantom limb sensation (PLS, described as tingling or itchy or the limb needing to be repositioned), and phantom limb pain (PLP; described as burning, cramping, shooting). In addition, there can be pain in the stump (*stump pain*). These sensations tend to begin within days of the amputation and usually decrease in frequency and duration over time. In a retrospective chart audit, Burgoyne et al. (2012) found that PLP after cancer-related amputation in children and young adults seems to be common (76%) but generally short-lived in most patients (with only 10% having PLP one year post-amputation). Clerici and colleagues (2012) found mirror therapy helped reduce PLP in children with amputations due to cancer treatment.

Pain Associated with Sickle Cell Disease

Sickle cell disease (SCD) is a genetic condition, characterised by abnormal haemo-globin molecules that distort the red blood cells into a crescent or sickle shape. People with SCD often experience acute severe pain crises caused by the sickled cells obstruct-ing small blood vessels thus disrupting oxygenation to tissues (Vijenthira et al. 2012). People with SCD are at risk of developing chronic pain due to tissue and end-organ damage and under-treatment of acute pain episodes (Ballas 2007; Taylor et al. 2010). Tissue damage may include musculoskeletal conditions such as avascular necrosis of humeral or femoral head, chronic arthritis or vertebral collapse, or it may be idio-pathic (pain for unknown reasons) (Johnson 2005). A thorough pain assessment is required to determine if the pain is neuropathic in nature, or musculoskeletal, as pharmacological treatment approaches may differ.

Optimal management of pain in the home and emergency department settings (or day treatment hospitals) can prevent admissions to hospital. Pain in SCD is often poorly managed, as evidenced by sub-therapeutic opioid dosage and moderate to high pain scores during hospitalisation (Vijenthira et al. 2012). Acute pain crises, which usually require hospitalisation, should be managed with a combination of opioids, NSAIDs and paracetamol (acetaminophen) (Dunlop and Bennett 2006). It is impor-tant for clinicians to be aware that children with SCD often have genetically increased clearance rates of morphine and may require higher doses as well as more frequent administration (Darbari et al. 2011). Many children with SCD use physical and psy-chological methods of pain-relief. In a study of 63 children with SCD, more than 70% were using some form of physical and psychological therapies including complemen-tary and alternative therapy (Yoon and Black 2006). Most commonly used therapies were prayer and spiritual healing, as well as physical (massage) and psychological (relaxation) therapies (Yoon and Black 2006).

In a study of parents (*n* = 53) of children with SCD, those children who had less adaptive coping strategies showed an increased use of the emergency department and increased hospital admissions (Mitchell et al. 2007). Referral to a multidisciplinary pain clinic to learn coping strategies and other pain management techniques decreased the number of hospitalisations for pain management in a group (*n* = 19) of children with sickle cell disease (Brandow et al. 2011). Thus, teaching children and their fami-lies active coping strategies and other physical and psychological pain management techniques may reduce hospitalisation and help families to manage pain crises at home (Mitchell et al. 2007). The National Institute for Health and Care Excellence in the England has recently published guidelines on the management of acute pain in SCD (see http://guidance.nice.org.uk/CG143).

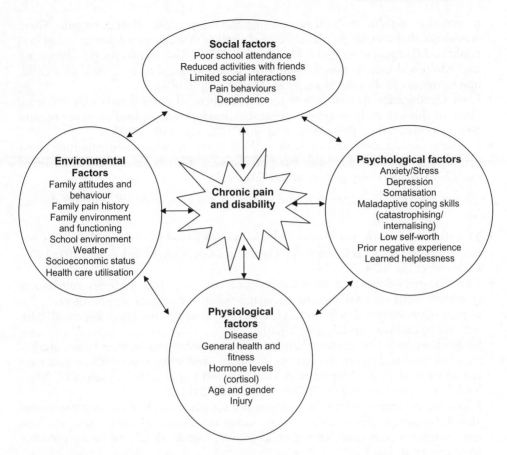

Figure 8.1 Factors associated with children's chronic pain.
Source: McGrath (2006). With kind permission from Springer Science + Business Media.

Factors Triggering and Maintaining Chronic Pain

As outlined in Chapter 3, many factors influence a child's perception of pain and ways in which they behave when in pain. Many studies have provided evidence (primarily using cross-sectional studies) that a few isolated biological, physical, psychological, family and social factors play an important role in chronic pain in children (Figure 8.1). However, little is known about which factors or combination of factors predispose children to chronic pain and disability. Research has shown that:

- Certain situational factors (Figure 8.1) can intensify pain and distress, while others can trigger pain episodes and prolong pain-related disability or maintain the cycle of repeated pain episodes in recurrent pain syndromes (McGrath 2006).
- Age, gender and psychosocial factors are now recognised as important aspects in the development of persistent pain and pain-related disability (McGrath 2006). For example, in a recent population-based Canadian study, being female and having high levels of depressive and anxiety symptoms at age 10 years were highly predictive of the likelihood to develop and maintain pain across adolescence (Stanford et al. 2008).
- Miró et al. (2007) conducted a Delphi study to establish consensus on the factors that predict chronic pain in children. Excessive use of healthcare services, a tendency

to somatise, and children's catastrophising had the greatest influence on pain. There is evidence that chronic pain in childhood persists throughout adolescence and into adulthood (Perquin et al. 2003; Mallen et al. 2006). Risk factors for pain persisting into adulthood include family history of pain, admission to a hospital as a child, and having more illnesses than peers (Mallen et al. 2006).

- Early identification of risk factors for development of chronic pain may influence outcome through early treatment to prevent development and maintenance of pain and pain-related disability (Miró et al. 2007; Walker et al. 2012).
- In a large population-based study ($n = 2230$) maternal anxiety and parenting stress identified in 10- to 12-year-olds were predictive of the presence of chronic pain at age 12–15 years (Darlington et al. 2012).

Coping styles of the child, parents and family have a significant influence on chronic pain:

- Maladaptive or ineffective coping styles have been linked to anxiety, depression and functional disability in children with chronic pain (Kashikar-Zuck et al. 2001, 2002; Eccleston et al. 2004).
- Pain catastrophising is a multidimensional construct that includes rumination (excessive focus on pain sensations), magnification (exaggerating the threat value of pain sensations) and helplessness (perceiving oneself as unable to cope with pain symptoms) (Sullivan and Adams 2006).
- Studies have found associations between catastrophising and increased pain, disability, depression and emotional distress in children and adolescents with chronic pain (Crombez et al. 2003; Merlijn et al. 2006; Vervoort et al. 2006; Lynch et al. 2007; Kashikar-Zuck et al. 2008a, 2008b; Guite et al. 2011).
- Following experimentally induced visceral discomfort in children with functional abdominal pain, higher levels of parents' symptom-related talk were associated with more symptom complaints among children with high levels of pain catastrophising (Williams et al. 2011).

Practice point

Education of both the child and family is essential to reduce fear and misconceptions related to chronic pain and to teach appropriate coping strategies (relaxation and cognitive restructuring).

As outlined in Chapter 3, *gender differences* are apparent in relation to chronic pain in older school-age children and adolescents. Chronic pain is more common in girls, who also report more intense, frequent and prolonged pain than boys (Martin et al. 2007; Stanford et al. 2008; King et al. 2011). Differences in coping styles also exist, with girls using more emotional coping styles such as catastrophising (Keogh and Eccleston 2006; Lynch et al. 2007). Differences in self-reported trigger factors are also present between boys and girls (Roth-Isigkeit et al. 2005).

Due to lack of knowledge of the psychosocial aspects and complexity of chronic pain, children with unexplained or persistent chronic pain are sometimes viewed as malingerers or attention seekers, or made to feel that the problem is *all in their head*.

This can further exacerbate the pain and increases the family's distrust of health professionals and leads them to doubt healthcare professionals' ability to diagnose and treat the pain.

> **Practice point**
>
> Once serious or treatable physical causes are ruled out, most children and parents need and are willing to accept an explanation based on both physical (sensitisation of pain receptors) and psychological (stress or worry) factors. This helps prevent or reduce the continued search for a cause for the pain (von Baeyer 2006).

Pain-Related Disability

The term *pain-related disability* is used to describe chronic pain in patients who regardless of the location or cause of their pain are unable to function effectively (e.g. they experience severe impairments in physical, social and role functioning). Many children and adolescents experience persistent or recurrent pain; however, only a small proportion become disabled by it (Gauntlett-Gilbert and Eccleston 2007). Outlined below are some key factors in the prevalence, development and maintenance of pain-related disability:

- Scharff et al. (2005) used a statistical technique to identify three levels of disability in children and adolescents ($n = 117$) with chronic pain. Thirty percent of the sample were classified as highly distressed (high anxiety, depression and escape/avoidance) and disabled, 18% were in the moderately distressed/disabled group, and 52% of the sample were comparatively well-functioning and not distressed.
- Miró et al. (2007) explored predictors of pain-related disability in children. Factors that had the greatest influence on long-term disability were children's self-concept as being disabled, a hesitance to perform exercise because of fear of potential injury, and children's catastrophising.
- Higher levels of functional disability have been found to be associated with greater pain intensity and depression (Gauntlett-Gilbert and Eccleston 2007).
- Zernikow and colleagues (2012a) conducted a retrospective review of children ($n = 2249$) assessed in their interdisciplinary chronic pain clinic to determine the level of disability. Fifty-five percent of children had more than one distinct pain diagnosis. They found clinically significant levels of depression and general anxiety. Those with extremely high pain-related disability were older in age, had multiple pain locations, increased depression and prior hospitalisations, and were at risk for developmental stagnation (e.g. not becoming independent from parents).
- Perceptions of self-worth seem to be important in reducing the relationship between pain and functional disability in children with chronic pain (Guite et al. 2009).

The Impact of Chronic Pain on the Child and Family

Chronic pain negatively impacts many aspects of the child's life and results in frequent use of healthcare services (Sleed et al. 2005; Ho et al. 2008). Recent studies demonstrate that chronic pain can severely affect the lives of children:

- Petersen et al. (2009) explored the impact of recurrent pain on health-related quality of life in school-age children ($n = 1455$) in Sweden. They found that all domains of health-related quality of life were impaired twice as much in children with recurrent pain compared to children without recurrent pain.

- Co-occurring chronic pain and obesity exacerbates the impact of chronic pain on the health-related quality of life of children and adolescents (Hainsworth et al. 2009).
- Meldrum et al. (2009) interviewed children and adolescents living with chronic pain ($n = 53$) and identified five common themes – isolation, altered self-perception, activity limitations, concerns and barriers about the future, and the lack of medical validation.
- Depression, emotional distress and anxiety are common in children with chronic pain (Konijnenberg et al. 2005).
- Psychiatric disorders are common in children with chronic pain. Knook et al. (2012) examined the 6-year clinical outcomes of children and adolescents ($n = 91$) referred to a chronic pain outpatient clinic. They found that comorbid psychiatric disorder at study entry was a predictor of psychiatric disorder, but not of persistent chronic pain in adolescents and young adulthood.
- Adolescents with chronic pain may avoid social situations when they perceive that their friends may not support them (Forgeron et al. 2011).
- Adolescents with chronic pain self-report being less socially developed than their peers (Eccleston et al. 2008).
- Simons et al. (2010a) explored how social functioning related to school impairment in a sample of 126 adolescents with chronic pain being followed at a multidisciplinary pain clinic. They found that lower social functioning was significantly associated with pain, physical limitations, somatic symptoms and school impairment. Social functioning was found to mediate the relationship between the teens' pain experience and school impairment.
- Children with chronic pain often have long periods of absence from school and their social and emotional functioning is affected. This can impact their long-term development and future role within society (Eccleston 2005).
- Chronic pain affects cognitive function but more research is required to determine long-term effects on the developmental trajectory (Dick and Pillai Riddell 2010).
- Chronic pain in adolescents has been found to be a risk factor for suicidal ideation, and in youths with comorbid depression this risk is increased (van Tilburg et al. 2011).

The parent–child relationship has a major influence on the child's response to pain. Chronic pain often occurs in early adolescents a stressful period for any parent–child relationship, and parents of children with chronic pain report high levels of parenting stress (Eccleston et al. 2004). Research has shown that the parent–child relationship affects the child's perception of and ability to cope with pain (Reid et al. 2005; Logan et al. 2006). Chronic pain is also more common in children who have a parent with a chronic pain condition (Evans et al. 2006; Evans and Keenan 2007; Saunders et al. 2007). Furthermore, children of mothers with chronic pain have been found to have more physical and psychological problems compared to having a father with a pain problem or parents without persistent pain (Evans and Keenan 2007). Figure 8.2 outlines a conceptual model of the psychosocial mechanisms linking child and parent pain.

Some key parental factors that influence the child's response to pain include:

- Parental protective responses to the adolescent's pain may promote increased disability and symptom complaints (Simons et al. 2008; Guite et al. 2011).
- Children whose parents catastrophise about their pain, and who exhibit protective responses, miss more school days and report more overall school impairment (Logan et al. 2011).

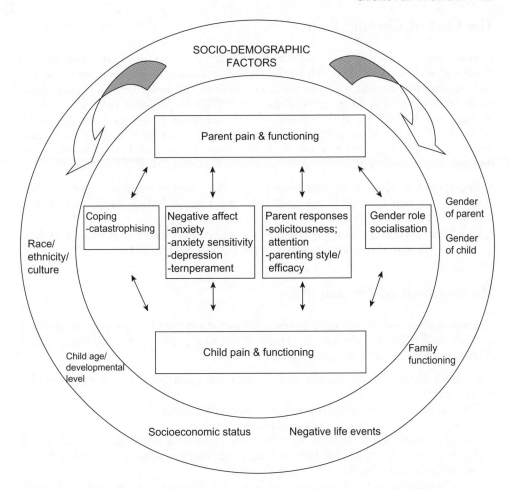

Figure 8.2   Conceptual model of psychosocial mechanisms linking parent and child pain.
Source: Evans et al. 2008

- Parental perceptions of child vulnerability are related to poor child functioning and more child pain-related healthcare utilisation regardless of the child's age, gender and duration of persistent pain (Connelly et al. 2012).
- Parents who worry, and who believe that their child's pain is 'medical only', use more pain-promoting behaviours, and their adolescents demonstrate more physical disability (Guite et al. 2009).
- Parents describe needing to continuously 'be on call' when caring for a child experiencing chronic pain, which leads to pain dominating the lives of not only the child, but also the parents (Maciver et al. 2010).
- Lewandowski et al. (2010) conducted a systematic review of family functioning in children with chronic pain. They found that families of children with chronic pain generally have poorer family functioning than healthy populations, and that pain-related disability is more consistently related to family functioning than pain intensity.

The Cost of Chronic Pain

Chronic pain in adults is costly (direct and indirect costs) to society in terms of both treatment and lost workdays. However, there has been little research regarding the cost of children's chronic pain. In the 3 months prior to being seen in a pain clinic, mean medical costs in American dollars were $8781.46; children spent 28 hours in medical appointments; and their family members missed 4 days of work (Ho et al. 2008). Parents of children with chronic pain often have to take time off work to care for their child, which also has an effect on the workforce and the economy. Other research has shown that:

- The cost of adolescent chronic pain in the UK has been estimated to be £3,840 million per year or £8,000 per adolescent per year, including direct and indirect costs (Sleed et al. 2005).
- Children with chronic pain have higher rates of healthcare consultation and medication use compared to a community sample (Wilson et al. 2011).

Management of Chronic Pain

The management of chronic pain involves the use of a range of psychological, physical and pharmacological interventions (Table 8.6). Key points in the management of chronic pain in children are outlined below.

- Many children and adolescents with chronic pain can be managed effectively by their family doctor.
- Referral to a multidisciplinary paediatric pain programme should be considered for children with complex or ongoing chronic pain.
- The main goal of treatment is to return the child to a functional state that will enable them to participate in daily activities and return to school, rather than focusing solely on reducing or controlling the pain.
- A multidisciplinary, multimodal approach that incorporates the 3 Ps (physical, psychological and pharmacological interventions) is likely to be most effective.

Table 8.6 An overview of interventions for chronic pain management in children

Pharmacological interventions	Physical interventions	Psychological interventions
• Simple analgesics • Opioid analgesics • Anticonvulsants • Antidepressants • Antiarrhythmics (alpha-adrenergic blockers) • Anxiolytics • Nerve blocks	• Exercise • Thermal stimulation (heat, cold, desensitisation) • Physiotherapy • Occupational therapy • Massage • TENS • Acupuncture	• Education (about pain diagnosis and coping) • Sleep hygiene • Relaxation • Biofeedback • Behavioural therapies • Cognitive therapies • Cognitive behavioural therapy (CBT) • Acceptance and commitment therapy (ACT) • Mindfulness therapy • Family therapy • Psychotherapy

- Decisions regarding the most appropriate treatments should be individualised and based on the assessment of the child.
- Interventions should be aimed at treating any trigger factors, as well as the underlying cause(s) of the pain wherever possible.
- Treatment should also address pain-related disability with the goal of maximising functioning and improving quality of life. This approach includes specific treatment targeting possible underlying pain mechanisms, as well as symptom-focused management addressing pain, sleep disturbance, anxiety or depressive feelings.
- Treatment must also address education and support of the parents' reactions to their child's pain and how they can best support their child (Palermo and Eccleston 2009).
- Parents of children seen in a paediatric pain clinic want information about the causes of their child's pain, information on the various treatment options, as well as effective strategies to help their child cope with the pain. In addition it is very important to them to have a pain team 'be there' for them (Reid et al. 2010).

The general goals of treatment are outlined in Box 8.3.

Practice point

Controlling pain is not merely *drug versus physical and/or psychological strategies* but rather an integrated approach to reduce or block nociceptive activity by attenuating responses in the peripheral afferents and central pathways, activating endogenous pain inhibitory systems and modifying situational factors that exacerbate pain (McGrath 2006).

Physical and psychological methods of pain relief

Using physical and psychological strategies in combination with pharmacological strategies optimises pain relief and improves functional outcomes. Physical and psychological methods of pain relief are discussed in Chapter 5 and are briefly outlined below.

Physical pain-relieving interventions

Chronic pain often leads children to avoid physical activities due to fear of re-injury or because it exacerbates the pain (fear of movement is called kinesiophobia). Lack

---

BOX 8.3

General treatment goals

1. Increasing independent function in terms of activities of daily living, school, social and physical activities
2. Facilitating adaptive problem-solving, communication and coping skills
3. Reducing specific symptoms, deficits, or problems revealed in a comprehensive biopsychosocial assessment (e.g. anxiety, depression, poor sleep)
4. Helping children and their families to understand the nature of pain, the pain condition, and its treatment from a holistic perspective

Source: Stinson (2006)

of muscle use leads to loss of muscle strength, flexibility and endurance and overall deconditioning. Physiotherapy (physical therapy) is, therefore, an integral component (Table 8.6), and in certain instances (e.g. with CRPS) it is the cornerstone of treatment for children with chronic pain (Engel and O'Rourke 2006).

Physiotherapy is usually administered on an outpatient basis with the ultimate goal of teaching the child to continue the programme at home. Regular exercise (e.g. 20 minutes three times per week) can also help improve sleep, mood, self-esteem and energy levels (McCarthy et al. 2003; Engel and O'Rourke 2006; Stinson 2006). Exercise programmes should be individually designed and tailored to the needs of the patient. However, for any benefit to be realised, a minimum of two sessions per week on non-consecutive days with a minimum duration of 20 minutes (broken up into two 10-minute sessions over the day for deconditioned patients) should be carried out (Wittink and Takken 2008).

Research has shown that:

- Adolescents with irritable bowel syndrome (n = 25) who participated in yoga reported less functional disability, and wanted to continue practising yoga (Kuttner et al. 2006).
- Iyengar yoga, which uses props for support and tailors poses to medical conditions, shows promise in current clinical trials (Evans et al. 2012).
- Fear avoidance beliefs were found to be related to greater activity limitations, above pain intensity and depressive symptoms, and were a mediator between parental protectiveness and activity limitations (Wilson et al. 2011). Therefore, fear avoidance beliefs are important to assess in order to target physical interventions to decrease activity limitations (Hestbaek and Stochkendahl 2010).

Physiotherapists (physical therapists) and occupational therapists are primarily, although not exclusively, involved in rehabilitation programmes for children with chronic musculoskeletal pain.
Physiotherapists apply a wide range of physical and behavioural interventions to reduce pain, to prevent impairment and disability as well as to promote function.
Occupational therapists are primarily concerned with the psychosocial and environmental factors that contribute to pain and have an impact on the individual's daily activities and participation (Engel and O'Rouke 2006).
Despite the recognised importance of physiotherapy in treating children with chronic pain, little research has been conducted to document treatment effects or evaluate different therapeutic techniques (Campos et al. 2011).

Psychological therapies

Many psychological therapies are used to manage chronic pain in children (Table 8.6). Often these therapies are integrated into a comprehensive cognitive behavioural therapy (CBT) programme that is directed at identifying and eliminating or reducing triggering factors that affect the child's pain and disability. Such programmes usually include:

- education about the pain;
- learning cognitive behavioural pain coping skills (e.g. imagery, distraction and relaxation);

- stress management (e.g. identifying and coping with stressful situations, using thought stopping, cognitive restructuring, assertiveness and problem-solving);
- relapse prevention.

(Hermann 2006)

A systematic review documented the efficacy of CBT for chronic headache and abdominal pain in children (Palermo et al. 2010). CBT has been found to be effective in treating juvenile fibromyalgia (Kashikar-Zuck et al. 2012) as well as abdominal pain (Levy et al. 2010). CBT is also useful in reducing the emotional component of pain in children with sickle cell disease (Anie and Green 2012).

There is strong evidence that CBT can be self-administered without a psychologist or nurse being physically present, using the Internet (Stinson et al. 2009; Palermo et al. 2010) or computer disks (CD-ROMs) (Connelly et al. 2006). A recent systematic review of computer-based psychological pain treatment programmes for children and adolescents with chronic pain (including four randomised controlled trials) found that self-administered treatments delivered over the Internet reduce pain intensity (Velleman et al. 2010). Biofeedback has also been found to be effective for the treatment of headaches in children (Hermann and Blanchard 2002). (CBT and biofeedback are discussed in more detail in Chapter 5.)

More recently, acceptance and commitment therapy (ACT) is being adopted as a treatment approach in chronic pain programmes (Wicksell et al. 2011). This emphasises the acceptance of or willingness to experience pain and other interfering experiences (fear of pain with activities) rather than trying to control or reduce symptoms. The goal is to achieve functionality even in the presence of interfering pain and distress. There is early evidence of the effectiveness of this approach in children with chronic pain (Wicksell et al. 2005 2007, 2011; Masuad et al. 2011).

Sleep hygiene

Sleep disturbances are common in children with chronic pain (Palermo and Kiska 2005). Adolescents with chronic pain report poorer sleep quality and increased insomnia and demonstrated more night-time wakenings as compared to healthy adolescents (Palermo et al. 2007). Pain can interfere with the quality and quantity of sleep, and insufficient sleep can cause daytime sequelae (behavioural and emotional changes) that undermine the coping skills necessary for effective pain management. Efforts should, therefore, be directed towards improving the sleep hygiene (good sleep habits) of children with chronic pain.

> For specific strategies to improve sleep hygiene, see the National Sleep Foundation at www.sleepfoundation.org.

Complementary and alternative medicine

Complementary and alternative medicine (CAM) has been defined as those interventions not generally provided by hospitals and clinics, nor widely taught in medical schools (Tsao and Zelter 2005). There are few high-quality empirical investigations that permit definitive conclusions to be drawn regarding the efficacy of CAM interventions for paediatric pain. For example, spinal pain is the most common reason that children and adolescents see chiropractors; however, there is no evidence that these therapies are effective (Hestbaek and Stochkendahl 2010).

For more information on CAM in chronic pain see the Centre for Complementary and Alternative Medicine at the National Institutes of Health (NIH) at http://nccam.nih.gov/health/pain/chronic .htm.

Pharmacological interventions

Pharmacological interventions are of benefit for some types of chronic pain; although research involving children is lacking. Few of the medications prescribed are licensed for use in children (Grégoire and Finley 2007) with the clinical indications and use extrapolated from research and clinical practice in adults with chronic pain. There is limited research supporting their use in children (World Health Organization 2012). This is discussed further in Chapter 4.

Invasive therapies

Non-invasive therapies are the mainstay of treatment of paediatric chronic pain conditions. A recent systematic review found no evidence that regional anaesthesia is effective compared to placebo for managing CRPS (Perez et al. 2010). Spinal cord stimulation has also been reported to be effective in a case series of seven female adolescents with severe, incapacitating and therapy-resistant CRPS type I (Olsson et al. 2008). However, more research is needed to determine their effectiveness using rigorous trials and determining which children would benefit most from these invasive therapies, given their risks.

Multidisciplinary approach

The key to the success of chronic pain management in children is adopting a multidisciplinary, multimodal rehabilitation approach (Kashikar-Zuck 2006). Because of the complexity of chronic pain, no single discipline has the expertise to assess and manage it independently. While not all children require a multidisciplinary approach, the services provided by multidisciplinary pain treatment programmes (chronic pain clinics) are considered the optimal therapeutic model for the management of chronic pain in children (Peng et al. 2007).

Chronic pain clinics

Specialised interdisciplinary chronic pain teams are now the standard of care for children with complex chronic pain conditions (Stinson 2006). Chronic pain teams for children generally include specialist physicians (e.g. anaesthetists, neurologists and psychiatrists), nurses and allied health professionals (e.g. psychologists, occupational therapists and physiotherapists) (Peng et al. 2007). More recently, teams may also include complementary and alternative therapists (e.g. acupuncturists and/or massage therapists). The specific team members involved are selected depending on the needs of the child and family (Stinson 2006).

A child's initial consultation includes either a joint interview and physical examination or separate interviews with each healthcare professional. Comprehensive physical and psychosocial assessments may typically last a few hours to a full day, depending on the child's previous diagnostic tests and the team's set of core assessment measures (e.g. standardised sensory testing, questionnaires). The team then meets to formulate the child's diagnosis and treatment plan and then discusses recommendations with the patient and their family (Figure 8.3).

1. *Evaluate child with chronic pain*

- Complete medical and pain history
- Assess pain location, onset, duration, quality, variability, exacerbating and alleviating factors
- Assess associated disability including impact of pain daily life such as sleep, school, eating, social and physical activities
- Physical and neurological exam including appearance, posture, gait, growth parameters and vital signs
- Complete appropriate diagnostic tests

2. *Diagnose the primary and secondary causes*

- Current nociceptive and neuropathic components
- Attenuating physical symptoms
- Contributing psychological factors, social factors and biological processes

3. *Select appropriate therapies to improve overall functioning and quality of life*

Pharmacological	Physical	Psychological
• Analgesics • Adjunct analgesics • Anaesthetics	• Graded exercise program • Regular daily activity (e.g., walking, swimming, stretching) • Pacing	• Relaxation strategies • CBT • School reintegration • Sleep hygiene • Teach parents adaptive responses to child's pain

4. *Implement pain management plan*

- Provide pain diagnosis, feedback on causes and contributing factors
- Provide rationale for integrated treatment program
- Develop mutually agreed upon treatment goals
- Measure child's pain and functional improvement regularly
- Evaluate effectiveness of treatment plan
- Revise plan as necessary

Figure 8.3   Treatment algorithm for children with chronic pain. Adapted from Brown (2006); APS (2012).

The treatment plan should include:

- diagnosis (underlying causes and contributing factors);
- rationale for rehabilitation approach with a clear description of the specific treatment options;
- opportunity for the family to help fine-tune the plan.

(Stinson 2006)

There are only a few chronic pain services for children internationally (Peng et al. 2007). A survey by Peng et al. (2007) found only five multidisciplinary chronic pain programmes in Canada and all were located in large urban centres. Children's chronic pain services typically offer outpatient programmes; however, some centres offer inpatient, day or residential treatment programmes (Berde and Solodiuk 2003; Eccleston et al. 2003; Logan and Simons 2010). Logan and Simons (2010) investigated the willingness to self-manage pain among children and parents (*n* = 157 children aged 10–18 years) undergoing an intensive interdisciplinary rehabilitation treatment programme and to determine whether increased willingness to self-manage pain influenced functional treatment outcomes. They found that the rehabilitation programme increased willingness to self-manage pain, which is associated with improvements in function and psychological wellbeing.

Ongoing assessment and re-evaluation of the treatment plan is essential. One way to monitor children with chronic pain is through the use of electronic pain diaries. Diaries can be used to obtain a better understanding of the impact of pain on their daily lives and activities as well as the pain intensity (Stinson et al. 2007). Diaries can also be a useful way to help children and adolescents keep track of improvements in their physical, social and psychological functioning. (Pain assessment is discussed in detail in Chapter 6.)

Practice point

Nurses play a key role in educating children and their families about the nature of chronic pain (different from acute pain where there is a single cause and treatment) and the factors that intensify it, as well as pharmacological and non-drug strategies used to control the pain.

Long-term outcomes

Little research has been conducted on long-term outcomes of children treated for chronic pain conditions. Only a small proportion of children who require an interdisciplinary chronic pain clinic can access one due to the paucity of programmes, and they may wait up to 8 months to be seen (Peng et al. 2007).

More research is required to understand longer-term outcomes in children with chronic pain, especially into adulthood. Outcomes have been explored in three studies:

- De Blecourt et al. (2008) reported on the outcomes of children (*n* = 70) who were admitted to an inpatient programme for a period of 3 months. They found a significant improvement in motor skills, school attendance and understanding of chronic pain, reduced pain scores and less medication use. These results were maintained for 3 months following discharge from the programme.

- Kozlowska and colleagues (2008) reported on the outcomes of 28 children with somatoform pain disorders being treated by an integrated pain team. At discharge, 82% of patients reported significant reduction in pain intensity and 71% had returned to school full-time.
- Simons et al. (2010b) examined the adherence to treatment recommendations from a multidisciplinary children's chronic pain programme. Seventy parents and 57 children participated in 3-month follow-up interviews and reported significantly fewer doctor visits, decreased somatic symptoms, fewer functional limitations and decreased pain compared to their initial evaluation. However, adherence rates to treatment recommendations ranged from 47 to 100%, with highest adherence to physical therapy and lowest for a new psychological treatment

Summary

- Chronic pain in children is the result of a dynamic integration of biological processes, psychological factors, and socio-cultural context, considered within a developmental trajectory.
- Chronic pain can occur as a result of a chronic medical condition, may develop following surgery, illness or injury, or may have no obvious cause.
- Persistent and recurrent pains in childhood are common.
- Chronic pain can negatively impact all aspects of life and lead to pain-related disability.
- Children's chronic pain can impact family functioning and result in significant economic costs.
- Those children at risk of pain-related disability should be referred to a multidisciplinary, multimodal rehabilitative programme.
- Most chronic pain conditions can be treated using a combination of pharmacological, physical and psychological therapies.

Additional information

Great Ormond Street Hospital: *Helping children with musculoskeletal chronic pain conditions.* Available at: www.ich.ucl.ac.uk/factsheets/families/F050225/index.html

National Children's Pain Centre at: www.pediatricpain.org/home.php

National Sleep Foundation at: www.sleepfoundation.org

SickKids Pain Resource Centre at www.aboutkidshealth.ca/en/resourcecentres/Pain/Pages/default.aspx

Assessment and Management of Children with Chronic Pain: A Position Statement from the American Pain Society available at: www.aboutkidshealth.ca/en/resourcecentres/Pain/Pages/default.aspx

YouTube video on webinar, called *Kids get chronic pain too: Assessment and Management of Paediatric Chronic Pain,* at: www.youtube.com/watch?v=H4NbgG77E-w

Key to Case Studies

See Box 8.4 and Box 8.5.

BOX 8.4

Suzie

A thorough assessment of Suzie's pain involves assessing: pain location, onset, duration, quality, variability, exacerbating and alleviating factors.

It is important to look for 'red flags' such as pain away from the umbilicus, fever, weight loss, significant emesis, blood in stool, jaundice or organomegaly.

In addition to pain, assess associated functional disability including impact of pain on daily life (e.g. sleep, school, diet, social and physical activities).

There is little evidence that medications provide benefit for chronic abdominal pain, although case reports have demonstrated that low dose tricyclic antidepressants may assist with sleep.

Suzie should be encouraged to increase her activity in a gentle paced manner, and to be active daily. Helpful activities include yoga, walking or swimming.

Suzie and her family would benefit from an explanation of the biopsychosocial nature of her pain.

Suzie should be taught relaxation strategies such as deep breathing, guided imagery and mindfulness. It is important that she return to school and she may need help establishing a back to school plan.

Suzie's parents would benefit from learning adaptive coping strategies to help Suzie, such as focusing on her functional goals, using distraction and encouraging her to use breathing techniques, mindfulness and imagery.

BOX 8.5

Amanda

Questions to ask Amanda about her pain include: pain location, onset, duration, quality, variability, exacerbating and alleviating factors. It is important to ask specific questions about any previous injury to her leg, even mild such as a fall.

In addition to her pain, assess Amanda's associated disability including impact of pain on her daily life (e.g. sleep, school, diet, social and physical activities).

Explaining the clinical diagnosis and the reasons for the treatment plan is important in order for Amanda to participate in treatment.

Amanda may benefit from:

- an anticonvulsant at bedtime, starting at low dose to prevent over sedation. Medication may then be titrated up if required;
- a referral to a physiotherapist experienced in managing CRPS. Exercises should aim to restore function of the leg as well as desensitise the leg to reduce allodynia and hyperalgesia. This can be done by having Amanda start to gently touch her own leg with different textures as tolerated;
- being taught to use distraction therapies and relaxation exercises, especially during physiotherapy sessions.

References

AAP (American Academy of Pediatrics) Subcommittee and NASPGHAN (North American Society for Pediatric Gastroenterology, Hepatology, and Nutrition) Committee on Chronic Abdominal Pain (2005) Chronic abdominal pain in children. *Pediatrics* **115**(3), e370–e381.

American Academy of Pediatrics (2005) Chronic abdominal pain in children. *Pediatrics* **115**, 812–815.

American Pain Society (2012) *Assessment and Management of Children with Chronic Pain: A Position Statement from the American Pain Society.* Available from: www.ampainsoc.org/advocacy/downloads/aps12-pcp.pdf (accessed September 2012).

American Psychiatric Association (2000) *Diagnostic and statistical manual of mental disorders, 4th ed, text revision* [Online]. Available from: www.behavenet.com/capsules/disorders/dsm4tr.htm (accessed September 2012).

Anie, K.A. and Green, J. (2012) Psychological therapies for sickle cell disease and pain. *Cochrane Database of Systematic Reviews* issue 2, CD001916.

Ballas, S. (2007) Current issues in sickle cell pain and management. *Hematology* 2007(1), 97–105.

Bejia, I., Abid, N., Ben Salem, K. et al. (2005) Low back pain in a cohort of 622 Tunisian school children and adolescents: An epidemiological study. *European Spine Journal* 14, 331–336.

Berde, C.B., Lebel, A.A. and Olsson, G. (2003) Neuropathic pain in children. In: *Pain in Infants, Children and Adolescents* (eds N.L. Schechter, C.B. Berde and M. Yaster), 2nd edition, pp. 620–641. Lippincott, Williams & Wilkins, Baltimore, MD.

Berde, C.B., and Solodiuk, J. (2003) Multidisciplinary programs for management of acute and chronic pain in children. In: *Pain in Infants, Children and Adolescents* (eds N.L. Schechter, C.B. Berde and M. Yaster), pp. 471–486. Lippincott Williams & Wilkins, Baltimore, MD.

Brandow, A., Weisman, S., and Panepinto, J. (2011) The impact of a multidisciplinary pain management model on sickle cell disease pain hospitalizations. *Pediatric Blood and Cancer* 56, 789–793.

Breau, L., McGrath, P. and Zabalia, M. (2006) Assessing pediatric pain and developmental disabilities. In: *Pain in Children and Adults with Developmental Disabilities* (eds T. Oberlander and F. Symons). Paul H. Brookes Publishing, Baltimore, MD.

Brown, S.C. (2006) Cancer pain: Palliative care in children. In: *Encyclopedic Reference of Pain* (eds R.F. Schmidt and W.D. Willis), pp. 220–224. Springer-Verlag, Heidelberg.

Bruehl, S. (2010) An update on the pathophysiology of complex regional pain syndrome. *Anesthesiology* 113, 713–725.

Burgoyne, L.L., Billups, C.A., Jirón, J.L et al. (2012) Phantom limb pain in young cancer-related amputees: Recent experience at St Jude Children's Research Hospital. *Clinical Journal of Pain* 28(3), 222–225.

Campos, A., Amaria, K., Campbell, F. and McGrath, P.A. (2011) Clinical impact and evidence base for physiotherapy in treating childhood chronic pain. *Physiotherapy Canada* 63(1), 21–23.

Clerici, C.A., Spreafico, F., Cavallotti, G. et al. (2012) Mirror therapy for phantom limb pain in adolescent cancer survivor. *Tumori* 98(1), 27–30.

Collins, J.J., Stevens, M.M. and Berde, C.B. (2008) Pediatric cancer pain. In: *Clinical Pain Management* (eds A. Rice, R. Howard, D. Justins and C. Miaskowski), pp. 345–358. Hodder Education, London.

Connelly, M., Rapoff, M.A. Thompson, N. and Connelly, W. (2006) Headstrong: A pilot study of a CD-ROM intervention for recurrent pediatric headache. *Journal of Pediatric Psychology* 31, 737–747.

Connelly, M. and Schanberg, L. (2006) Latest developments in the assessment and management of chronic musculoskeletal pain syndromes in children. *Current Opinion in Rheumatology* 18(5), 496–502.

Connelly, M., Anthony, K.K., and Schanberg, L.E. (2012) Parent perceptions of child vulnerability are associated with functioning and health care use in children with chronic pain. *Journal of Pain and Symptom Management* 43, 953–9660.

Crombez, G., Bijttebier, P., Eccleston, C. et al. (2003) The child version of the pain catastrophizing scale (PCS-C): A preliminary validation. *Pain* 104(3), 639–446.

Darbari, D., Neely, M., van den Anker, J. and Rana, S. (2011) Increased clearance of morphine in sickle cell disease: Implications for pain management. *Journal of Pain* 12(5), 531–538.

Darlington, A., Verhulst, F., De Winter, A., Ormel, J., Passchler, J., and Hunfeld, J. (2012) The influence of maternal vulnerability and parenting stress on chronic pain in a general population sample: The TRAILS study. *European Journal of Pain* 16(1), 150–159.

De Blecourt, A., Schiphorst Preuper, H.R., Van Der Schans, C.P., Groothoff, J.W. and Reneman, M.F. (2008) Preliminary evaluation of a multidisciplinary pain management program for children and adolescents with chronic musculoskeletal pain. *Disability and Rehabilitation* 30, 13–20.

Dick, B.D. and Pillai Riddell, R. (2010) Cognitive and school functioning in children and adolescents with chronic pain: A critical review. *Pain Research and Management* 15, 238–244.

Diepenmaat, A.C.M., Van der Wal, M.F., de Vet, H.C.W. and Hirasing, R.A. (2006) Neck/shoulder, low back, and arm pain in relation to computer use, physical activity, stress, and depression among Dutch adolescents. *Pediatrics* 117, 412–416.

Dhroove, G., Chogle, A. and Saps, M. (2010) A million-dollar workup for abdominal pain: Is it worth it? *Journal of Pediatric Gastroenterology and Nutrition* 51(5), 579–583.

Dunlop, R. and Bennett, D. (2006) Pain management in sickle cell disease. *Cochrane Database of Systematic Reviews* issue 2, CD003350.

Eccleston, C., Malleson, P.N., Clinch, J., Connell, H. and Sourbut, C. (2003) Chronic pain in adolescents: Evaluation of a programme of interdisciplinary cognitive behaviour therapy. *Archives of Disease in Childhood* 88, 881–885.

Eccleston, C., Crombez, G., Scotford, A., Clinch, J. and Connell, H. (2004) Adolescent chronic pain: Patterns and predictors of emotional distress in adolescents with chronic pain and their parents. *Pain* 108(3), 207–208.

Eccleston, C. (2005) Managing chronic pain in children: The challenge of delivering chronic care in a 'modernising' health care system. *Archives of Disease in Childhood* 90, 332–333.

Eccleston, C., Bruce, E. and Carter, B. (2006) Chronic pain in children and adolescents. *Paediatric Nursing* 18(10), 30–33.

Eccleston, C., Wastell, S., Crombez, G. and Jordan, A. (2008) Adolescent social development and chronic pain. *European Journal of Pain* 12, 765–774.

El-Metwally, A., Salminen, J.J., Auvinen, A., Kautiainen, H. and Mikkelsson, M. (2004) Prognosis of non-specific musculoskeletal pain in preadolescents: A prospective 4-year follow-up study till adolescence. *Pain* 110, 550–559.

El-Metwally, A., Salminen, J.J., Auvinen, A., Kautiainen, H. and Mikkelsson, M. (2005) Lower limb pain in a preadolescent population: Prognosis and risk factors for chronicity – a prospective 1- and 4-year follow-up study. *Pediatrics* 116, 673–681.

El-Metwally, A., Salminen, J.J., Macfarlane, G. and Mikkelsson, M. (2007). Risk factors for development of non-specific musculoskeletal pain in preteens and early adolescents: A prospective 1-year follow-up study. *BMC Musculoskeletal Disorders* 8, 46–53.

Engel, J.M. and O'Rouke, D.A. (2006) Chronic pain in children, physical medicine and rehabilitation. In: *Encyclopedic Reference of Pain* (eds R.F. Schmidt and W.D. Willis), pp. 368–371. Springer-Verlag, Heidelberg.

Engel, J., Kartin, D., Carter, GT., Jensen M.P., and Jaffe, KM. (2009) Pain in youths with neuromuscular disease. *American Journal of Hospice and Palliative Care* 26(5), 405–412.

Evans, S. and Keenan, T.R. (2007) Parents with chronic pain: are children equally affected by fathers as mothers in pain? A pilot study. *Journal of Child Health* 11, 143–157.

Evans, S., Shipton, E.A. and Keenan, T. (2006) The relationship between maternal chronic pain and child adjustment: The role of parenting as a mediator. *Journal of Pain* 7, 236–243.

Evans, S., Tsao, J.C., Lu, Q., Myers, C., Suresh, J. and Zeltzer, L.K. (2008) Parent–child pain relationships from a psychosocial perspective: A review of the literature. *Journal of Pain Management* 1(3), 237–246.

Evans, S., Moieni, M., Sternlieb, B., Tsao, J. and Zeltzer, L. (2012) Yoga for youth in pain: The UCLA pediatric pain program model. *Journal of Holistic Nursing* 26(5), 262–271.

Forgeron, P.A., McGrath, P., Stevens, B. et al. (2011) Social information processing in adolescents with chronic pain: My friends don't really understand me. *Pain* 152(12), 2273–2280.

Gauntlett-Gilbert, J. and Eccleston, C. (2007) Disability in adolescents with chronic pain: Patterns and predictors across different domains of functioning. *Pain* 131, 132–141.

Gieteling, M., Bierma-Zeinstra, S., Passchier, J. and Berger, M. (2008) Prognosis of chronic or recurrent abdominal pain in children. *Journal of Pediatric Gastroenterology and Nutrition* 47, 316–327.

Grégoire, M.C. and Finley, G.A. (2007) Why were we abandoned? Orphan drugs in pediatric pain. *Paediatrics and Child Health* 12, 95–96.

Guite, J.W., Logan, D.E., McCue, R., Sherry, D.D. and Rose, J.B. (2009) Parental beliefs and worries regarding adolescent chronic pain. *Clinical Journal of Pain* 25(3), 223–232.

Guite, J., McCue, R., Sherker, J., Sherry, D. and Rose, J. (2011) Relationships among pain, protective parental responses, and disability for adolescents with chronic musculoskeletal pain: The mediating role of pain catastrophizing. *Clinical Journal of Pain* 27(9), 775–781.

Hainsworth, K.R., Davies, W.H., Khan, K.A. and Weisman, S.J. (2009) Co-occuring chronic pain and obesity in children and adolescents: The impact on health-related quality of life. *Clinical Journal of Pain* 25, 715–721.

Harden, R., Bruehl, S., Stanton-Hicks, M. and Wilson, P. (2007) Proposed new diagnostic criteria for complex regional pain syndrome. *Pain Medicine* 8, 327–331.

Hermann, C. (2006) Psychological treatment of pain in children. In: *Encyclopedic Reference of Pain* (eds R.F. Schmidt and W.D. Willis), pp. 2037–2039. Springer-Verlag, Heidelberg.

Hermann, C. and Blanchard, E.B. (2002) Biofeedback in the treatment of headache and other childhood pain. *Applied Psychophysiology Biofeedback* 27, 143–162.

Hestbaek, L. and Stochkendahl, J. (2010) The evidence base for chiropractic treatment of musculoskeletal conditions in children and adolescents: The emperor's new suit? *Chiropractic and Osteopathy* 18, 15.

IHS Classification ICHD-II (2012) *Part II: The Secondary Headaches. International Headache Society* [Online]. Available from: http://ihs-classification.org/en/02_klassifikation/03_teil2/ (accessed December 2012).

Ho, I., Goldschneider, K., Kashikar-Zuck, S., Kotegal, U., Tessman, C. and Jones, B. (2008) Health care utilization and indirect burden among families of pediatric patients with chronic pain. *Journal of Musculoskeletal Pain* 16, 155–164.

Huguet, A, and Miró, J. (2008) The severity of chronic pediatric pain: An epidemiological study. *Journal of Pain* 9, 226–236.

Johnson, L. (2004) The nursing role in recognizing and assessing neuropathic pain. *British Journal of Nursing* 13(18), 1092–1097.

Johnson, L. (2005) Managing acute and chronic pain in sickle cell disease. *Nursing Times* 101(8), 40–43.

Jones, D.S. and Walker, L.S. (2006) Recurrent abdominal pain in children. In *Encyclopedic Reference of Pain* (eds R.F. Schmidtand W.D. Willis), pp. 359–363. Springer-Verlag, Heidelberg.

Jones, G.T. and Macfarlane, G.J. (2009) Predicting persistent low back pain in schoolchildren: A prospective cohort study. *Arthritis and Rheumatism* 61(10), 1359–1366.

Kashikar-Zuck, S., Goldschneider, K.R., Powers, S.W., Vaught, M.H. and Hershey, A.D. (2001) Depression and functional disability in chronic pediatric pain. *Clinical Journal of Pain* 17, 341–349.

Kashikar-Zuck, S., Vaught, M.H., Goldschneider, K.R., Graham, T.B. and Miller J.C. (2002) Depression, coping, and functional disability in juvenile primary fibromyalgia syndrome. *Journal of Pain* 3(5), 412–419.

Kashikar-Zuck, S. (2006) Treatment of children with unexplained chronic pain. *Lancet* 367, 380–382.

Kashikar-Zuck, S., Parkins, I.S., Graham, T.B. et al. (2008a) Anxiety, mood, and behavioral disorders among pediatric patients with juvenile fibromyalgia syndrome. *Clinical Journal of Pain* 24(7), 620–626.

Kashikar-Zuck, S., Lynch, A.M., Slater, S., Graham, T.B., Swain, N.F. and Noll, R.B. (2008b) Family factors, emotional functioning, and functional impairment in juvenile fibromyalgia syndrome. *Arthritis and Rheumatism* 59(10), 1392–1398.

Kashikar-Zuck, S., Ting, T.V., Arnold, L.M. et al. (2012) Cognitive-behavioral therapy for the treatment of juvenile fibromyalgia: A multisite, single-blind, randomized, controlled clinical trial. *Arthritis and Rheumatism* 64(1), 297–305.

Keogh, E. and Eccleston, C. (2006) Sex differences in adolescent chronic pain and pain-related coping. *Pain* 123(3), 275–284.

King, S., Chambers, C.T., Huguet, A. et al. (2011) The epidemiology of chronic pain in children and adolescents revisited: A systematic review. *Pain* 152, 2729–2738.

Knook, L.M., Lijmer, J.G., Konijnenberg, A.Y., Taminiau, B. and van Engeland, H. (2012) The course of chronic pain with and without psychiatric disorders: A 6-year follow-up study from childhood to adolescence and young adulthood. *Journal of Clinical Psychiatry* 73(1), e134–139.

Konijnenberg, A.Y., Uiterwaal, C.S., Kimpen, J.L., van der Hoeven. J., Buitelaar, J.K. and de Graeff-Meeder, E.R. (2005) Children with unexplained chronic pain: Substantial impairment in everyday life. *Archives of Disease in Childhood* 90(7), 680–686.

Kopek, J.A. and Sayre, E.C. (2005) Stressful experiences in childhood and chronic back pain in the general population. *Clinical Journal of Pain* 21, 478–483.

Kozlowska, K., Rose, D., Khan, R., Kram, S., Lane, L. and Collins, J. (2008) A conceptual model and practice framework for managing chronic pain in children and adolescents. *Harvard Review of Psychiatry* 16(2), 136–150.

Kuttner, L., Chambers C., Hardial, J., Israel, D., Jacobson, K. and Evans, K. (2006) A randomized trial of yoga for adolescents with irritable bowel syndrome. *Pain Research and Management* 11(4), 217–224.

Levy, R.L., Langer, S.L., Walker, L.S. et al. (2010) Cognitive-behavioral therapy for children with functional abdominal pain and their parents decreases pain and other symptoms. *American Journal of Gastroenterology* 105(4), 946–956.

Lewandowski, A., Palermo, T.M., Stinson, J., Handley, S. and Chambers, C. (2010) Systematic review of family functioning in families of children and adolescents with chronic pain. *Journal of Pain* 11(11), 1027–1038.

Lewis, D.W. (2009) Pediatric migraine. *Neurologic Clinics* 27(2), 481–501.

Logan, D.E., Guite, J.W., Sherry, D.D. and Rose, J.B. (2006) Adolescent–parent relationships in the context of adolescent chronic pain conditions. *Clinical Journal of Pain* 22(6), 576–583.

Logan, D.E., Simons, L.E. and Carpino, E.A. (2011) Too sick for school? Parent influences on school functioning among children with chronic pain. *Pain* 153(2), 437–443.

Logan, D.E. and Simons, L.E. (2010) Development of a group intervention to improve school functioning in adolescents with chronic pain and depressive symptoms: A study of feasibility and preliminary efficacy. *Journal of Pediatric Psychology* 35, 823–836.

Low, A.K., Ward, K. and Wines, A.P. (2007) Pediatric complex regional pain syndrome. *Journal of Pediatric Orthopedics* 27, 567–572.

Lu, Q., Krull, K.R., Leisenring, W. et al. (2011) Pain in long-term adult survivors of childhood cancers and their siblings: A report from the childhood cancer survivor study. *Pain* 152(11), 2616–2624.

Lynch, A.M., Kashikar-Zuck, S., Goldschneider, K.R. and Jones, B.A. (2007) Sex and age differences in coping styles among children with chronic pain. *Journal of Pain and Symptom Management* 33(2), 208–216.

Maciver, D., Jones, D. and Nicol, M. (2010) Parent's' experiences of caring for a child with chronic pain. *Qualitative Health Research* 20(9), 1272–1282.

Mallen, C.D., Peat G., Thomas, E. and Croft, P.R. (2006) Is chronic pain in adulthood related to childhood factors? A population-based case-study of young adults. *Journal of Rheumatology* 33(11), 2286–2290.

Martin, A.L., McGrath, P.A., Brown S.C. and Katz, J. (2007) Children with chronic pain: Impact of sex and age on long-term outcomes. *Pain* 128, 13–19.

Masuad, A., Cohen, L.L., Wicksell, R.K., Kemani, M.K. and Johnson, A. (2011) A case study: Acceptance and commitment therapy for pediatric sickle cell disease. *Journal of Pediatric Psychology* 36, 398–408.

McCarthy, C.F., Shea, A.M. and Sullivan, P. (2003) Physical therapy management of pain in children. In: *Pain in Infants, Children and Adolescents* (eds N.L. Schechter, C.B. Berde and M. Yaster), 2nd edition, pp. 434–448. Lippincott, Williams & Wilkins, Baltimore, MD.

McGrath, P.A. (2006) Pain in children. In: *Encyclopedic Reference of Pain* (eds R.F. Schmidt and W.D. Willis), pp. 1665–1669. Springer-Verlag, Heidelberg.

Meldrum, M., Tsao, J. and Zeltzer, L. (2009). 'I can't be what I want to be': Children's narratives of chronic pain experiences and treatment outcomes. *Pain Medicine* 10(6), 1018–1034.

Merlijn, V.P.B.M., Hunfield, J.A.M., van der Wouden, J.C., Hazebroek-Kamschreur, A.A.J.M., Passchier, J. and Koes, B.W. (2006) Factors related to quality of life in adolescents with chronic pain. *Clinical Journal of Pain* 22, 306–315.

Miró, J., Huguet, A. and Nieto, R. (2007) Predictive factors of chronic pediatric pain and disability. *Journal of Pain* 8, 774–792.

Mitchell, M., Lemanek, K., Palermo, T., Crosby, L., Nichols, A. and Powers, S. (2007) Parent perspectives on pain management, coping, and family functioning in sickle cell disease. *Clinical Pediatrics* 46(4), 311–319.

Mullick, M.S.I. (2002) Somatoform disorders in children and adolescents. *Bangladesh Medical Research Council Bulletin* 28, 112–122.

Olsson, G.L., Meyerson, B.A. and Linderoth, B. (2008) Spinal cord stimulation in adolescents with complex regional pain syndrome type 1 (CRPS-I). *European Journal of Pain.* 12, 53–59.

O'Sullivan, P., Beales, D., Jensen, L., Murray, K. and Myers, T. (2011) Characteristics of chronic non-specific musculoskeletal pain in children and adolescents attending a rheumatology outpatients clinic: A cross-sectional study. *Pediatric Rheumatology Online Journal* 9(1), 3–11.

Palermo, T. and Eccleston, C. (2009) Parents of children and adolescents with chronic pain. *Pain* 146, 15–17.

Palermo, T.M. and Kiska, R. (2005) Subjective sleep disturbances in adolescents with chronic pain: Relationship to daily functioning and quality of life. *Journal of Pain* 6, 201–207.

Palermo, T., Toliver-Sokol, M., Fonareva, I. and Koh, J. (2007) Objective and subjective assessment of sleep in adolescents with chronic pain compared to healthy adolescents. *Clinical Journal of Pain* **23**, 812–820.

Palermo, T.M., Eccleston, C., Lewandowski, A.S., Williams, A.C. and Morley, S. (2010) Randomized controlled trials of psychological therapies for management of chronic pain in children and adolescents: An updated meta-analytic review. *Pain* **148**(3), 205–213.

Pavone, V., Lionetti, E., Gargano, V., Evola, F.R., Costarella, L. and Sessa, G. (2011) Growing pains: A study of 30 cases and a review of the literature. *Journal of Pediatric Orthopedics* **31**(5), 606–609.

Peng, P., Stinson, J., Choiniere, M. et al. and STOP PAIN Investigator Group (2007) Dedicated multidisciplinary pain management centres for children in Canada: The current status. *Canadian Journal of Anesthesia* **54**, 963–968.

Perez, R.S., Zollinger, P.E., Dijkstra, P.U. et al. and CRPS I task force (2010) Evidence-based guidelines for complex regional pain syndrome type 1. *BMC Neurology* **10**, 20–33.

Perquin, C.W., Hunfled,, J.A.M., Hazebroek-Kampschreur, A.A.J.M. et al. (2003) The natural course of chronic benign pain in childhood and adolescence: A two-year population-based follow-up study. *European Journal of Pain* **7**(6), 551–559.

Petersen, S., Haglof, B.L. and Bergstrom, E.I. (2009) Impaired health-related quality of life in children with recurrent pain. *Pediatrics* **124**, 759–767.

Pillai Riddell, R., Stevens, B., McKeever, P. et al. (2009) Chronic pain in hospitalized infants: Health professionals' perspectives. *Journal of Pain* **10**(12), 1217–1225.

Ramstad, K, Jahnsen, R., Skjeldal, O.H. and Diseth, T.H. (2011) Characteristics of recurrent musculoskeletal pain in children with cerebral palsy aged 8 to 18 years. *Developmental Medicine and Child Neurology* **53**, 1013–1018.

Reid, G.J., McGrath, P.J. and Lang, B.A. (2005) Parent–child interactions among children with juvenile fibromyalgia, arthritis, and healthy controls. *Pain* **113**(1), 201–210.

Reid, K., Lander, J., Scott, S. and Dick, B. (2010) What do the parents of children who have chronic pain expect from their first visit to a pediatric chronic pain clinic? *Pain Research and Management* **15**(3), 158–162.

Roth-Isigkeit, A., Thyen, U., Stoven, H., Schwarzenberger, J. and Schumaker, P. (2005) Pain among children and adolescents: Restrictions in daily living and triggering factors. *Pediatrics* **115**(2), 152–162.

Saunders, K., Korff, M.V., LeResche, L. and Mancl, L. (2007) Relationship of common pain conditions in mothers and children. *Clinical Journal of Pain* **23**(3), 204–213.

Scharff, L., Langan, N., Rotter, N. et al. (2005) Psychological, behavioural and family characteristics of pediatric patients with chronic pain. A 1-year retrospective study and cluster analysis. *Clinical Journal of Pain* **21**, 432–438.

Scholl, J. and Allen, P. (2007) A primary care approach to functional abdominal pain. *Pediatric Nursing* **33**(3), 247–259.

Shashi, S.S. (2012) Chronic daily headache in children and adolescents. *Current Pain and Headache Report* **16**(1), 60–72.

Simons, L.E., Claar, R.L. and Logan, D.L. (2008) Chronic pain in adolescence: Parental responses, adolescent coping, and their impact on adolescent's pain behaviors. *Journal of Pediatric Psychology* **33**(8), 894–904.

Simons, L.E., Logan, D.E., Chastain, L. and Stein, M. (2010a) The relation of social functioning to school impairment among adolescents with chronic pain. *Clinical Journal of Pain* **26**, 16–22.

Simons, L., Logan, D.E., Chastain, L. and Cerullo, M. (2010b) Engagement in multidisciplinary interventions for pediatric chronic pain: Parental expectations, barriers and child outcomes. *Clinical Journal of Pain* **26**, 291–299.

Sleed, M., Eccleston, C., Beecham, J., Knapp, M. and Jordan, A. (2005) The economic impact of chronic pain in adolescence: Methodological considerations and a preliminary costs-of-illness study. *Pain* **119**(1–3), 183–190.

Stanford, E.A., Chambers, C.T., Biesanz, J.C. and Chen, E. (2008) The frequency, trajectories and predictors of adolescent recurrent pain: A population-based approach. *Pain* **138**, 11–21.

Stinson, J.N. (2006) Complex chronic pain in children, interdisciplinary treatment. In: *Encyclopedic Reference of Pain* (eds R.F. Schmidt and W.D. Willis), pp. 431–434. Springer-Verlag, Heidelberg.

Stinson, J., Stevens, J., Feldman, B. et al. (2007) Construct validity of a multidimensional electronic pain diary for adolescents with arthritis. *Pain* **136**(3), 281–292.

Stinson, J, Wilson, R, Gill, N., Yamada, J. and Holt, J. (2009) A systematic review of internet-based self-management interventions for youth with health conditions. *Journal of Pediatric Psychology* 34(5), 495–510.

Subcommittee on Chronic Abdominal Pain (2005) Chronic abdominal pain in children. *Pediatrics* 115(3), 812–815.

Sullivan, M.J.L. and Adams, H. (2006) Castrophizing. In: *Encyclopedic Reference of Pain* (eds R.F. Schmidt and W.D. Willis), pp. 297–298. Springer-Verlag, Heidelberg.

Tan, E., Zijlstra, B., Essink, M.L., Goris, R. and Severijnen, R. (2008) Complex regional pain syndrome type 1 in children. *Acta Paediatrica* 97, 875–879.

Taylor, S. and Garralda, E. (2003) The management of somatoform disorder in childhood. *Current Opinion in Psychiatry* 16, 2227–2231.

Taylor, L.E.V, Stotts, N.A., Humphreys, J., Treadwell, M.J. and Miaskowski, C. (2010) A review of the literature on the multiple dimensions of chronic pain in adults with sickle cell disease. *Journal of Pain and Symptom Management* 40, 416–435.

Tsao, J.C. and Zelter, L.K. (2005) Complementary and alternative medicine approaches for pediatric pain: A review of the state-of-the-science. *Evidence Based Complementary and Alternative Medicine* 2(2), 149–159.

van Cleve, L., Munoz, C.E., Riggs, M.L., Bava, L. and Savedra, M. (2012) Pain experience in children with advanced cancer. *Journal of Pediatric Oncology Nursing* 29(1), 28–36.

Van Den Kerkhof, E. and van Dijk, A. (2006) Prevalence of chronic pain disorders in children. In: *Encyclopedic Reference of Pain* (eds R.F. Schmidt and W.D. Willis), pp. 1972–1974. Springer-Verlag, Heidelberg.

van Gessel, H., Gaβmann, J. and Kröner-Herwig, B. (2011) Children in pain: Recurrent back pain, abdominal pain, and headache in children and adolescents in a four-year period. *Journal of Pediatrics* 158(6), 977–983.

van Tilburg, M., Spence N.J., Whitehead, W.E., Bangdiwala, S. and Goldston, D.B. (2011) Chronic pain in adolescents is associated with suicidal thoughts and behaviors. *Journal of Pain.* 10, 1032–1039.

Velleman, S., Stallard, P. and Richardson, T. (2010) A review and meta-analysis of computerized cognitive behaviour therapy for the treatment of pain in children and adolescents. *Child: Care Health and Development* 36(4), 465–472.

Vervoort, T., Goubet, L., Eccleston, C., Bijttebier, P. and Crombez, G. (2006) Catastrophic thinking about pain is independently associated with pain severity, disability and somatic complaints in school children and children with chronic pain. *Journal of Pediatric Psychology* 31, 674–683.

Vijenthira, A., Stinson, J., Friedman, J. et al. (2012) Benchmarking pain outcomes from children with sickle cell disease hospitalized in a tertiary referral pediatric hospital. *Pain Research and Management* 17(4), 291–296.

Von Baeyer, C. (2006) Understanding and managing children's recurrent pain in primary care: A biopsychosocial perspective. *Paediatrics and Child Health* 12, 121–125.

Walco, G.A., Dworkin, R.H., Krane, E.J., LeBel, A.A. and Treede, R.D. (2010) Neuropathic pain in children: Special considerations. *Mayo Clinic Proceedings* 85(3_suppl), S33–S41.

Walker, L.S., Dengler-Crish, C.M., Rippel, S. and Bruehl, S. (2010) Functional abdominal pain in childhood and adolescence increases risk for chronic pain in adulthood. *Pain* 150(3), 568–572.

Walker, L.S., Sherman, A.L., Bruehl, S., Garber, J. and Smith, C.A. (2012) Functional abdominal pain patient subtypes in childhood predict functional gastrointestinal disorders with chronic pain and psychiatric comorbidities in adolescence and adulthood. *Pain* 153(9), 1798–1806.

Watson, K.D., Papageorgiou, A.C., Jones, G.T. et al. (2002) Low back pain in schoolchildren: Occurrence and characteristics. *Pain* 97, 87–92.

Wicksell, R., Dahl, J., Magnusson, B. and Olsson, G. (2005) Using acceptance and commitment therapy in the rehabilitation of an adolescent female with chronic pain: A case example. *Cognitive Behavioural Practitioner* 12, 415–423.

Wicksell, R., Melin, L. and Olsson, G. (2007) Exposure and acceptance in the rehabilitation of adolescents with idiopathic chronic pain: A pilot study. *European Journal of Pain* 11, 267–274.

Wicksell, R., Olsson, G. and Hayes, S (2011) Mediators of change in acceptance and commitment therapy for pediatric chronic pain. *Pain* 152, 2792–2801.

Williams, S., Smith, C., Bruel, S., Gigante, J. and Walker, L. (2009) Medical evaluation of children with chronic abdominal pain: Impact of diagnosis, physician practice orientation, and maternal trait anxiety on mothers' responses to the evaluation. *Pain* 146, 283–292.

Williams, S.E., Blount, R.L. and Walker, L.S. (2011) Children's pain threat appraisal and catastrophizing moderate the impact of parent verbal behaviour on children's symptom complaints. *Journal of Pediatric Psychology* 36(1), 55–63.

Wilson, A.C., Lewandowski, A.S. and Palermo, T.M. (2011) Fear-avoidance beliefs and parental responses to pain in adolescents with chronic pain. *Pain Research Management* 16(3), 178–182.

Wittink, H. and Takken, T. (2008) Exercise testing and training in patients with (chronic) pain. *Integrative Pain Medicine* 11, 173–191.

Wood, J. (2008) Functional abdominal pain: The basic science. *Journal of Pediatric Gastroenterology and Nutrition* 47(5), 688–693.

World Health Organization (2012) WHO *guidelines on the pharmacological treatment of persisting pain in children with medical illness* [Online]. Available from: http://whqlibdoc.who.int/publications/2012/9789241548120_Guidelines.pdf (accessed May 2012).

Yoon, S. and Black, S. (2006) Comprehensive, integrative management of pain for patients with sickle cell disease. *Journal of Alternative and Complementary Medicine.* 12(10), 995–1001.

Zernikow, B., Wager, J., Hechler, T. et al. (2012a) Characteristics of highly impaired children with severe chronic pain: A 5-year retrospective study on 2249 pediatric pain patients. *BMC Pediatrics* 12(1), 54–66.

Zernikow, B., Gerhold, K., Burk, G. et al. (2012b) Definition, diagnosis and therapy of chronic widespread pain and so-called fibromyalgia syndrome in children and adolescents: Systematic literature review and guideline. *Schmerz (Berlin)* 26, 318–330.

CHAPTER 9

Palliative Care in Children

Stephanie Dowden

Paediatric Palliative Care, Princess Margaret Hospital for Children, Australia

Introduction

This chapter provides an overview of paediatric palliative care (PPC) with a particular focus on controlling pain and other distressing symptoms. After defining PPC, causes of death in childhood will be identified. Conditions requiring PPC will be described and best practice will be reviewed together with the key aims for quality outcomes. Finally, there will be detailed discussion about pain and symptom management during palliative care and particularly at end-of-life (EOL). Physical, psychological and pharmacological methods will be included.

What is Palliative Care?

The World Health Organization (WHO 2006) defines palliative care as encompassing the following:

- providing relief of pain and other distressing symptoms;
- affirming life and regarding dying as a normal process;
- intending to neither hasten nor postpone death;
- integrating psychological and spiritual aspects of care;
- supporting people to live fully before they die;
- using a team approach to address the needs of patients and their families;
- supporting the family to cope during the illness and after the death.

Managing Pain in Children: A Clinical Guide for Nurses and Healthcare Professionals, Second Edition.
Edited by Alison Twycross, Stephanie Dowden, and Jennifer Stinson.
© 2014 John Wiley & Sons, Ltd. Published 2014 by John Wiley & Sons, Ltd.

What is Paediatric Palliative Care?

Paediatric palliative care definition

Children's palliative care is an active and total approach to care, from the point of diagnosis or recognition, throughout the child's life, death and beyond. It embraces physical, emotional, social and spiritual elements and focuses on the enhancement of quality of life for the child or young person and support for the whole family. It includes the management of distressing symptoms, provision of short breaks and care through death and bereavement (Together for Short Lives 2012).

Paediatric palliative care combines key palliative care ideals with child-specific considerations:

- developmental, ethical and legal concerns;
- small patient numbers with a diverse range of conditions;
- rare conditions and diseases not seen in adulthood;
- palliative care involvement ranging from days to years;
- parental involvement and family dynamics;
- impact of the death of a child on parents and siblings.

(Craig et al. 2007; Mellor et al. 2011)

Knowledge of PPC developed following the publication of *Cancer Pain Relief and Palliative Care in Children* (WHO 1998), which proposed that all children should have access to a minimum standard of pain relief and palliative care. Internationally PPC provision is limited with 65% of countries having no PPC services, and only 16% having localised or national services (Knapp et al. 2011). Palliative care terminology is defined in Table 9.1.

Death in Childhood

Causes of death in childhood

- Worldwide, the majority of childhood deaths occur in the first year of life, with two-thirds in the first month of life (WHO 2012a).
- In high-income countries (e.g. North America, Europe, Australia and New Zealand) accidents are the primary cause of death, with most remaining deaths due to congenital anomalies, perinatal causes, neurological conditions and cancers (Fraser et al. 2012; McNamara-Goodger and Feudtner 2012).
- In the USA there are 50,000 deaths per year in the under-19 age group (Friebert 2009).
- In England and Wales there are 5,000 deaths per year in the under-15 age group (Office for National Statistics 2010).
- In low-income countries (e.g. South-East Asia, Africa and Central America), 50% of deaths (approximately 4 million per year) in the under-5 age group are due to preventable or treatable conditions, perinatal events and accidents (WHO 2012a).
- In Africa, HIV/AIDS rates have slowed since 2010 but contribute to 50% of childhood deaths, with more than 230,000 children under 15 dying of AIDS in 2011 (Kippenberg and Thomas 2010; United Nations Joint Programme on HIV/AIDS 2012).

Table 9.1 Paediatric palliative care terminology

Term	Definition
Chronic complex condition (CCC)	Medical condition lasting more than 12 months with several systems involved requiring specialist care
Death	Death is not the endpoint of palliative care. The family is supported in their bereavement
End-of-life (EOL)	The final days or weeks of life
Hospice	A service that cares for a person at EOL (often in their own home) or a place to provide EOL care. (In the US 'hospice' also refers to a funding category for people who are terminally ill)
Life limiting illness (LLI) or condition (LLC)	An illness or condition that cannot be cured and the child or young person will die early
Life-sustaining treatment	Medical treatment directed at sustaining life (e.g. mechanical ventilation, cardiopulmonary resuscitation)
Life-threatening condition	Where curative treatments may be feasible but can fail (e.g. cancer)
Premature or early death	Where the child is expected to die before their parents (e.g. in childhood or early adulthood)
Technology-dependent children	Children who are dependent on medical technology for survival and to prevent an early death
Terminal care	Care during the EOL phase. Terminal care is just one component of palliative care
Terminally ill	The final days to months of an illness

Source: Data from Wolfe et al. (2011); McNamara-Goodger and Feudtner (2012)

Where do children die?

Despite evidence that families, if offered a choice, would prefer their children to die at home, most die in hospital:

- In studies from the US, UK, Mexico, Singapore and Taiwan, rates of in-hospital childhood deaths range from 60% to 85% (Cardenas-Turanzas et al. 2008; Friebert 2009; Tzuh Tang et al. 2011; Chong et al. 2012; Fraser et al. 2012).
- Shah et al. (2011) reviewed children (*n* = 1,864) in the UK who were diagnosed and died of cancer between 1999 and 2006. Death at home and in hospital was evenly split (45%/47%) with death at hospice increasing from 2% to 10% over this period.
- Devanney et al. (2012) reviewed 33 of 35 UK children's hospice providers in 2011–12; 7,638 children were supported. There were 701 deaths: 40% died in hospital, 33% at home and 21% in a hospice.
- Of in-hospital deaths fewer than 15% of children die in ward areas, with 80–90% dying in critical care areas (e.g. in paediatric intensive care units [PICU] or neonatal intensive care units) (Ramnarayan et al. 2007; Fraser et al. 2011).

The majority of PICU deaths occur in children with life-limiting conditions (Ramnarayan et al. 2007). Despite the expectation that PICU will improve outcomes and

Table 9.2 Factors influencing place of death

Factors increasing likelihood of death at home/hospice	Factors increasing likelihood of death in hospital
• Child aged over 1 year • Discussions about health status with family and multidisciplinary team • Referral to palliative care • Availability of community-based palliative or hospice services • Paediatric support available • Cancer diagnosis • Funding to support home-based care • Racial majority groups • Comfort-focused treatment • Easy access to health services	• Child aged under 1 year • No or limited discussions about health status with family and multidisciplinary team • No referral to palliative care • No or limited community-based palliative or hospice services • Specific cancers: leukaemia, lymphoma or expected short duration of survival • Chronic complex conditions with high medical needs • Socially deprived background • Racial minority groups • Cure-focused treatment • Geographical isolation from health services

Source: Data from Vickers et al. (2007); Widger et al. (2007); Dussel et al. (2009); Wolff et al. (2010); Feudtner (et al. 2011); Chong et al. (2012)

restore health, for many children with life-limiting conditions this may not be possible. Significantly, discussions and planning reduce deaths from life-limiting conditions in intensive care and increase the likelihood of death at home or hospice (Dussel et al. 2009; Fraser et al. 2011).

Place of death is strongly influenced by diagnosis, complexity of care, palliative care referral and community support available (Table 9.2). Ideally, when death is anticipated, families should be offered all the options available in their local area and be able to change from one to another as desired or as circumstances change.

How Many Children Need Palliative Care?

The number of children, aged 0–19 years, with palliative care needs in high-income countries is estimated at 15–30 per 10,000 (Friebert 2009; Fraser et al. 2012). In low-income countries the need for PPC is difficult to estimate (Amery 2009). Further, limited access to medical treatments means that the need for palliative care services exceeds that of high-income countries (Amery 2009; Kippenberg and Thomas 2010).

Conditions Requiring Paediatric Palliative Care

A joint working party of the Association for Children with Life-threatening or Terminal Conditions and their Families (ACT) and the Royal College of Paediatrics and Child Health (RCPCH) identified four groups of conditions (Table 9.3) for which children and young people require palliative care (ACT (2009).

Of children and young people with life-limiting conditions about 20–30% have cancer and 70–80% have non-cancer conditions (McNamara-Goodger and Feudtner 2012). Importantly, about 50% of children with palliative care needs have cognitive impairment and significant physical disability, and 47% are reliant on medical technology (Feudtner et al. 2011).

Table 9.3 Conditions requiring paediatric palliative care

Group 1	Life-threatening conditions for which treatment is possible, but may fail (e.g. cancer, irreversible organ failure)
Group 2	Conditions requiring intensive treatment aimed at prolonging life, where premature death is inevitable (e.g. cystic fibrosis, Duchenne muscular dystrophy)
Group 3	Progressive conditions without curative options, where treatment is palliative after diagnosis (e.g. Batten disease, progressive metabolic disorders)
Group 4	Non-progressive conditions with severe neurologic disability causing vulnerability to health complications (e.g. severe cerebral palsy, brain or spinal cord injury)

Source: ACT (2009)

Table 9.4 Types of paediatric palliative care delivery

Place of care	Services offered
Hospital-based care with community outreach	• Multidisciplinary PPC teams in tertiary children's hospitals (specialty or consultative service) providing comprehensive care • Emergency, acute care, respite or end-of-life care • Dedicated palliative care beds or end-of-life suite • Bereavement support • Paediatric beds in secondary/local hospitals for acute, respite or end-of-life care • Tele-video and tele-audio conference link-ups to external sites • Liaison, education and training with secondary hospitals, community teams, disability services, schools, residential respite units • Home visits for symptom management
Community-based care	• Community-based PPC nurses or (disease-specific) liaison nurses • (Adult-focused) community palliative care teams or community nurses supporting paediatric patients • At-home emergency care, symptom management, end-of-life care • At-home art, music, play therapy, complementary therapies • Domiciliary services (cleaning, shopping, childminding), practical support • Volunteer or lay carers, respite • Sibling/family support • Bereavement support
Hospice care	• Hospice at home or free-standing children's hospice or child area in adult hospice • Respite, emergency care, symptom management, end-of-life care • Sibling/family support • Bereavement support

Source: Data from Foster et al. (2010); Devanney et al. (2012); McNamara-Goodger and Feudtner (2012)

Where is Palliative Care for Children Delivered?

Palliative care for children has a combined hospital and community focus (Table 9.4). Increasingly, PPC teams offer consultative models and work across hospital and community-based settings.

Challenges of home-based palliative care

Although many families prefer their child to die at home, this is not without challenges. For home-based care to be successful it must be desired by the child and parents and supported by their healthcare team. Access to 24-hour advice and clinical review is crucial, with easy access to PPC experts desirable. The family needs to be supported with respite and non-medical care services, and rapid admission to hospital should be available if required.

There are many hidden burdens of providing *at-home palliative care* including:

- emotional and psychological cost (e.g. social isolation, sleep disruption/deprivation, uncertainty, fatigue, grief and stress);
- balancing need for assistance with loss of privacy (e.g. impact of health and support staff coming into the home);
- financial costs (e.g. loss of wages, cost of consumables and hiring equipment, child care);
- skills and knowledge required (e.g. learning nursing tasks, managing medications and medical technology, dual role of being a nurse and a parent);
- low skill or knowledge in community healthcare professionals, especially of children with rare conditions.

(Carroll et al. 2007; Vickers and Chrastek 2012)

When Should Palliative Care be Implemented?

When considering referral to PPC, several issues need addressing (Table 9.5). Barriers to referral include: confusion about PPC, uncertain prognosis, clinician indecision,

Table 9.5 Factors to consider before making a paediatric palliative care referral

Factor	Points to consider
Timeliness	• Recognising opportunities to discuss palliative care • Making referral at most useful time for the child and family • Early referral leads to improved symptom control, fewer medical interventions and reduced likelihood of unhelpful treatments
Illness trajectory	• Is a slow or rapid decline expected? • Has there been significant change in function (swallowing, feeding, mobility)? • Are there increasing episodes of serious illness? • Are life-threatening events anticipated?
Goals of care	• Acknowledging cure is unlikely • Balancing cure-based care versus comfort-focused care • Considering quality of life • Conversations about benefits versus burdens of treatment • Advance care planning discussions or decisions
Maintaining hope	• Encouraging families to view palliative care not as giving up but as offering different hopes for their child • Allowing reality to be accepted and new openness between child, family and clinicians

Source: Data from Klick and Hauer (2010); Bergstraesser (2013)

BOX 9.1

Challenges to carrying out research in paediatric palliative care

Ethical concerns
Fear of intruding in a child's last weeks/days
Burden of research participation
Attrition rates due to early death
Definition of end-of-life/palliative phase
Recruitment issues due to overprotective clinicians, families and ethics committees
Small patient numbers and diverse diagnoses
Unpredictable time course
Lack of appropriate outcome measures or research endpoints
Lack of funding
Randomisation issues and lack of ability to have a control group

Source: Data from Hynson et al. (2006); Mongeau and Liben (2007); Wolfe and Siden (2012)

---

family reluctance, cultural beliefs, discrepancies in treatment goals, and poor communication (Davies et al. 2008a; Bergstraesser 2013).

> Earlier referral to PPC avoids inappropriate or futile interventions and facilitates a more peaceful death.

Evidence Base for Palliative Care

Obtaining evidence about care at the end of life is challenging (Box 9.1) (Rapoport 2009). This is further complicated by PPC being a relatively new clinical specialty and the added responsibility of research with children (Wolfe and Siden 2012). (See Chapter 11 for additional information about research with children.) To address some of these issues PPC clinicians have established national and international collaborative networks (Feudtner et al. 2011).

Research priorities in paediatric palliative care

Steele et al. (2008) and Malcolm et al. (2009) identified a number of research priorities in PPC: bereavement and end-of-life care, symptom management interventions and symptom assessment. The WHO (2012b) identified the following areas as requiring attention in caring for children with palliative care needs: safety and dosing of non-opioids and opioids in different age groups, dose conversion of opioids; and development of specific pain assessment tools.

Quality in Palliative Care

Measuring quality in PPC has improved over the last decade as policies and tools (Table 9.6) for best practice have been developed (Knapp and Madden 2010). Kane and Baker (2012) identified key areas as quality improvement targets:

- integrating palliative care practices into the care of severely ill children;
- implementing advance care planning;

Table 9.6 Paediatric palliative care standards, policies and quality tools

Organisation and publication details	Location	Document type
International Children's Palliative Care Network (ICPCN) www.icpcn.org.uk	International	Advocacy Education
African Palliative Care Association *Standards for quality palliative care across Africa (2010)* www.africanpalliativecare.org	Africa	Standards
Department of Health, Western Australia *Paediatric and Adolescent Palliative Model of Care (2009)* www.healthnetworks.health.wa.gov.au/cancer/providers/ hp_palliative.cfm#resources	Australia	Model of care
Canadian Hospice and Palliative Care Association (CHPCA) *Pediatric Hospice Palliative Care: Guiding principles and norms of practice. (2006)* www.chpca.net/	Canada	Standards
European Association for Palliative Care *International Meeting for Palliative Care in Children, Trento (IMPaCCT): standards for paediatric palliative care in Europe (2007)* www.eapcnet.eu	Europe	Standards
National Health Service (NHS) Scotland *PPC Guidelines (2009)* www.palliativecareguidelines.scot.nhs.uk/paediatric_ palliative_care/	Scotland	Standards
Together for Short Lives (Formerly ACT and Children's Hospices UK) *Care Pathways* *Family companion (2011)* *End of life planning (2012)* www.togetherforshortlives.org.uk	United Kingdom	Standards Care pathways
Association for Paediatric Palliative Medicine (APPM) *Children's Palliative Care Handbook for GPs (2011)* *Basic Symptom Control in PPC, 8th edition (2011)* *Master Formulary for PPC (2012)* www.appm.org.uk	United Kingdom	Clinical guidelines
American Academy of Pediatrics (AAP) *Palliative Care for Children (2000)* www2.aap.org/sections/palliative/	United States	Policy statement Standards
Initiative for Pediatric Palliative Care (IPPC) www.ippcweb.org/	United States	Quality improvement tools Education
National Consensus Project (NCP) *Clinical practice guidelines for quality palliative care (2009)* www.nationalconsensusproject.org	United States	Clinical guidelines
National Hospice Palliative Care Organisation (NHPCO) *Standards for Pediatric Palliative and Hospice Care (2009)* *Facts and Figures for Pediatric Palliative and Hospice Care in America (2009)* www.nhpco.org	United States	Standards Data

- improving symptom control;
- supporting family centred-care;
- promoting enhanced communication;
- care coordination.

> The key to effectiveness in PPC is family and patient satisfaction with care, quality of life and symptom management (Knapp and Madden 2010; Wolfe and Siden 2012).

Symptoms in Children Receiving Palliative Care

Children receiving palliative care experience a range of symptoms. The most frequent symptoms irrespective of diagnosis are *pain, fatigue, dyspnoea* and *anorexia* (Lavy 2007; Theunissen et al. 2007; Hendricks-Ferguson 2008; Heath et al. 2010). Gastrointestinal symptoms are also prevalent with all diagnoses (Friedrichsdorf et al. 2011). Children with cancer may also have low mood and psychological distress (Collins et al. 2011). Children with neurological conditions tend to have excessive secretions, swallowing difficulty, seizures and agitation (Collins et al. 2011; Friedrichsdorf 2011).

Pain and Symptom Management

Symptom management is a fundamental component of palliative care (Klick and Hauer 2010). In palliative care, more than most other areas of pain management, there is a strong interconnection between physical and psychological symptoms with one having considerable effect on the other. Thus it is vital to combine physical and psychological interventions with pharmacological approaches. High levels of suffering from pain and non-pain symptoms continue to be reported, especially in the last months and weeks of life (Friedrichsdorf 2010; Heath et al. 2010; Klick and Hauer 2010).

Types of pain seen in PPC

All types of pain are seen in children receiving palliative care.

- Nociceptive pain is common, due to medical procedures, surgical interventions or when nearing the end of life.
- Neuropathic pain is predominately seen in children with neurological conditions and children with solid tumours or as a consequence of cancer treatment.
- Thalamic or *central pain* is seen in children with severe neurological impairment who may have associated autonomic nervous system dysfunction.

> *Total pain* is a concept referred to in adult palliative care. describing the combined physical, emotional and spiritual components of pain. There is limited discussion of this concept in PPC literature (Klepping 2012).

Sources of pain in different patient groups requiring palliative care are discussed in Tables 9.7, 9.8, 9.9 and 9.10.

Table 9.7 Sources of pain in conditions with neurological impairment

System	Pain source or presentation
Head, eyes, ears, nose, throat (HEENT)	Headaches, VP shunt malfunction, otitis media, corneal abrasion, sinusitis, pharyngitis, dental pain
Musculoskeletal (MS)	Chronic/acute musculoskeletal pain, spasticity, hip dislocation, fracture, osteomyelitis
Gastrointestinal (GI)	Gastro-oesophageal reflux, oesophagitis, pancreatitis, ulcer, gallstones, ileus
Renal	Urinary tract infection/pyelonephritis, nephrolithiasis

Source: Friedrichsdorf (2011)

Table 9.8 Sources of pain in cardiac and respiratory conditions

Cause	Pain source or presentation
Cardiac	Chest pain, reduced coronary perfusion, decreased myocardial blood supply, pulmonary hypertension, pericarditis, myocarditis
End-stage cardiac failure	Ascites, chronic dyspnoea, peripheral oedema, angina/ischemia pain
Respiratory	Chronic dyspnoea, headache, costochondritis Musculoskeletal pain: back and chest pain, joint and limb pain Fractures: ribs, vertebrae
End-stage respiratory failure	Chronic cough and dyspnoea, chest wall pain, abdominal pain

Source: Data from Sermet-Gaudelus et al.(2009); Reddy and Singh (2010); Sands et al. (2011); WHO (2012b)

Table 9.9 Sources of pain in HIV/AIDS

Cause	Pain source or presentation
Pain-related to HIV/AIDS	Dysphagia and gingivitis HIV neuropathy and myelopathy Kaposi's sarcoma Secondary infections, organomegaly Arthritis, vasculitis Myopathy, myositis, myalgia, arthralgia Chest pain, generalised pain
HIV-related conditions causing pain	Meningitis and sinusitis Gastroenteritis and abdominal pathology Infections/Sepsis: focal, systemic, candidiasis Spasticity associated with encephalopathy

Source: Data from Amery (2009); WHO (2012b)

Table 9.10 Sources of pain in cancer

Cause	Pain source or presentation
Treatment-related pain	Chemotherapy: mucositis, ulceration, severe vomiting/diarrhoea, myalgia, neuralgia Radiotherapy: fibrosis, inflammation, skin reactions Medical procedures Infections/Sepsis: focal, systemic, candidiasis
Tumour-related pain	Tissue or viscera distension, compression or infiltration Hollow organ obstruction Bone and joint pain, pathologic fractures Bone marrow infiltration Metastases: secondary tumours
Neuropathic pain	Neuropathies: treatment-related (vincristine neuralgia) Spinal cord or peripheral nerve compression or infiltration

Source: Data from Collins et al. (2011); WHO (2012b)

Case study: Sam

Sam is a 3-year-old boy with a neurodegenerative condition. He has low muscle tone in his trunk with spasticity in his limbs and frequent dystonic posturing of his arms, legs and head. His mother reports he gets very distressed with the dystonia.

• What pharmacological, physical and psychological strategies would be helpful in relieving Sam's symptoms?

Pain Assessment

Pain assessment is described in Chapter 6. Many of the pain history questions for children with chronic pain are also appropriate in palliative care. For some children a pain diary may be helpful. However, for others self-report is not possible and tools for non-verbal and/or cognitively impaired children should be used.

To ensure a global pain assessment, direct and indirect causes of pain must be considered including:

• child report (where possible);
• parent/family and/or clinician report;
• behavioural components (e.g. impact on activities, sleep and energy levels);
• physiological components (e.g. organ function, disease progression, consequences of illness or treatment);
• affective components (e.g. emotions, self-image);
• cognitive components (e.g. understanding, past experience, developmental stage, beliefs and coping, sense of control, meaning of pain);
• sensory components (e.g. pain aetiology, location, quality, relieving and aggravating factors, duration, frequency);
• previous and current pain management (e.g. efficacy, acceptability, preferences);
• social factors (e.g. family structure, relationships, social and community support).

(Wrede-Seaman 2005; Klick and Hauer 2010)

Frequency of pain assessment

Regular pain assessment can be impractical and onerous in PPC. The most useful strategy is to encourage the child or request a parent to use a pain diary and increase assessment if there are changes in:

- pain level or quality;
- analgesia requirements;
- behaviour or function.

Choosing pain-relieving interventions

The pain-relieving interventions chosen will depend on:

- findings from the global pain assessment;
- pain location, type and severity;
- other medications the child is receiving;
- stage of disease or condition;
- nearness to death.

The core principles and aims of pain management in PPC are:

- follow the WHO two-step strategy individualised to the child (see Chapter 4);
- procedural pain should be anticipated and prevented (see Chapter 10);
- analgesia should allow the child restful sleep and participation in activities;
- the appropriate opioid dose is the one that effectively relieves pain;
- adverse effects of medications should be anticipated and treated;
- opioid tolerance should be anticipated (see Chapter 4);
- include physical and psychological therapies (see Chapter 5).

(Craig et al. 2007; WHO 2012b)

These aims can be achieved by:

- explaining pain assessment findings and management options to the child and family;
- addressing pain first, then other issues (e.g. mood);
- developing a plan based on *all* the information gathered;
- working together with the child and family to meet their needs;
- educating the child and family about analgesics;
- assisting the child and family to identify and manage pain exacerbations.

(Wrede-Seaman 2005)

The different analgesic and adjuvant drugs used in PPC are discussed in Chapters 4 and 7. Delivery routes need consideration, aiming for simplicity and child or family preference. Intramuscular injections should be avoided; instead the oral, nasogastric tube or gastric tube routes are preferred. Additionally, some analgesics are given by transdermal, intranasal or buccal routes. Subcutaneous or intravenous routes are reserved for the end-of-life period unless the child cannot receive medicines by the enteral route (WHO 2012b). (For detail of different routes see Chapter 4.)

Practice point

If the child's pain or medical condition changes, the route of administration may need to be altered.

Table 9.11 Palliative care pain and analgesia terminology

Term	Definition
Breakthrough pain	Temporary/episodic pain that *breaks through* the baseline pain level
Controlled-release/prolonged-release/modified-release/slow-release/sustained-release	Long-acting formulation of medicines, to allow less frequent dosing and more stable pain control
Incident pain	Pain induced by an action or activity that would not normally cause pain
Rescue dose	A dose of analgesia given to enable rapid control of breakthrough pain
Switching/rotation of opioids	Changing from one opioid to another to reduce dose-related adverse effects and/or improve analgesia
Short-acting/normal-release/immediate-release	Immediate acting medicines

Source: Data from Klick and Hauer (2010); WHO (2012b)

Managing Pain in Palliative Care

Palliative care pain and analgesia terminology is explained in Table 9.11.

Practice point

Children with life-limiting conditions who have seizure disorders commonly receive a complex regime of anti-epilepsy drugs that can interfere with drug metabolism or increase the risk of adverse drug reactions when combined with analgesics and sedatives.

Management of intermittent/episodic pain

For intermittent or episodic pain, as needed (PRN) doses of analgesia are usually sufficient.

Management of persistent pain

If pain occurs around the clock, analgesia needs to be given regularly. PPC analgesia regimes commonly use opioids. Other analgesics (e.g. paracetamol, nonsteroidal anti-inflammatory drugs [NSAIDs] or adjuvant analgesics) may be administered unless contraindicated (e.g. if the child has thrombocytopenia or hepatic dysfunction) (Zernikow et al. 2009; Collins et al. 2011). Combination analgesics (e.g. combined paracetamol or NSAID and opioid) are not advocated in PPC due to the risk of exceeding recommended doses of the non-opioid component (Friedrichsdorf 2010).

For opioid-naïve patients, starting doses of opioids should be calculated using appropriate dose per kilogram guidelines (see Chapter 4). If the child is already receiving opioids, the ongoing dose is calculated based on existing requirements. Once the opioid requirements have been established, the amount used in 24 hours is calculated and given in divided doses:

- every 3–4 hours for immediate-release formulations;
- usually every 12 hours for controlled-release formulations.

> Some children require controlled-release formulations to be given every 8 hours if they have regular breakthrough pain before the next dose is due.

Practice point

Immediate-release morphine is inexpensive, thus affordable in resource-poor settings. Controlled-release opioid formulations allow for less frequent dosing and more stable pain control and are well tolerated by children, but are not available in all countries.

Case study: Jade

You are looking after Jade, an 8-year-old girl who was diagnosed with an osteosarcoma in her femur 15 months ago. Despite aggressive chemotherapy and amputation of her leg, the cancer has spread and is incurable. A recent scan shows bony metastases to six ribs, lumbar spine, scalp and two lung lesions. Jade is currently taking paracetamol (acetaminophen) 500 mg 6-hourly and oxycodone 5 mg 4-hourly.

- What type of pain is to be expected?
- What pain-relieving options should be considered for Jade?

Managing common opioid adverse drug effects

It is important to be alert for and treat opioid-induced adverse effects (Table 9.12 and Chapters 4 and 7). Educating the child and family about symptoms and their management will help resolve problems early.

Managing breakthrough pain

For pain that occurs between the regular opioid doses, an additional or *rescue dose* (calculated as **5–10%** of the total daily dose) is administered every 1–4 hours as required (Zernikow et al. 2009; Collins et al. 2011; WHO 2012b). For children on *around the clock* analgesia, regular assessment determines if more analgesia is required. The child and/or family should be asked:

- Is the current analgesia sufficient for normal function?
- Is the pain waking the child or restricting activities?
- Is the pain impacting on mood or interactions with others?
- Does the long-acting dose wear off before the next dose is due?
- Is the dose of rescue analgesia sufficient?
- How many rescue doses are needed in 24 hours?

> Before any changes are made to the analgesia regime, check:
>
> - Is the child taking all their analgesia?
> - Is the analgesia regime easy to follow?
> - Has the pain changed?
>
> *Source:* Wrede-Seaman (2005)

Table 9.12 Opioid-induced adverse effects and their management

Symptom	Comment
Constipation	Most patients will need aperients: stool softener and a bowel stimulant for the duration of their opioid therapy
Nausea, vomiting, pruritis, sedation, dysphoria or fatigue	Some or all of these may occur at commencement of opioids and with dose increases but usually settle within 72 hours • Treat nausea and vomiting using antiemetic protocols • Pruritis can be treated with low-dose opioid antagonists • Sedation and dysphoria are usually self-limiting • Fatigue may be treated with stimulant medication If symptoms persist, opioid rotation may be required
Myoclonus, persistent dysphoria, hyperalgesia or delirium	More common with high doses of opioids Consider opioid rotation
Urinary retention	Manage constipation and other treatable causes Consider opioid rotation
Respiratory depression	Very rare with appropriate dosing, may be due to concurrent medications Consider dose reduction or opioid rotation Opioid antagonists must be used with caution to avoid acute withdrawal syndrome
Tolerance	May be a problem for some patients and require dose increases Consider opioid rotation
Opioid withdrawal	At risk: if rapid weaning, changing to another opioid, missing doses or interruption to opioid supply

Source: Klick and Hauer (2010)

Practice point

Buccal and intranasal opioids (usually fentanyl) are administered to infants and children with episodic pain or dyspnoea and offer rapid-onset, minimally invasive relief of distress (Harlos et al. 2012).

Adjusting analgesia regimes

Ideally dose changes should not occur more often than every 48 hours, to enable the opioid to reach a steady state. If the child requires more than three doses per 24 hours of rescue analgesia for breakthrough pain, the following changes should be made:

- increase the total daily dose of (long-acting) opioid in 25–50% steps;
- the rescue dose should be adjusted accordingly (remaining 5–10% of the total daily dose);

- some children may require smaller or larger rescue doses;
- increases to the total daily dose can be made every 2–3 days, if needed sooner; rapid titration may need to occur in hospital;
- if dose escalation is frequent, the opioid may need to be switched (see below);
- adjuvant analgesics may be added to improve pain control (see Chapter 4).
  (Zernikow et al. 2009; Regnard and Dean 2010; Collins et al. 2011)

Practice point

Frequent dose changes are not suitable with transdermal opioids so the child may need opioids by a different route until the pain stabilises.

Pain crisis

Some children experience episodes of severe pain escalation or pain crisis. McCulloch and Collins (2006) suggest that if this occurs the following steps are taken:

- treat the crisis as an emergency;
- diagnose the primary cause of pain if possible;
- titrate IV bolus doses of opioid at 10- to 15-minute intervals until pain relief is achieved;
- increase the bolus dose by 50 to 100% if no response;
- adjust analgesia regime to meet the new needs, including adjuvant analgesics;
- consider invasive approaches to treat the pain if the above steps are insufficient (e.g. regional anaesthesia or neurosurgical techniques);
- consultation with paediatric pain or palliative care specialists is beneficial.

Practice point

Some children require exceedingly high doses of opioids (up to 100 times the standard dose) to control severe pain (Friedrichsdorf 2010).

Opioid rotation or switching

Changing from one opioid to an alternative is required for a small number of patients in order to manage dose-limiting side-effects or ongoing dose escalation, but this is not a routine strategy (Collins et al. 2011). There is limited data on opioid dose conversion in children. Due to variation in cross-tolerance, the dose of the new opioid may need to be reduced by up to 50% to avoid adverse effects (Zernikow et al. 2009; Collins et al. 2011). Opioid rotation or switching should be done in consultation with paediatric pain or palliative care specialists if possible.

Practice point

Methadone

Methadone is used in PPC to treat neuropathic pain or nociceptive pain unresponsive to other opioids.

There is limited data about efficacy and safety in children.

Due to its complex pharmacokinetics and need for careful titration and monitoring, methadone should only be prescribed in consultation with paediatric pain or palliative care specialists.

Source: Davies et al. (2008b); Anghelescu et al. (2011)

Transdermal opioids

Fentanyl and buprenorphine can be administered via transdermal patches.

These must only be used for children already receiving opioids and with stable pain, as they are difficult to titrate and have prolonged action. Patches are changed every 48–72 hours.

There is limited experience using buprenorphine in children, with fentanyl used more commonly.

Transdermal opioids should only be prescribed in consultation with clinicians experienced in their use to minimise adverse events.

Source: Zernikow et al. (2007, 2009)

Intractable pain and palliative sedation

Pain that is resistant to standard analgesia regimes is referred to as refractory or intractable pain (McCulloch and Collins 2006; Collins et al. 2011). The incidence of intractable pain in children is low, most commonly occurring in children with cancer at the end of life. Palliative sedation is required only rarely (McCulloch and Collins 2006) but, if this is being considered, advice should be sought from a paediatric palliative care or pain specialist.

Additional information

Recommendations about the use of palliative sedation from the European Association for Palliative Care can be found in:

Cherny, N.I., Radbruch, L. and Board of the European Association for Palliative Care (2009) European Association for Palliative Care (EAPC) recommended framework for the use of sedation in palliative care. *Palliative Medicine* **23**(7), 581–593.

An overview of end-of-life care sedation for children is provided in:

Kiman, R., Wuiloud, A.C. and Requena, M.L. (2011) End-of-life care sedation for children. *Current Opinion in Supportive and Palliative Care* **5**, 285–290.

An institution's experience of developing and using an algorithm for palliative sedation can be found in:

Anghelescu, D.L., Hamilton, H., Faughnan, L.G., Johnson, L.M. and Baker, J.N. (2012) Pediatric palliative sedation therapy with propofol: Recommendations based on experience in children with terminal cancer. *Journal of Palliative Medicine* **15**(10), 1082–1090.

Other Pain-Relieving Interventions

Table 9.13 summarises other pain-relieving interventions principally used for children with cancer, although in rare cases they may be used for non-cancer conditions.

Table 9.13 Other pain-relieving interventions

Modality	Use	Comments
Radiotherapy	• Reduces tumour-related: pain, bleeding, obstruction or compression • Treats pain from bony metastases, pathological fractures, spinal cord compression, soft tissue lesions and headache from brain tumours	Significant pain relief is usually achieved, thus opioid doses may need reducing
Palliative chemotherapy	• Treat pain from metastases, local tumour infiltration and reduces tumour size • Decrease proliferation of immature cancer cells in the bone marrow	Adverse effects may lead to further medical interventions and hospitalisation
Regional anaesthesia	• Targets pain in specific regions of the body • Administered as short-term infusions or implantable delivery devices for long-term management	Benefits need to outweigh risks, additional monitoring and reduction in mobility. See Chapter 7
Bisphosphonates	• Reduces pain of osteopenia and bone metastases	See Chapter 4
Corticosteroids	• Reduces pain of organ distension or tumour infiltration, raised intracranial pressure (ICP) and headache	See Chapter 4
Surgery	• Reduces tumour bulk, management of hydrocephalus or ascites and fixation of fractures	Surgery is rarely used unless the benefits outweigh less-invasive interventions

Source: Zaki (2005); Anghelescu et al. (2010); Klick and Hauer (2010); Tucker et al. (2010); Shelton and Jackson (2011); McCulloch (2012)

Management of Non-Pain Symptoms

Symptoms other than pain cause significant distress and suffering to children and may worsen at the end of life (Klick and Hauer 2010). The varied causes of common non-pain symptoms seen in PPC and their management are reviewed in Table 9.14.

Assessing non-pain symptoms

Using the strategies for pain assessment discussed earlier in this chapter may assist in assessing non-pain symptoms. Two multidimensional symptom assessment tools are available:

- Memorial Symptom Assessment Scale (MSAS) rates the severity, prevalence and impact of cancer-related symptoms in children (Collins et al. 2000);
- Therapy-Related Symptom Checklist–Children (TRSC-C) rates symptoms and severity, functional status and quality of life for children with cancer (Williams et al. 2012).

Table 9.14 Management of distressing non-pain symptoms

Symptom	Possible causes	Considerations/Education	Pharmacological	Physical/Psychological
Fatigue and/ or drowsiness	• Disease process • Raised ICP • Anaemia • Hypoxia • Medication • Mood related • Inactivity • Deconditioning • Renal/hepatic failure	• Review activity and sleep regime • Educate that opioid tolerance improves in time • May be a normal part of disease process or progression • May indicate decline if other signs of dying are present	• Adjust medications • Add non-opioids • Consider morning psychostimulants • Consider medication for sleep cycle, e.g. melatonin • Treat anaemia if present	• Schedule a.m. activities and p.m. naps • Keep active/mild exercise and avoid inactivity • Review mood • Consider trial of caffeinated beverages • Emotional support
Dyspnoea and/or cough	• Disease process • Anxiety • Anaemia • Secretions • Medication • Pulmonary oedema • Hypoxia • Infection • Ascites • Pain • Organ failure	• Review mood • Educate and reassure • May be a normal part of disease process or progression	• Trial low-dose opioid (25–50% analgesic dose) • Consider nebulised opioid • Topical local anaesthetic • Benzodiazepines, if anxiety component • Trial anticholinergic, e.g. glycopyrrolate, atropine, hyoscine • Consider antibiotics • Consider bronchodilator • Treat anaemia if present	• Positioning • Try fan, breeze • Trial wafting/blow-by oxygen • Emotional support • Distraction, play, hypnosis • Relaxation, music • Calm environment • Sip iced water • Suctioning • Breathing exercises • Humidification • Saline nebulisers • Airway management • Psychological support • Spiritual support
Anorexia and/or weight loss (cachexia)	• Disease process • Medication • Bowels/nausea-related • Ileus/obstruction • Pain • Mucositis • Inactivity • Depressed mood • Metabolic	• Educate and reassure • May be a normal part of disease process or progression • Review current food intake • Review mood	• Consider appetite stimulants or steroids • Consider food supplements or hydration depending on goals of care	• Small, frequent, high-calorie meals as desired • Mouth care • Relaxation, hypnosis • Emotional support

Symptom	Causes			
Seizures	• Epilepsy • Disease process • Metabolic • Hypoxia • Haemorrhage • Raised ICP • Infection • Tumour growth • Hypoglycaemia • Medications • Acute drug withdrawal	• Educate about seizures and safety • Ensure seizure management plan • Ensure safe environment	• Adjust/review epilepsy drugs • Benzodiazepines for prolonged seizures, e.g. diazepam, midazolam or clonazepam • Ketogenic diet	• Consider use of helmet • Emotional support • Decrease environmental stimulation if contributing to seizures
Restlessness, agitation, confusion	• Medications • Disease process • Pain • Raised ICP • Haemorrhage • Infection • Metabolic • Hypoxia • Renal/hepatic failure • Fear/anxiety • Urinary retention • Acute drug withdrawal	• Educate and reassure • Review mood • Review environment stimulus • Review medications	• Rotate opioids Consider: • Benzodiazepines, e.g. lorazepam, diazepam • Neuroleptics, e.g. haloperidol • Antipsychotics, e.g. respiridone, chlorpromazine • Other medications: clonidine, chloral hydrate	• Decrease environmental stimulation • Regular orientation • Relaxation, massage • Emotional support • Calm and safe environment • Music • Aromatherapy
Anxiety, distress, sadness and/or depression	• Pain • Hypoxia • Sleep • Mood • Secrecy • Poor communication • Loss of hope • Collusion • Spiritual distress	• Educate and reassure • Assess child's and family knowledge of the situation • Review mood • Review parent mood	• Consider mood-elevating drugs • Consider benzodiazepines for anxiety	• Calm and safe environment • Open communication • Emotional support • Relaxation, play, hypnosis • Massage • Music, aromatherapy • Psychological support • Spiritual support

Continued

Table 9.14 Continued

Symptom	Possible causes	Considerations/Education	Pharmacological	Physical/Psychological
Nausea and/or vomiting (including feeding intolerance)	• Medications • Constipation • Reduced motility • Tumour growth • Disease process • Neurological • Raised ICP • Metabolic • Renal/hepatic failure • Pain • Anxiety • Secretions • Ileus/obstruction	• Educate family • Review environmental stimulus • Assess hydration status • Specialist review with surgeon or gastroenterologist • Consider hydration depending on goals of care	• Antiemetics, e.g. metoclopramide, ondansetron, dexamethasone, promethazine • Prokinetic agents, e.g. domperidone, metoclopramide • Anticholinergics, e.g. scopolamine • Sedation, e.g. benzodiazepines, haloperidol, clonidine • Opioid rotation • Cortocosteroids	• Peppermint • Ginger • Ginger ale • Acupressure bands • Iced drinks • Acupuncture • Relaxation • Distraction • Hypnosis • Small, bland meals • Jejunal feeds • Continuous feeds or comfort feeds • Minimise environmental smells • Mouth care
Constipation	• Medication • Inactivity • Muscle weakness • Neurological • Tumour growth • Reduced intake • Metabolic • Ileus/obstruction	• Educate • Prevention is the best treatment • Begin laxative regime when opioids commence • Monitor bowel actions	• Stool softeners • Bowel stimulants • Osmotic agents • Bulking agents • Enema	• Increase fluid and diet intake • High fibre • Activity • Abdominal massage • Heat packs
Secretions and/or swallowing difficulty	• Disease process • Medication • Cough • Intake • Bulbar palsy • Neurological • Infection	• Educate family about signs of deteriorating swallow • Assess if safe to have oral intake • Non-oral feeding	• Trial drying secretions, e.g. glycopyrrolate, atropine, hyoscine • BoTox to salivary glands • Saline nebulisers • Artificial saliva • Consider sedation if distressed	• Suctioning • Positioning • Mouth care • Ice chips • Diet as tolerated • Citrus sweets • Position upright or on side

Source: Sourkes et al. (2005); Wrede-Seaman (2005); Poltorak and Benore (2006); Kersun and Shemesh (2007); Santucci and Mack (2007); Wusthoff et al. (2007); Kersun & Shemesh (2007); Siden et al. 2009; Regnard and Dean (2010); Friedrichsdorf et al. (2011)

In addition, there are some unidimensional symptom assessment tools, namely:

- PedsQL Multidimensional Fatigue Scale (Varni et al. 2002);
- Dalhousie Dyspnea Scale (DDS) (McGrath et al. 2005);
- Pediatric Nausea Assessment Tool (PeNAT) (Dupuis et al. 2006).

The majority of these tools are intended for cancer diagnoses and currently all are patient-rated, excluding children with non-cancer conditions or who are unable to self-report.

When to treat non-pain symptoms

When considering which symptoms need treating the following points should be considered:

- impact of the symptoms;
- interference with life;
- degree of distress and suffering to the child and family;
- effect of the child's symptoms on parental mood and coping.

Physical and Psychological Methods to Relieve Pain and Other Distressing Symptoms

Research into the use of physical and psychological methods to relieve pain in the PPC setting is limited (Kelly 2007). Therapies focusing on stress reduction and promotion of wellbeing are used. Vickers et al. (2007) found that two-thirds of children ($n = 160$) with cancer at end-of-life used methods including relaxation (30%), massage (43%), physiotherapy (30%) and hypnosis (2.5%); 54% of children were using one method at time of death whileh 32% were using more than two. Complementary and alternative medicine (CAM) techniques (e.g. prayer, homeopathy, herbal remedies, Reiki) are extensively used for children with cancer as an adjunct to curative therapies or during the end-of-life stage (Sencer and Kelly 2007; Bishop et al. 2010; Tomlinson et al. 2011; Heath et al. 2012).

Many of the methods that relieve pain are also effective for non-pain symptoms and are outlined in Table 9.14 (see also Chapter 5). Although there is limited research, which on the whole relates to children with cancer, several authors recommend methods for use in PPC such as cognitive behavioural approaches and sensory therapies:

- Brown and Sourkes (2006) recommend relaxation, guided imagery and hypnosis in PPC to give the child sense of control over anxiety, nausea and pain, to decrease emotional and physical distress and to increase their sense of wellbeing.
- Poltorak and Benore (2006) suggest the benefits of cognitive behavioural therapy (CBT) seen in children with chronic illness could be extrapolated to PPC to manage fear and anxiety, increase self-efficacy and improve overall coping.
- Rheingans (2007) in a systematic review of non-pharmacological therapies for symptom management in children with cancer concluded the most efficacious methods were CBT, distraction and hypnosis.
- Russell and Smart (2007) in a small case series ($n = 4$) found hypnosis and guided imagery a useful tool in a paediatric hospice to augment other analgesic strategies.
- Van Breeman (2009) considered that the use of play therapy in palliative care assisted with psychological support for the child and family.

Table 9.15 Misconceptions affecting care at end of life

Issue	Reason	Consequence	Reality
Pain is often under-treated at end of life due to misconceptions about the use of opioids	Clinicians': • fear of giving too much analgesia • fear of hastening death with opioids • uncertainty about correct dosing for analgesia or sedation at end of life Clinician and family fear of opioid addiction or tolerance	• Pain is poorly treated • Underuse of opioids • High levels of family anxiety • The child suffers unnecessarily • Family and staff distress	• Exaggerated fears of adverse effects limit opioid use • There is no upper dose for opioids • Improved analgesia often prolongs life and improves quality of life • The risk of addiction is extremely low (Chapter 4) • Utilising pain and palliative care experts enables better outcomes at end of life
Cultural, philosophical or religious reasons (of clinicians or family)	• Fear of 'giving up' on curative therapy too soon • Belief that opioids should be reserved until all curative options have failed • Causing drug-induced respiratory depression is the same as euthanasia • Beliefs that suffering brings you closer to God	• Refusal to consider palliative care referral • Avoidance of opioids • Futile treatment offered • The child suffers unnecessarily • Avoidance of opioids • The child suffers unnecessarily	• Ceasing curative therapy does not imply failure • Relief of pain and suffering does not mean the treating team has given up on curative therapies • Respiratory depression is rare in opioid-tolerant patients • The intent of analgesia is to reduce pain and suffering, not to cause death • Religious beliefs should not be used to allow suffering • Involving religious advisors is vital to resolve any impasse
Clinician expertise issues	• Clinician expertise [in specialty area] and refusal to refer to palliative care or pain specialists • Clinicians used to managing non-complex pain • Staff not accepting the child's impending death • Futile treatment at all cost	• Impedes clinicians from seeking advice • Clinician may not know the best management for complex symptoms • Parents assume all is being done or nothing more can be done • No open discussions with family • No referral to palliative care • Focus on goal of cure • Inability to accept reality	• Pain and other distressing symptoms are often under-treated by primary clinicians • Parents should be encouraged to always ask for pain relief • Clinical burden of failure • Acknowledging that a cure is unlikely allows the family to consider other choices • Curative goals should never override the child's best interest

Source: Friedrichsdorf (2010); Klick and Hauer (2010)

- Moody et al. (2010) in a case series of children ($n = 20$) with cancer or sickle cell disease found yoga contributed to overall reduction in both pain and anxiety scores.
- Buttle et al. (2011) discussed the use of massage in the PPC setting.
- The use of music therapy in PPC has been explored in several studies. The effect on pain is unclear; however, benefits included stress reduction, relaxation and parental satisfaction (Knapp et al. 2009; Lindenfelser et al. 2012).

An overview of different physical and psychological methods and their application in treating different EOL symptoms can be found in:

Sourkes, B., Frankel, L., Brown, M. et al. (2005) Food, toys and love: Pediatric palliative care. *Current Problems in Pediatric and Adolescent Health Care* **35**, 350–386.

Wrede-Seaman, L. (2005) *Pediatric Pain and Symptom Management Algorithms for Palliative Care* Intellicard Inc., Washington.

Further research is needed, particularly for non-oncology conditions.

Case study: Jackson

You are on a home visit to Jackson, a 4-month-old infant with spinal muscular atrophy type 1. He has severe muscle weakness and deteriorating respiratory function with tachypnoea and intermittent air hunger. His family have declined technology to assist his breathing and wish to care for him at home. Jackson has been prescribed morphine; however, his parents are afraid that they will hasten his death if they give it.

- How would you explain the use of morphine in this context and reassure Jackson's parents?
- How could you ensure that Jackson's respiratory distress is relieved?

Misconceptions Relating to Paediatric Palliative Care

A number of misconceptions exist in relation to PPC, which contribute to poor symptom management and child and family suffering. These are discussed in Table 9.15.

To overcome these misconceptions and enable delivery of optimal palliative care these issues must be dealt with openly, involving the child, family and clinicians, by:

- addressing the fears;
- clarifying any misconceptions and providing written information;
- explaining the current understanding about opioids;
- the use of policies and guidelines to direct clinical practice;
- having proformas or templates to enable rapid titration of medication to manage symptoms.

Practice point

Reassure parents that:

- saving opioids until pain worsens is unnecessary;
- the child is *not* a drug addict if they require opioids;
- there is *no need* for the child to suffer severe and prolonged pain;
- strong opioids are best for severe pain.

Ethical and Legal Issues in Paediatric Palliative Care

Caring for children at EOL presents ethical challenges to clinicians. Different views about value and quality of life, religion, beliefs and moral standards can cause conflict between individual clinicians and between clinicians and families (Larcher and Carnevale 2012).

A summary and discussion about ethical issues in PPC is provided by:

Larcher, V. and Carnevale, F. (2012) Ethics. In: *The Oxford Textbook of Palliative Care for Children* (eds A. Goldman, R. Hain and S. Liben), 2nd edition, pp 35–46. Oxford University Press, Oxford.

Rowse, V. and Smith, M. (2011) Palliative care of children: Some ethical dilemmas. In: *Ethical and Philosophical Aspects of Nursing Children and Young People* (eds G.M. Brykczynska and J. Simons), pp 187–198. Wiley-Blackwell, Oxford.

Futility in medical management

- The difficulty some clinicians and families have in accepting the untimely death of a child can lead to futile medical treatments being continued, sometimes until the moment of death.
- Uncertainty about illness trajectory, treatment efficacy, prognosis, defining the terminal phase and illnesses with mixed phases (e.g. cystic fibrosis) can play a key role also.
- The consequence of continuing futile treatments can lead to the child's best interests being overlooked, which can be compounded by clinicians with poor skills in communication, decision-making and the ability to be objective.

(Davies et al. 2008a; Puckey and Bush 2011)

Additional information

Advance care planning allows children and their families to take control of decisions that affect their care (Zinner 2008; Fraser et al. 2010).

Guidance about advance care planning can be found at:

A guide to EOL care (2012): www.togetherforshortlives.org.uk/

Children and Young Persons Acute Deterioration Management (CYPADM): www.scotland.gov .uk/Topics/Health/Quality-Improvement-Performance/Living-Dying-Well/CYPADM

Advance care planning guides for children, *My Wishes*, and adolescents, *Voicing my Choices*: www.agingwithdignity.org

---

Euthanasia versus double effect

It is important *all* healthcare professionals clearly understand the differences between *euthanasia* and *treatment to relieve pain and suffering* and *the principle of double effect*.

- Euthanasia and physician-assisted suicide are defined as intentional or deliberate acts with the *primary intent* being to cause death and the *secondary effect* being pain relief or end to suffering. Euthanasia and physician-assisted suicide are illegal in many countries.
- Euthanasia or physician-assisted suicide is not part of palliative care practice, even if requested by the patient or family.

- In palliative care the *primary intent* is to relieve intolerable suffering and the *secondary effect* of this may be respiratory depression or early death. Analgesia given to relieve suffering is thus considered a morally good and legally justified act.
- There is a philosophical and legal difference between the intended and unintended outcomes of these actions, known as the *principle of double effect*.
- The principle of double effect is defined as: *the actions resulting in unfavourable results are forgiven if the consequences are foreseen but unintended.*

(Wellesley and Jenkins 2009; Puckey and Bush 2011; Larcher and Carnevale 2012)

Additional information

Further information about withholding or withdrawing medical treatment in children can be found in: Royal College of Paediatrics and Child Health (2004) *Withholding or Withdrawing Life Sustaining Treatment in Children: A framework in practice*, available from: www.rcpch.ac.uk/what-we-do/rcpch-publications/publications-list-title/publications-list-title

Royal Australasian College of Physicians (2008) *Decision Making at the End of Life in Infants, Children and Adolescents*, available from: www.racp.edu.au/page/paediatrics-and-child-health-division/online-resources/paediatric-policy/

British Association of Perinatal Medicine (2010) *Palliative care (supportive and end-of-life care): A framework for clinical practice in perinatal medicine*, available from: www.bapm.org/publications/documents/guidelines/Palliative_Care_Report_final_%20Aug10.pdf

---

End-of-Life Care

Causes of pain and distressing symptoms at EOL

A range of factors can contribute to pain and other distressing symptoms at end-of-life:

- disease progression (e.g. cancer metastases);
- end-stage disease (e.g. respiratory failure in cystic fibrosis or neuromuscular disease);
- muscle spasms, contractures, joint pain;
- headache, sleeplessness;
- dyspnoea, hypoxia, secretions;
- oedema;
- feeding intolerance, constipation;
- pressure areas;
- fear and anxiety.

Diagnosing dying

The diagnosis and physical process of dying causes enormous distress to many clinicians, who in their attempts to support families or reduce their own anxiety can unwittingly make the situation worse (Brook and Hain 2008). The family is often unaware that death is imminent, because of confusing and conflicting information and poor communication. This leads to:

- false hopes;
- distrust;
- concerns about withholding or withdrawing treatment;
- uncontrolled symptoms;
- futile interventions;

- inappropriate resuscitation;
- child's and family's needs not being met;
- family regrets after the death.

(Ellershaw and Ward 2003; Brook and Hain 2008)

All these factors place families at increased risk of complex bereavement. Ellershaw and Ward (2003) and Wolfe (2011) recommend overcoming these issues by clinicians:

- identifying and regularly reporting signs of dying to the family;
- communicating clearly and unambiguously;
- planning care based on clinical findings.

> Skills for talking with families of dying children are discussed in:
> Kuttner, L. (2007) Talking with families when their children are dying. *Medical Principles and Practice* **16**(Suppl 1), 16–20.

Management of dying

It can be difficult to determine *when* a child is dying, and it is often not clear until the last one or two days of life (Brook and Hain 2008; Wolfe 2011). Clinicians should not be too definitive in making a prognosis if they are uncertain, as some children may have several *near-death* episodes before finally dying. It is also important to have early discussions with the family about the preferred place of death so that timely arrangements are made.

During the final days of life the following steps should be taken:

- ensure that *do not resuscitate* (DNR) or *allow natural death* (AND) orders are made;
- ongoing assessment of symptoms;
- regular identification of the child's and family's wishes;
- frequent update about the clinical condition with the family;
- have rescue plans for symptom control (adequate for severe escalation);
- identify a key contact person for 24-hour support (regardless of the location of death);
- offer food and fluids as desired and tolerated;
- administer medications by the most simple *and* effective route: oral or gastric tube (if gut is functioning), subcutaneous or intravenous;
- discontinue less-necessary medications, e.g. simple analgesics, laxatives, antibiotics, steroids, cardiac drugs;
- cease or minimise tests, observations, interventions, monitoring, turning regimes;
- continue comfort care: mouth and eye care, repositioning;
- provide emotional support to the child, parent, siblings and extended family;
- support spiritual and cultural practices requested by the family;
- offer discussions about autopsy, organ and tissue donation and funerals.

Practice point

Continuous subcutaneous infusions (CSI) of analgesics (sometimes combined with other drugs for symptom control) may be used at end-of-life when other routes are not available. CSI is usually administered via small portable infusion pumps.

Signs of dying vary in children, depending on the underlying disease process. Commonly children display respiratory and circulatory signs:

- breathing changes: rapid/laboured breathing with pauses, progressing to irregular slow breathing with apnoea (*Cheyne-Stokes respirations*);
- airway secretions;
- cardiac: irregular rhythm or tachycardia, hypotension;
- skin colour changes, decreased peripheral perfusion;
- temperature decreases;
- progressive weakness;
- increased sleeping;
- incontinence, oliguria or anuria;
- loss of appetite, slowed gut function, paralytic ileus;
- restlessness, agitation, confusion or coma;
- decreased speaking, loss of interest, withdrawal.

(Wolfe 2011)

After Death

Family bereavement care

The death of a child causes intense grief and distress for the whole family. Parental grief may be more severe, profound and longer lasting than other types of grief. This makes psychosocial care of families during the palliative phase of a child's illness particularly important. It has been recognised that support is crucial in the time leading up to the child's death as well as following the death (Bartell and Kissane 2005; Wender et al. 2012).

No consensus has been reached about the best way to support bereavement, but factors that promote recovery are:

- family-focused psychological support prior to the death;
- providing information about normal grief and what to expect;
- encouraging strong social support systems;
- offering additional support for those with very high levels of distress and at risk for complicated grief.

(Bartell and Kissane 2005; Wender et al. 2012)

Staff support

Clinicians involved in paediatric palliative care may experience trauma responses, particularly secondary traumatic stress (Rourke 2007). Witnessing pain, suffering and family anguish can cause high levels of distress. To continue working in this area, clinicians need to care for themselves in a systematic way for self-preservation, satisfaction and most importantly to ensure their patients and families are optimally supported (Rourke 2007; Keene et al. 2010).

Summary

- Palliative care encompasses relief of pain and other symptoms by providing total care for the child and family while aiming for the best quality of life.
- Most children die in hospital receiving high levels of invasive medical care.

- Two-thirds of children requiring palliative care do not have an oncology diagnosis.
- Evidence and quality in PPC has improved considerably in the last decade.
- Children are highly symptomatic at end-of-life and experience considerable distress from pain and non-pain symptoms.
- Holistic family-centred care utilising pharmacological, physical and psychological strategies is the best way to achieve symptom control.
- Opioids are commonly used for pain control. Severe pain should be treated as an emergency and dealt with rapidly.
- Confusion about euthanasia and sedation leads to concerns about opioid use.
- Misconceptions about opioids and end-of-life care should be dealt with promptly to avoid these impacting negatively on the child.
- Open, honest discussions about death and dying reduce futile treatments, relieve family distress and decrease the risk of complex bereavement.
- Family bereavement should be addressed before and after the death of a child.
- Clinicians involved in PPC risk burnout unless preventive measures are implemented.

Key to Case Studies

See Boxes 9.2, 9.3 and 9.4.

BOX 9.2

Sam

Dystonia can cause severe and distressing pain.
Antispasmodic drugs and anti-epilepsy drugs are somewhat effective.
Benzodiazepines can benefit but may contribute to low muscle tone or sedation.
Positioning, splinting, calming, warm baths and massage can all reduce dystonia and distress.

BOX 9.3

Jade

Disseminated bone tumours can cause severe nociceptive and neuropathic pain. Multiple metastases were identified on Jade's scan, thus pain escalation should be expected.
Use a multidimensional pain scale to discern the type, location and quality of pain. Consider the impact of pain on mood, sleep and functioning.
Both pharmacological and non-drug methods will be useful. Consider the effect of her current analgesia. Can she perform her usual daily activities and is she having breakthrough pain?
Jade may need the opioid dose increased now or rapid titration if her pain worsens. NSAIDs may be useful, if her blood counts permit.
Adjuvants, e.g. steroids, chemotherapy, radiotherapy and regional anaesthesia, may assist to reduce pain and diminish the need for opioid analgesia.

BOX 9.4
Jackson

SMA is characterised by progressive muscle weakness. Most infants with SMA are cognitively normal and become distressed and anxious as their condition advances.

Dosing of morphine for respiratory distress is 25–50% of the usual starting opioid analgesic dose. This should relieve respiratory distress and air hunger and give feelings of wellbeing.

Describe/show the parents (on Jackson) signs of respiratory distress: nasal flaring, rapid breathing, head bobbing, tense posture and distressed face.

If required assist the parents to administer morphine. If not required at this time, plan to have a clinician available (e.g. hospice nurse, visiting nurse, family doctor) to administer the first dose. Explain that if they are uncertain about the effect they can give a smaller initial dose.

Monitor the response and describe this to parents: less distress, more interactive, breathing eased, happier.

Educate about constipation prevention.

Liaise with the prescriber for dose changes if:

- Jackson is too sedated;
- dyspnoea is relieved but only for a short period;
- dyspnoea is relieved but Jackson is still distressed (low-dose benzodiazepine may assist).

Additional information

Together for Short Lives: www.togetherforshortlives.org.uk
The Canadian Network for Palliative Care for Children: www.cnpcc.ca
International Children's Palliative Care Network (ICPCN): www.icpcn.org.uk/
Children's International Project on Palliative/Hospice Services (ChIPPS): www.nhpco.org
Initiative for Pediatric Palliative Care: www.ippcweb.org/
The Royal Children's Hospital, Melbourne, PPC programme: www.rch.org.au/rch_palliative/index.cfm?doc_id=1650

References

Amery, J. (2009) *Children's Palliative Care in Africa*. Oxford University Press, Oxford.

Anghelescu, D.L., Faughnan, L.G., Baker, J.N., Yang, J. and Kane, J.R. (2010) Use of epidural and peripheral nerve blocks at the end of life in children and young adults with cancer: The collaboration between a pain service and a palliative care service. *Paediatric Anaesthesia* 20(12), 1070–1077.

Anghelescu, D.L., Faughnan, L.G., Hankins, G.M., Ward, D.A. and Oakes, L.L. (2011) Methadone use in children and young adults at a cancer center: A retrospective study. *Journal of Opioid Management* 7(5), 353–361.

Association for Children with Life-threatening or Terminal Conditions and their Families (ACT) (2009) *A Guide to the Development of Children's Palliative Care Services*, 3rd edition. ACT, Bristol.

Bartell, A.S. and Kissane, D.W. (2005) Issues in pediatric palliative care: Understanding families. *Journal of Palliative Care* 21(3), 165–172.

Bergstraesser, E. (2013) Pediatric palliative care: When quality of life becomes the main focus of treatment. *European Journal of Pediatrics* 172(2), 139–150.

Bishop, F.L., Prescott, P., Chan, Y.K., Saville, J., von Elm, E., and Lewith, G.T. (2010) Prevalence of complementary medicine use in pediatric cancer: A systematic review. *Pediatrics* 125(4), 768–776.

Brook, L. and Hain, R. (2008) Predicting death in children. *Archives of Disease in Childhood* 93(12), 1067–1070.

Brown, M.R. and Sourkes, B. (2006) Psychotherapy in pediatric palliative care. *Child and Adolescent Psychiatric Clinics of North America* 15, 585–596.

Buttle, S.G., McMurtry, M. and Marshall, S. (2011) Massage for pain relief in pediatric palliative care: Potential benefits and challenges. *Pediatric Pain Letter* 13(3), 24–29.

Cardenas-Turanzas, M., Tovalín-Ahumada, H., Carrillo, M.T., Paez-Aguirre, S. and Elting, L. (2008) The place of death of children with cancer in the metropolitan areas of Mexico. *Journal of Palliative Medicine* 11(7), 973–979.

Carroll, J.M., Torkildson, C. and Winsness, J.S. (2007) Issues related to providing quality pediatric palliative care in the community. *Pediatric Clinics of North America* 54(5), 813–827.

Chong, P.H., Chan, M.Y. and Yusri, L.I. (2012) Do children die? A retrospective review of deaths in a children's hospital. *Singapore Medical Journal* 53(3), 192–195.

Collins, J.J., Byrnes, M.E., Dunkel, I.J. et al. (2000) The measurement of symptoms in children with cancer. *Journal of Pain and Symptom Management* 19(5), 363–377.

Collins, J.J., Berde, C.B. and Frost, J.A. (2011) Pain assessment and management. In: *Textbook of Interdisciplinary Pediatric Palliative Care* (eds J. Wolfe, P.S. Hinds and B.M. Sourkes), pp. 284–299. Elsevier Saunders, Philadelphia.

Craig, F., Abu-Saad, H., Benini, F. et al. EAPC Taskforce Steering Group (2007) IMPaCCT: Standards for paediatric palliative care in Europe. *European Journal of Palliative Care* 14(3), 109–114.

Davies, B., Sehring, S.A., Partridge, J.C. et al (2008a) Barriers to palliative care for children: Perceptions of pediatric health care providers. *Pediatrics* 121(2), 282–288.

Davies, D., DeVlaming, D. and Haines, C. (2008b) Methadone analgesia for children with advanced cancer. *Pediatric Blood Cancer.* 51(3), 393–397.

Devanney, C., Bradley, S. and Together for Short Lives (2012) Count Me In: Children's Hospice Service Provision 2011/12. Available from: http://childhospiceuk.dumu.org.uk (accessed January 2013).

Dupuis, L.L., Taddio, A., Kerr, E.N., Kelly, A. and MacKeigan, L. (2006) Development and validation of the pediatric nausea assessment tool for use in children receiving antineoplastic agents. *Pharmacotherapy* 26(9), 1221–1231.

Dussel, V., Kreicbergs, U., Hilden, J.M., Watterson, J., Moore, C., Turner, B.G., Weeks, J.C. and Wolfe, J. (2009) Looking beyond where children die: determinants and effects of planning a child's location of death. *Journal of Pain and Symptom Management* 37(1), 33–43.

Ellershaw, J. and Ward, C. (2003) Care of the dying patient: the last hours or days of life. *British Medical Journal* 326, 30–34.

Feudtner, C., Kang, T.I., Hexem, K.R., Friedrichsdorf, S.J., Osenga, K., Siden, H., Friebert, S.E., Hays, R.M., Dussel, V., and Wolfe, J. (2011) Pediatric palliative care patients: a prospective multicenter cohort study. *Pediatrics* 127(6), 1094–1101.

Foster, T.L., Lafond, D.A., Reggio, C. and Hinds, P.S. (2010) Pediatric palliative care in childhood cancer nursing: from diagnosis to cure or end of life. *Seminars in Oncology Nursing* 26(4), 205–221.

Fraser, J., Harris, N., Berringer, A.J., Prescott, H. and Finlay, F. (2010) Advanced care planning in children with life-limiting conditions - the Wishes Document. *Archives of Disease in Childhood* 95(2), 79–82.

Fraser, L.K., Miller, M., Draper, E.S., McKinney, P.A. and Parslow, R.C. (2011) Place of death and palliative care following discharge from paediatric intensive care units. *Archives of Disease in Childhood* 96(12): 1195–1198.

Fraser, L.K., Miller, M., Hain, R., Norman, P., Aldridge, J., McKinney, P.A. and Parslow R.C. (2012) Rising national prevalence of life-limiting conditions in children in England. *Pediatrics* 129(4), e923–e929.

Friebert, S. (2009) NHPCO *Facts and Figures: Pediatric Palliative and Hospice Care in America.* National Hospice and Palliative Care Organization, Alexandria, VA. Available from: www.nhpco.org/sites/default/files/public/quality/Pediatric_Facts-Figures.pdf (accessed February 2013).

Friedrichsdorf, S.J. (2010) Pain management in children with advanced cancer and during end-of-life care. *Pediatric Hematolgy and Oncology* 27(4): 257–261.

Friedrichsdorf, S.J. (2011) Palliative care for children in paediatric neurology. *Neuropädiatrie in Klinik und Praxis* 10(1), 5–6.

Friedrichsdorf, S.J., Drake, R. and Webster, M.L. (2011) Gastrointestinal symptoms In: *Textbook of Interdisciplinary Pediatric Palliative Care* (eds J. Wolfe, P.S. Hinds and B.M. Sourkes), pp. 311–334. Elsevier Saunders, Philadelphia.

Harlos, M.S., Stenekes, S., Lambert, D., Hohl, C. and Chochinov, H.M. (2012) Intranasal fentanyl in the palliative care of newborns and infants. *Journal of Pain and Symptom Management,* online early.

Heath, J.A., Clarke, N.E., Donath, S.M., McCarthy, M., Anderson, V.A. and Wolfe, J. (2010) Symptoms and suffering at the end of life in children with cancer: An Australian perspective. *Medical Journal of Australia* 192(2), 71–75.

Heath, J.A., Oh, L.J., Clarke, N.E. and Wolfe, J. (2012) Complementary and alternative medicine use in children with cancer at the end of life. *Journal of Palliative Medicine* 15(11), 1218–1221.

Hendricks-Ferguson, V. (2008) Physical symptoms of children receiving pediatric hospice care at home during the last week of life. *Oncology Nursing Forum* 35(6), E108–E115.

Hynson, J.L., Aroni, R., Bauld, C. and Sawyer, S.M. (2006) Research with bereaved parents: A question of how not why. *Palliative Medicine* 20, 805–811.

Kane, J.R. and Baker, J.N. (2012) Quality improvement. In: *Oxford Textbook of Palliative Care for Children* (eds A. Goldman, R. Hain and S. Liben), 2nd edition, pp. 430–440. Oxford University Press, Oxford.

Keene, E., Hutton, N., Hall, B. and Rushton, C. (2010) Bereavement debriefing sessions: An intervention to support health care professionals in managing their grief after the death of a patient. *Pediatric Nursing* 36(4), 185–189.

Kelly, K.M. (2007) Complementary and alternative medicines for use in supportive care in pediatric cancer. *Supportive Care in Cancer* 15, 457–460.

Kersun, L.S. and Shemesh, E. (2007) Depression and anxiety in children at the end of life. *Pediatric Clinics of North America* 54, 691–708.

Kippenberg, J., and Thomas, L. (2010). *Needless Pain: Government Failure to Provide Palliative Care for Children in Kenya.* Human Rights Watch. Available from: www.hrw.org/reports/2010/09/09/needless-pain-0 (accessed February 2013).

Klepping, L. (2012) Total pain: A reflective case study addressing the experience of a terminally ill adolescent. *International Journal of Palliative Nursing* 18(3), 121–127.

Klick, J.C., and Hauer, J. (2010) Pediatric palliative care. *Current Problems in Pediatric and Adolescent Health Care* 40(6), 120–151.

Knapp, C., Madden, V., Wang, H., Curtis, C., Sloyer, P. and Shenkman, E. (2009) Music therapy in an integrated pediatric palliative care program. *American Journal of Hospice and Palliative Care* 26(6), 449–455.

Knapp, C. and Madden, V. (2010) Conducting outcomes research in pediatric palliative care. *American Journal of Hospice and Palliative Care* 27(4), 277–281.

Knapp, C., Woodworth, L., Wright, M. et al. (2011) Pediatric palliative care provision around the world: A systematic review. *Pediatric Blood Cancer* 57, 361–368.

Kuttner, L. (2007) Talking with families when their children are dying. *Medical Principles and Practice* 16(Suppl 1), 16–20.

Larcher, V. and Carnevale, F. (2012) Ethics. In: *The Oxford Textbook of Palliative Care for Children* (eds A. Goldman, R. Hain and S. Liben), 2nd edition, pp 35–46. Oxford University Press, Oxford.

Lavy, V. (2007) Presenting symptoms and signs in children referred for palliative care in Malawi. *Palliative Medicine* 21, 333–339.

Lindenfelser, K.J., Hense, C. and McFerran, K. (2012) Music therapy in pediatric palliative care: Family-centered care to enhance quality of life. *American Journal of Hospice and Palliative Care* 29(3), 219–226.

Malcolm, C., Knighting, K., Forbat, L. and Kearney, N. (2009) Prioritization of future research topics for children's hospice care by its key stakeholders: A Delphi study. *Palliative Medicine* 23(5), 398–405.

McCulloch, R. and Collins, J.J. (2006) Pain in children who have life-limiting conditions. *Child and Adolescent Psychiatric Clinics of North America* 15(3), 657–682.

McCulloch, R. (2012) Pharmacological approaches to pain. 3: Adjuvants for neuropathic and bone pain. In: *Oxford Textbook of Palliative Care for Children* (eds A. Goldman, R. Hain and S. Liben), 2nd edition, pp. 247–259. Oxford University Press, Oxford.

McGrath, P.J., Pianosi, P.T., Unruh, A.M. and Buckley, C.P. (2005) Dalhousie dyspnea scales: Construct and content validity of pictorial scales for measuring dyspnea. *BMC Pediatrics*, 5, 33.

McNamara-Goodger, K. and Feudtner, C. (2012) History and epidemiology. In: *Oxford Textbook of Palliative Care for Children* (eds A. Goldman, R. Hain and S. Liben), 2nd edition, pp. 3–12. Oxford University Press, Oxford.

Mellor, C., Heckford, E., and Frost, J. (2011) Developments in paediatric palliative care. *Paediatrics and Child Health* 22(3), 115–120.

Mongeau, S. and Liben, S. (2007) Participatory research in pediatric palliative care: Benefits and challenges. *Journal of Palliative Care* 23(1), 5–13.

Moody, K., Daswani, D., Abrahams, B. and Santizo, R. (2010) Yoga for pain and anxiety in pediatric hematology-oncology patients: Case series and review of the literature. *Journal of the Society for Integrative Oncology* 8(3), 95–105.

Office for National Statistics (2010) Mortality in the United Kingdom 2010. Available from: www.ons.gov.uk/ons/rel/mortality-ageing/mortality-in-the-united-kingdom/mortality-in-the-united-kingdom–2010/mortality-in-the-uk-2010.html (accessed January 2013).

Poltorak, D.Y. and Benore, E. (2006) Cognitive-behavioral interventions for physical symptom management in pediatric palliative medicine. *Child and Adolescent Psychiatric Clinics of North America* 15, 683–691.

Puckey, M. and Bush, A. (2011) 'Passage to Paradise' ethics and end-of-life decisions in children. *Paediatric Respiratory Reviews* 12(2), 139–143.

Rapoport, A. (2009) Addressing ethical concerns regarding pediatric palliative care research. *Archives of Pediatric and Adolescent Medicine* 163(8), 688–691.

Ramnarayan, P., Craig, F., Petros, A. and Pierce, C. (2007) Characteristics of deaths occurring in hospitalised children: Changing trends. *Journal of Medical Ethics* 33, 255–260.

Reddy, S.R., and Singh, H.R. (2010) Chest pain in children and adolescents. *Pediatric Reviews* 31(1): e1–e9.

Regnard, C. and Dean, M. (2010) *A Guide to Symptom Relief in Palliative Care*. Radcliffe Publishing, Oxford.

Rheingans, J.I. (2007) A systematic review of nonpharmacologic adjunctive therapies for symptom management in children with cancer. *Journal of Pediatric Oncology Nursing* 24(2), 81–94.

Rourke, M.T. (2007) Compassion fatigue in pediatric palliative care providers. *Pediatric Clinics of North America* 54, 631–644.

Russell, C. and Smart, S. (2007) Guided imagery and distraction therapy in paediatric hospice care. *Paediatric Nursing* 19(2), 24–25.

Sands, D., Repetto, T., Dupont, L.J., Korzeniewska-Eksterowicz, A., Catastini, P. and Madge, S. (2011) End-of-life care for patients with cystic fibrosis. *Journal of Cystic Fibrosis* 10(Suppl 2), S37–S44.

Santucci, G. and Mack, J.W. (2007) Common gastrointestinal symptoms in pediatric palliative care: Nausea, vomiting, constipation, anorexia, cachexia. *Pediatric Clinics of North America* 54, 673–689.

Sencer, S.F. and Kelly, K.M. (2007) Complementary and alternative therapies in pediatric oncology. *Pediatric Clinics of North America* 54(6), 1043–1060; xiii.

Sermet-Gaudelus, I., De Villartay, P., de Dreuzy, P. et al. (2009) Pain in children and adults with cystic fibrosis: A comparative study. *Journal of Pain and Symptom Management* 38(2), 281–290.

Shah, A., Diggens, N., Stiller, C., Murphy, D., Passmore, J. and Murphy, M.F. (2011) Place of death and hospital care for children who died of cancer in England, 1999–2006. *European Journal of Cancer* 47(14), 2175–2181.

Shelton, J. and Jackson, G.P. (2011) Palliative care and pediatric surgery. *Surgical Clinics of North America* 91(2), 419–428, ix.

Siden, H., Tucker, T., Derman, S. et al. (2009) Pediatric enteral feeding intolerance: A new prognosticator for children with life-limiting illness? *Journal of Palliative Care* 25(3), 213–217.

Sourkes, B., Frankel, L., Brown, M. et al. (2005) Food, toys and love: Pediatric palliative care. *Current Problems in Pediatric and Adolescent Health Care* 35, 350–386.

Steele, R., Bosma, H., Johnston, M.F. et al. (2008) Research priorities in pediatric palliative care: A Delphi study. *Journal of Palliative Care* 24(4), 229–239.

Theunissen, J.M., Hoogerbrugge, P.M., van Achterberg, T., Prins, J.B., Vernooij-Dassen, M.J. and van den Ende, C.H. (2007) Symptoms in the palliative phase of children with cancer. *Pediatric Blood Cancer*, 49(2),160–165.

Together for Short Lives (2012) What is children's palliative care? Available from: www.togetherforshortlives.org.uk/families/faqs (accessed January 2013).

Tomlinson, D., Hesser, T., Ethier, M.C. and Sung, L. (2011) Complementary and alternative medicine use in pediatric cancer reported during palliative phase of disease. *Supportive Care in Cancer*, 19(11), 1857–1863.

Tucker, T.L., Samant, R.S. and Fitzgibbon, E.J. (2010) Knowledge and utilization of palliative radiotherapy by pediatric oncologists. *Current Oncology* 17(1), 48–55.

Tzuh Tang, S., Hung, Y.N., Liu, T.W. et al. (2011) Pediatric end-of-life care for Taiwanese children who died as a result of cancer from 2001 through 2006. *Journal of Clinical Oncology* 29(7), 890–894.

United Nations Joint Programme on HIV/AIDS (UNAIDS) (2012) Global Report: UNAIDS Report on the Global AIDS Epidemic. Available from: www.unaids.org/en/resources/documents/2012/ (accessed February 2013).

Van Breeman, C. (2009) Using play therapy in paediatric palliative care: Listening to the story and caring for the body. *International Journal of Palliative Nursing* 15, 510–514.

Varni, J.W., Burwinkle, T.M., Katz, E.R., Meeske, K. and Dickinson, P. (2002) The PedsQL in pediatric cancer: Reliability and validity of the Pediatric Quality of Life Inventory Generic Core Scales, Multidimensional Fatigue Scale, and Cancer Module. *Cancer* 94(7), 2090–2106.

Vickers, J. and Chrastek, J. (2012) Place of care. In: *Oxford Textbook of Palliative Care for Children* (eds A. Goldman, R. Hain and S. Liben), 2nd edition, pp. 391–401. Oxford University Press, Oxford.

Vickers, J., Thompson, A., Collins, G.S., Childs, M. and Hain, R. (2007) Place and provision of palliative care for children with progressive cancer. *Journal of Clinical Oncology* 25(28), 4472–4476.

Wellesley, H. and Jenkins, I.A. (2009) Withholding and withdrawing life-sustaining treatment in children. *Paediatric Anaesthesia* 19(10), 972–978.

Wender, E. and the Committee on Psychosocial Aspects of Child and Family Health (2012) Supporting the family after the death of a child. *Pediatrics* 130(6), 1164–1169.

Widger, K., Davies, D., Drouin, D.J. et al. (2007) Pediatric patients receiving palliative care in Canada: Results of a multicenter review. *Archives of Pediatrics and Adolescent Medicine* 161(6), 597–602.

Williams, P.D., Williams, A.R., Kelly, K.P. et al. (2012) A symptom checklist for children with cancer: The Therapy-Related Symptom Checklist–Children. *Cancer Nursing* 35(2), 89–98.

Wolfe, J. (2011) Easing distress when death is near. In: *Textbook of Interdisciplinary Pediatric Palliative Care* (eds J. Wolfe, P.S. Hinds and B.M. Sourkes), pp. 368–384. Elsevier Saunders, Philadelphia.

Wolfe, J. and Siden, H. (2012) Research in pediatric palliative care. In: *Oxford Textbook of Palliative Care for Children* (eds A. Goldman, R. Hain and S. Liben), 2nd edition, pp. 441–457. Oxford University Press, Oxford.

Wolff, J., Robert, R., Sommerer, A. and Volz-Fleckenstein, M. (2010) Impact of a pediatric palliative care program. *Pediatric Blood and Cancer* 54(2), 279–283.

Wolfe, J. Hinds, P.S. and Sourkes, B.M. (2011) The language of pediatric palliative care. In: *Textbook of Interdisciplinary Pediatric Palliative Care* (eds J. Wolfe, P.S. Hinds and B.M. Sourkes), pp. 3–6. Elsevier Saunders, Philadelphia.

World Health Organization (1998) *Cancer Pain Relief and Palliative Care in Children*. World Health Organization, Geneva.

World Health Organization (2006) *Definition of palliative care*. Available from: www.who.int/cancer/palliative/definition/en/ (accessed January 2013).

World Health Organization (2012a) Children: reducing mortality. Fact sheet No.178. Available from: www.who.int/mediacentre/factsheets/fs178/en/index.html (accessed January 2013).

World Health Organization (2012b) *WHO Guidelines on the pharmacological treatment of persisting pain in children with medical illnesses*. World Health Organization, Geneva.

Wrede-Seaman, L. (2005) *Pediatric Pain and Symptom Management Algorithms for Palliative Care*. Intellicard Inc, Washington.

Wusthoff, C.J., Shellhaas, R.A. and Licht, D.J. (2007) Management of common neurologic symptoms in pediatric palliative care: Seizures, agitation and spasticity. *Pediatric Clinics of North America* 54, 709–733.

Zaki, B.I. (2005) Palliative and pain medicine: Radiation oncology. *Techniques in Regional Anesthesia and Pain Management* 9, 177–183.

Zernikow, B. Michel, E. and Anderson, B. (2007) Transdermal fentanyl in childhood and adolescence: A comprehensive literature review. *Journal of Pain* 8(3), 187–207.

Zernikow, B., Michel, E., Craig, F. and Anderson, B.J. (2009) Pediatric palliative care: Use of opioids for the management of pain. *Paediatric Drugs* 11(2), 129–151.

Zinner, S.E. (2008) The use of pediatric advance directives: A tool for palliative care physicians. *American Journal of Hospice and Palliative Care* 25(6), 427–430.

CHAPTER 10

Management of Painful Procedures

Kathy Reid

Paediatric Chronic Pain Program, Stollery Children's Hospital, Canada

Alison Twycross

Department for Children's Nursing and Children's Pain Management,
London South Bank University, United Kingdom

Dianne Tuterra

Child Life Department, Stollery Children's Hospital, Canada

Introduction

This chapter discusses best practice in the management of procedural pain in children, including the importance of planning and preparation. The chapter outlines the evidence for pharmacological interventions that can be used to manage procedural pain with a particular focus on needle-related pain, pain related to cancer investigations, immunisation pain, and pain associated with burns wound care. The management of procedural pain in neonates will also be discussed. Physical and psychological interventions are outlined briefly as they are discussed in depth in Chapter 5. The principles of procedural pain management apply to all healthcare settings where children are cared for including the emergency department (ED).

Procedure-Related Pain: Definition and Prevalence

Definition

'Procedures include all medical interventions which have the potential to cause pain, or to cause distress or anxiety' (Royal Children's Hospital, Melbourne 2011)

Managing Pain in Children: A Clinical Guide for Nurses and Healthcare Professionals, Second Edition.
Edited by Alison Twycross, Stephanie Dowden, and Jennifer Stinson.
© 2014 John Wiley & Sons, Ltd. Published 2014 by John Wiley & Sons, Ltd.

Children in hospitals undergo painful procedures on a regular basis. In a recent study of children ($n = 3822$) in paediatric hospitals in Canada, 78% of patients had experienced at least one painful procedure in the previous 24 hours (Stevens et al. 2011). In 2010, an estimated 109 million infants received the three diphtheria and tetanus immunisation series (World Health Organization [WHO] 2011). Indeed, children in developed nations receive up to 18 separate needles for immunisation before they are 16 years old (Curtis et al. 2012). Despite this, and the evidence to guide practice being readily available, these painful procedures are not always managed as effectively as they could be:

- Few children undergoing procedures such as venepuncture, intravenous (IV) cannulation, capillary sampling, nasogastric tube placement or urethral catheterisation received any pain-relieving interventions (Maclaren and Cohen 2007).
- Pain management strategies for lumbar punctures remain unsatisfactory (Ellis et al. 2007; Fein et al. 2010; Gorchynski and McLaughlin 2011; Hoyle et al. 2011).
- Needle phobia is a consequence of undertreated procedural pain and affects up to 10% of the population (Zempsky 2008a).

> Children continue to experience painful procedures without adequate management despite a large body of evidence and the availability of clinical guidelines on how to manage procedural pain.

Common paediatric painful procedures are outlined in Box 10.1. Several best practice guidelines exist in relation to managing procedural pain in children (Box 10.2).

Why is it Important to Manage Procedural Pain Effectively?

Much is known about the existence of pain response in early life, and the long-term consequences of unmanaged pain (Taddio et al. 1997; Grunau et al. 2009). These issues are discussed in more depth in Chapter 1. It is worth noting that in the context of procedural pain there is an increasing body of evidence suggesting that children's

---

BOX 10.1

Common paediatric painful procedures

- Immunisations
- Venepuncture
- Capillary sampling
- Intravenous cannulation
- Laceration repair
- Fracture reduction
- Diagnostic tests
- Dressing changes or wound care
- Insertion or removal of tubes (e.g. urinary catheters, nasogastric tubes, drains)
- Subcutaneous reservoir access (e.g. port-a-cath®)
- Lumbar puncture (LP)
- Bone marrow aspiration (BMA)

BOX 10.2

Best practice guidelines for procedural pain management

Association of Paediatric Anaesthetists of Great Britain and Ireland (APA) (2012) *Good Practice in Postoperative and Procedural Pain*, 2nd edition. Available from: http://onlinelibrary.wiley .com/doi/10.1111/pan.2012.22.issue-s1/issuetoc#group1

Czarnecki, M. et al. (2011) for the **American Society for Pain Management Nursing**. *Best Practice Guidelines on Procedural Pain Management*. Available from: www.aspmn.org/ Organization/documents/ProceduralPainMgt.PositionStatement.pdf

Fein, J.A. et al. (2012) for the **American Academy of Pediatrics**. *Relief of Pain and Anxiety in Pediatric Patients in the Emergency Medical Systems*. Available from: http://pediatrics .aappublications.org/content/130/5/e1391.full.pdf+html

Royal Australasian College of Physicians Paediatrics and Child Health Division (RACP) (2006) Guideline Statement: Management of procedure-related pain in children and adolescents. *Journal of Paediatrics and Child Health* **12**(1), S2–S29. Available from: http://onlinelibrary .wiley.com/doi/10.1111/j.1440-1754.2006.00798_2.x/abstract?systemMessage=Wiley+Onlin e+Library+will+be+disrupted+on+8+December+from+10%3A00-12%3A00+GMT+%2805% 3A00-07%3A00+EST%29+for+essential+maintenance

---

memories (past experiences) of pain affect how they react to future painful interventions (von Baeyer et al. 2004; Summer et al. 2007; Noel et al. 2012).

The effective management of pain is what matters to children:

- Children ($n = 44$), aged 4–11 years, describe needle-related pain as one of the worst kinds of pain they experienced when in hospital (Kortesluoma and Nikkonen 2004).
- Adolescents with a chronic illness ($n = 988$) ranked not having too much pain or discomfort as most important when hospitalised (van Staa et al. 2011).
- Children with cancer report experiencing more pain from procedures and cancer treatment than from the disease itself (Blount et al. 2006; Zernikow et al. 2006).

Managing procedural pain effectively is clearly important to children. Children's first experience with needle pain or other painful procedures sets the stage for future interventions.

Factors that Influence a Child's Response to Painful Procedures

A child's ability to cope with painful procedure is based on many variables. These include the child's:

- age and developmental level (McCarthy et al. 2010; Esteve and Marquina-Aponte 2012);
- temperament (Rocha et al. 2009);
- culture (Kristjansdottir et al. 2012);
- ability to cope in new and challenging situations (McCarthy et al. 2010);
- prior healthcare experiences and previous exposure to painful procedures (von Baeyer et al. 2004; Noel et al. 2012).

Parental anxiety appears to increase children's anxieties and affects their ability to cope with painful procedures (McCarthy et al. 2010; Bearden et al. 2012). (See Chapter 3 for additional information about the factors that impact on children's experiences of pain.)

Managing Procedural Pain: General Principles

Managing procedure-related pain requires the combined use of pharmacological, physical and psychological strategies (Czarnecki et al. 2011; Curtis et al. 2012). Details about key steps that should be followed before, during and after the procedure are now outlined.

Before the procedure

Assessment

A thorough assessment is essential to determine the amount of pain, fear and anxiety the procedure is likely to invoke (McMurtry et al. 2011). This assessment should determine the level of anticipatory pain, anxiety and fear as well as the child's current pain status. Pain assessment tools are described in Chapter 6. The FLACC scale (see Chapter 6) has been found to be particularly useful for assessing pain during painful procedures (Nilsson et al. 2008; Babl et al. 2012). The revised-FLACC can be used for children too young to use self-report or when self-report might be invalid, for example, due to a fear of needles. There is currently no gold standard tool for assessing children's fear and anxiety (Nilsson and Renning 2012). Some of the tools available are outlined in Box 10.3.

Preparing the child and parents

Children and their families benefit from advance knowledge and having the opportunity to prepare themselves for painful procedures (Jaaniste et al. 2007a; APA 2012). Children are less upset by known stressors than by unknown ones, and effective preparation has shown to be a successful means of promoting coping behaviour and decreasing stress levels (Jaaniste et al. 2007a; Gursky et al. 2010). A play therapist (child life specialist) can help prepare children for procedures and support the healthcare team in setting the stage for a successful intervention (American Academy of Pediatrics [AAP] 2006; Bandstra et al. 2008). If there is no play therapist this role should be undertaken by nursing staff or another healthcare professional.

> Further information about the role of play therapists (child life specialists) can be seen in:
> A day in the life of a Child Life Specialist: www.youtube.com/watch?v=OrFzwpAhijE
> BC Children's Child Life Specialists: www.youtube.com/watch?v=IJumvoJmzTl

Information needs to be provided in a developmentally appropriate manner and timeframe to allow the child the opportunity to process information, while not increasing anxiety by giving them too much time to dwell on it (Jaaniste et al. 2007a; Cohen 2008; Hockenberry et al. 2011). The appropriate timeframe will vary depending on

---

BOX 10.3

Tools for assessing a child's fear and anxiety

- State-Trait Anxiety Inventory (Marteau and Bekker 1992)
- Facial Affective Scale (McGrath et al. 1996)
- Multidimensional Anxiety Scale for Children (March et al. 1997)
- Child Pain Anxiety Symptoms Scale (Page et al. 2010)
- Children's Fear Scale (McMurtry et al. 2011)

Table 10.1 Information needs of children

Age/developmental stage	Type of information
Pre-school-age and young children	• Include information about what they will see, hear, smell and feel during procedure, e.g. let them know it will feel cold when their skin is cleaned, that when the needle is inserted it 'will pinch for a little while but this will go away'
School-aged children	• Provide clear concrete explanations, e.g. 'it may tingle', 'you might notice a cold feeling when the medicine goes in' • Discuss why the procedure is necessary and how long it will take • Use analogies to explain things – e.g. describing a cannula as being 'like a plastic straw that is in your hand' • Explain function and operation of medical equipment in concrete terms • Allow medical play with equipment beforehand • Allow time before and after the procedure for questions and discussion
Adolescents	• Discuss why the procedure is necessary and how the results will be used • Explain long-term consequences of procedures including information about body systems working together • Discuss how the procedure may affect appearance (e.g. scar) and what can be done to minimise this • Emphasise any physical benefits of the procedure • Use models or computer images to aid understanding

Source: Jaaniste et al. (2007a); Cohen (2008); Hockenberry et al. (2011)

BOX 10.4

Timing of physical and psychological interventions before a procedure

• Preparation: 60 minutes
• Relaxation: 30 minutes
• Breathing: 2 minutes
• Distraction: 2 minutes
• Encouraging coping: 2 minutes
• Comfort positioning: 2 minutes

Source: Zempsky (2008a)

---

the age of the child and the type of procedure to be undertaken (Jaaniste et al. 2007a; Cohen 2008; Zempsky 2008a).

The information provided to children should include sensory information (i.e. what the procedure will feel like) as well as information about why the procedure is necessary (Jaaniste et al. 2007b; Cohen 2008; Hockenberry et al. 2011). The information needs of children of different ages are outlined in Table 10.1. There is very little information available about the appropriate timings for providing children with information prior to a painful procedure. Suggested timings for physical and psychological interventions before a procedure can be seen in Box 10.4. Some of the actions healthcare professionals can take to help children and parents prepare for a painful procedure are outlined in Box 10.5. How children perceive the cause and effect of pain at different developmental stages is discussed in Chapter 3.

BOX 10.5

Helping children cope with pain: What health professionals can do

- Give step-by-step information about what will happen during the procedure, including what the child will see, hear and feel, and why the procedure is necessary
- Provide children with coping strategies they can use during the procedure
- Children need truthful information to build trust in the healthcare professionals working with them
- Use age- or developmentally appropriate language and avoid medical jargon
- Use medical play with young children - this allows them to use the equipment and adopt different roles such as the nurse or doctor
- Avoid making promises that you cannot keep, e.g. *'it won't hurt'* or *'it feels like a mosquito bite'*
- Avoid high anxiety words such as *pain, hurt, cut, needle* or *shot*
- Use words such as *poking, freezing* and *squeezing* instead
- Do not suggest that the procedure will definitely hurt
- Be aware of possible misinterpretations of words and phrases such as *dye* or *put to sleep*
- Address children's concerns (e.g. *taking all my blood*)
- Consider using books or web-based resources describing the procedure for the child and/or parent

Adapted from Young (2005); Jaaniste et al. (2007a); Kuttner (2010)

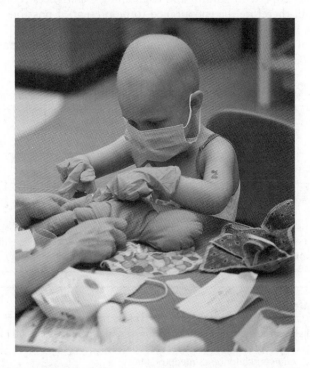

Figure 10.1   An example of medical play prior to a bone marrow aspiration.

The use of teaching dolls and real medical supplies to play with and act out the procedure helps children's understanding, enables expression of feelings and may clarify any misconceptions (Figure 10.1) (RACP 2006; Hockenberry et al. 2011). A variety of coping techniques should be selected beforehand and offered to children during the procedure. These are discussed in Chapter 5.

Children should be given choices that are appropriate for their age and the situation (Hockenberry et al. 2011). They should be able to choose the person to comfort them, which distraction item they want, and if possible where the procedure will be performed. Often a range of distraction items is needed, especially for younger children. (See Chapter 5 for more information about distraction.) Provide choices whenever possible without creating a situation where the procedure cannot be performed. For example, children can choose which arm is used for venepuncture, but should not be asked 'do you want a blood test?'

Practice point

Children should be given choices appropriate for their age and situation. This will increase their sense of control and help them cope with the painful procedure.

Involving parents in painful procedures

Over the past decade several studies have explored how parents can help support their child during painful procedures. We now know that:

- Children have identified parental presence as the single most important factor that helps them cope with painful and frightening experiences (Polkki et al. 2003). Parents should, therefore, be encouraged to be present, if possible, but should not be made to feel guilty if they are unable to stay.
- Parents' use of language when supporting their child through a painful procedure is important (Cohen 2008; McMurtry et al. 2010).

Examples of suggested language to use during painful procedures can be found in: Cohen, L. (2008) Behavioural approaches to anxiety and pain management for pediatric venous access. *Pediatrics* **122**(S3), S134–S139.

Practice point

Parents often want to reassure their child during a procedure but this may increase the child's distress.
Parents should be taught language for supporting their child through a painful procedure.
Parents should be instructed to use coping-promoting behaviours (e.g. distraction, encouragement) and to avoid distress-promoting behaviours (e.g. reassurance, sympathy).

Additional information

Information to help parents prepare their child for painful procedures can be found at:
www.youtube.com/watch?v=x32NIZWXym0&noredirect=1
www.med.umich.edu/yourchild/topics/medproc.htm
www.kidshealth.org.nz/childrens-painful-procedures-and-operations-how-can-parents-help
www.sch.edu.au/health/factsheets/joint/?painful_procedures_and_operations.htm

---

During the procedure

The following need to be considered when undertaking a painful procedure:

- The environment in which the procedure happens is important (RACP 2006; APA 2012).

- Some hospitals have assigned treatment rooms where children's procedures are completed. These rooms, if available, should be used wherever possible (Young 2005).
- Children and families in hospital need to have safe places where procedures will never be performed, such as play areas. For many children, their safe place needs to be their bed so procedures should be avoided while they are in their bed (Young 2005).
- A quiet, calm environment with as few people and voices as possible is optimal; several people giving information can lead to confusion for the child and family (APA 2012).
- Allow children to have their comfort items (e.g. favourite stuffed animal or comfort blanket) (Young 2005).
- If parents have chosen to be actively involved they can support their child by coaching, using distraction techniques, and assisting with comfort positioning (Czarnecki et al. 2011).
- Parents can encourage positive behaviours with phrases like 'You are doing a great job of staying still' or 'I like the way you let us know how you are feeling' (Cohen 2008; McMurtry et al. 2010).
- If the child becomes overly distressed during a procedure it should be discontinued until more appropriate management interventions, including the use of sedation, can be implemented (Czarnecki et al. 2011; APA 2012).
- The chosen distraction techniques should continue for the duration of the procedure (Zempsky 2008a).

Restraining a child and therapeutic holding
- Restraining a child for a painful procedure should be a last resort and only used in emergency situations. The need to restrain a child suggests a lack of preparation and that sufficient pain and anxiety-relieving interventions have not been used (Royal College of Nursing [RCN] 2010).
- Therapeutic holding or comfort holding includes immobilisation, which may be by splinting, or by using limited force. It may be a method of helping children, with their permission, to manage a painful procedure quickly or effectively (RCN 2010).
- Clinicians should be aware that therapeutic holding if applied inappropriately and without the child's consent or assent can result in the child or young person feeling out of control, anxious and distressed (Lambrenos and McArthur 2003).

Additional information

The RCN in the UK has written a guideline on *Restrictive physical intervention and therapeutic holding for children and young people* (RCN 2010). This is available from: www.rcn.org .uk/__data/assets/pdf_file/0016/312613/003573.pdf

---

After the procedure
Following the procedure it is important to:

- acknowledge the successful completion of the procedure with children;
- celebrate their achievement with validation of positive behaviours to build confidence for future procedures;

- answer any questions the child and family might have about what happened and provide honest explanations of what will happen next;
- discuss with the child and family what went well and whether any changes need to be made to the comfort plan for future procedures;
- use positive reinforcement.

(Cohen 2008; Czarnecki et al. 2011)

Using medical play after the procedure can help the child work through what has happened to them (Oakes 2011).

Additional information

Information about medical play can be found at:
www.chop.edu/service/child-life-education-and-creative-arts-therapy/childrens-needs-and
-helping-kids-cope/goals-of-medical-play-to-ease-anxiety-during-medical-experiences.html
www.choc.org/childlife/index.cfm?id=P00598

Practice point

Not all children are able to be brave when faced with highly stressful situations; removing the focus from bravery to achievement assists with mastery for future procedures.
Some hospitals have prizes or certificates for children to choose after a painful procedure.
Many children's hospitals participate in programmes such as *treasure beads*, which allow children to choose a bead each time they undergo a painful medical procedure, and create bead strings. (For additional information see: www.sickkids.ca/WomensAuxiliary/Our-programs/bravery-bead-program/index.html).
Medical play can give the child a voice to express any fears and misconceptions they may have about their experience.

An algorithm illustrating how procedural pain should be managed is provided in Figure 10.2.

Using Nitrous Oxide to Manage Procedural Pain

Nitrous oxide is an anaesthetic gas that provides analgesia, anxiolysis and sedation via action at GABA and NMDA receptors.
Once inhaled it provides rapid onset analgesia (within three to five breaths) as well as rapid offset once discontinued.
Nitrous oxide is available as compressed gas in cylinders or via medical gas supply in hospital. It comes premixed with oxygen as 50% nitrous oxide and 50% oxygen (Entonox®), which can be self-administered via a demand valve system.
Nitrous oxide can also be given via a continuous flow system (delivering up to 70% nitrous oxide). This high concentration achieves greater levels of sedation and requires managing by suitably trained clinicians.
Souce: Emmanouil and Quock (2007); Wilson-Smith (2011); APA (2012)

Nitrous oxide can been used alone or in combination with other analgesic drugs for paediatric procedural pain management (Babl et al. 2008a). Its rapid onset and offset

Prior to the procedure:
Assess pain, fear and anxiety
Use valid pain assessment tools
Make a comfort plan
Prepare the child and family
Consider timing of different strategies to optimise effects

During the procedure:
Pharmacological strategies
Apply topical local anaesthetics
Administer analgesic drugs
Use sucrose for infants under 12 months
Consider sedation for moderate to severely painful or distressing procedures

During the procedure:
Physical strategies
Comfort positioning
Use heat/cold as appropriate
For infants consider using non-nutritive sucking or kangaroo care (see Chapter 5)

During the procedure:
Psychological strategies
Provide distraction
Parental presence
Calm environment
Breathing techniques
Encourage coping
Appropriate language and choices
Competent healthcare professionals
Listen to the child

After the procedure:
Assess pain, fear and anxiety
Acknowledge the child's achievement
Reflect on the comfort plan and suggest changes for future procedures
Offer medical play

Figure 10.2   Algorithm for management of procedural pain.

make it a useful alternative to other analgesic agents. The effectiveness of nitrous oxide in managing procedural pain has been explored in several studies:

- When nitrous oxide is used alone it has limited efficacy for very painful procedures such as bone marrow aspiration and chest drain removal (Bruce et al. 2006; Babl et al. 2008a).
- Nitrous oxide has been used in combination with morphine or fentanyl to manage very painful procedures such as fracture reduction, laceration repair and abscess drainage (Ozil et al. 2010; Seith et al. 2012).
- A review of 7,802 cases in children over a 5-year period at one hospital demonstrated that high concentration (>50%) nitrous oxide administered by nasal mask is safe, especially for short (<15-minute) procedures (Zier and Liu 2011).
- 50% nitrous oxide was found to reduce procedural pain such as IV cannulation, intramuscular (IM) injection, lumbar puncture and bone marrow aspiration by approximately 50% when compared to placebo inhalation in children ($n = 100$), aged 1–18 years (Reinoso-Barbero et al. 2011).
- Nitrous oxide 50% plus EMLA® enabled shorter procedure time, improved success and less distress for IV cannulation for children ($n = 90$) compared to midazolam plus EMLA® (Ekbom et al. 2011).
- The analgesic and sedative effect of nitrous oxide was equivalent to IV ketamine for paediatric laceration repair in an emergency department setting ($n = 32$) with the advantage of faster recovery time (Lee et al. 2012).

Nitrous oxide is an effective pain-relieving strategy for procedure-related pain.
For severe pain, it is most effective when used in combination with other analgesic drugs.

Nitrous oxide 50% is normally only offered to children who are able to cooperate in administration by holding the mask/mouthpiece and breathing the gas themselves (Wilson-Smith 2011; APA 2012). This is usually around 5 or 6 years of age. The level of sedation is self-limiting for this method as, if the child becomes too sleepy, they will stop inhaling the gas.

For high concentration (>50%) nitrous oxide delivery a mask/mouthpiece is used with the clinician controlling the administration. Hospital guidelines and staff training should be available regarding the use of nitrous oxide (National Institute of Health and Care Excellence [NICE] 2010).

Side-effects are rare, and include:

- nausea and/or vomiting;
- hallucinations and/or confusion;
- diaphoresis (sweating);
- agitation or crying.

(Babl et al. 2008b; Zier and Liu 2011)

There are several **contra-indications** and **cautions** to consider. Nitrous oxide expands air-filled cavities, so should not be used in patients with:

- pneumothorax;
- bowel obstruction;
- head injury or raised intracranial pressure;
- chronic respiratory disease or acute asthma;
- some cardiac conditions and pulmonary hypertension;
- intoxication/drug overdose.

Source: Harvey and Morton (2007); Wilson-Smith (2011)

Several other factors need to be considered when using nitrous oxide:

- Prolonged exposure or frequent use can interfere with vitamin B12 metabolism and cause bone marrow suppression (Connor-Ballard 2009a; Wilson-Smith 2011; APA 2012).
- Nitrous oxide should not be used more often than every 4 days without careful monitoring (Wilson-Smith 2011; APA 2012).
- Although nitrous oxide is a valuable tool for managing procedural pain, it does have drawbacks, including exposure risks to healthcare professionals such as decreased fertility, as well as possible environmental effect as a greenhouse gas (APA 2012; Baum et al. 2012).

Additional information

Staff administering nitrous oxide should be appropriately trained.
The British Oxygen Company (BOC) provides an online training course about the use of Entonox®. This is available from: www.entonox.co.uk/en/discover_enotonox/training-support/online-training/entonox_online_training.shtml
Royal Children's Hospital, Melbourne has a nitrous oxide accreditation programme: www.rch.org.au/comfortkids/for_health_professionals

---

BOX 10.6

Best practice guidelines: Sedation of children

American Academy of Pediatrics (AAP), the American Academy of Pediatric Dentistry, Cote, C.J. and Wilson, S. (2006): www.aapd.org/media/policies_guidelines/g_sedation.pdf

The National Institute of Health and Care Excellence (NICE) (2010): http://publications.nice.org .uk/sedation-in-children-and-young-people-cg112

Using Sedation to Manage Procedural Pain

The addition of sedation is useful for procedures that are expected to cause moderate to severe pain, last for extended time, and that are distressing or anxiety provoking (APA 2012). However, most sedatives do not provide analgesia, and analgesic drugs should also be administered (Czarnecki et al. 2011). Sedation should only be provided by healthcare professionals experienced in airway management (NICE 2010). Details about the best practice guidelines relating to sedating children for painful procedures are provided in Box 10.6.

Practice point

Procedural sedation is commonly used in emergency departments (ED) for procedures including laceration repair, fracture reduction, abscess drainage, joint injection and lumbar puncture. Outside the ED, sedation is used for procedures including bone marrow aspiration, wound care, lumbar puncture and diagnostic procedures.

A range of drugs have been shown to be safe and effective in providing sedation and analgesia to children. These drugs can be given alone (e.g. dexmedetomidine, ketamine, nitrous oxide) or in combination (e.g. dexmedetomidine, ketamine, nitrous oxide, opioids, propofol). Drug selection depends of the degree and depth of sedation and analgesia required and length of the procedure. The different analgesic drugs are discussed further in Chapter 4.

Greater than minimal sedation has serious associated risks, including hypoventilation, apnoea, airway obstruction and laryngospasm (AAP et al. 2006). Healthcare professionals must be aware of the adverse effects of sedative drugs and monitor children appropriately (AAP et al. 2006; NICE 2010). This is particularly important; a recent study found that minor adverse events such as awakening prior to the procedure being completed, failure to sedate, problems with IV, and vomiting afterwards are under-reported (Lightdale et al. 2009). Levels of sedation are described in Box 10.7. Sedation monitoring guidelines are outlined in Box 10.8.

At least two healthcare professionals must be present when administering sedation, with one solely focused on monitoring the patient. In particular, healthcare professionals:

- should ensure that the environment is appropriate, with resuscitation equipment available;
- must have the skills to determine the level of sedation and provide rescue therapy if sedation is deeper than the intended level;

BOX 10.7

Levels of sedation

Minimal: the child responds normally to commands
Moderate: the child responds purposefully to commands such as 'open your eyes' but is sleepy
Conscious sedation: drug-induced depression of consciousness, similar to moderate sedation, except that verbal contact is always maintained with the patient
Deep: the child is asleep and does not respond to commands but responds purposefully to painful stimuli

(*Note:* deep sedation may impair the child's ability to maintain their own airway.)
Source: NICE (2010)

BOX 10.8

Sedation monitoring guidelines

Prior to the Procedure

- Perform a baseline assessment including health history, vital signs, current weight, fasting status
- Evaluation of the child's airway
- Fasting is required for moderate to deep sedation
- Prepare the child psychologically by providing information as well as coping strategies

During the Procedure

Monitor:
- airway, vital signs and depth of sedation
- oxygen saturation
- pain, coping and level of distress
(For deep sedation, in addition to the above, monitor BP, continuous ECG, capnography)

After the Procedure

- Monitor until the child remains awake for at least 20 minutes
- Longer monitoring may be required depending on the drugs administered and the child's response

Adapted from AAP et al. (2006); NICE (2010)

- require, at minimum, basic life support skills and advanced skills required for deep sedation as well as knowledge and competency in the administration of pharmacological agents.

(AAP et al. 2006; NICE 2010)

Fasting protocols vary depending on the degree of sedation, drugs used and institutional guidelines. For minimal sedation fasting is not usually required. Usual general anaesthesia guidelines are followed for moderate to deep sedation. As pharmacological agents aimed at both sedation and analgesia are effective in managing pain, few physical or psychological interventions are required.

Issues Relating to the Management of Specific Types of Procedural Pain

Best practice in relation to needle-related pain, pain due to burn wound care, pain related to cancer investigations, immunisation pain, and procedural pain in neonates will now be discussed.

Needle-related pain

Case study: Sophia

Sophia is a 3-year-old girl admitted to the hospital with fever and dehydration. She has a 2-day history of cough, rhinitis, lethargy and poor oral intake. On admission her oxygen saturation (pulse oximetry) is 92%, her temperature is 39.8°C, her respiratory rate is 38/min and her heart rate is 142/min. She requires an IV for parenteral antibiotics.

- How would you assess Sophia's fear and anxiety?
- What pharmacological strategies would you use to reduce Sophia's pain and anxiety related to this procedure (IV cannulation)?
- What physical strategies would you use to reduce Sophia's pain and anxiety related to this procedure?
- What psychological strategies would you use to reduce Sophia's pain and anxiety related to this procedure?

Pharmacological strategies

Healthcare professionals must plan in advance when using pharmacological agents and allow time for these drugs to work before carrying out a procedure (APA 2012). Some analgesic drugs take longer to be effective than others but with careful planning this should not be a barrier to successful management.

Topical local anaesthetics

Topical anaesthetics are the mainstay of pharmacological interventions for managing needle-related pain in children (Pershad et al. 2008; Zempsky 2008b; Curtis et al. 2012). In addition to pain relief they improve procedure success, decrease movement and increase accuracy (Zempsky 2008b). (For further information about local anaesthetics see Chapter 4.) Research in this area has demonstrated that:

- *All* transdermal forms of topical local anaesthetic creams and patches (e.g. EMLA®, amethocaine [tetracaine], liposomal lignocaine [lidocaine] 4% or 5%) are effective in reducing needle pain (Crowley et al. 2011).
- Amethocaine (tetracaine) is superior to EMLA® in reducing needle-related pain (Stinson et al. 2008) and the pain associated with IV cannulation (Curtis et al. 2012).
- Liposomal lignocaine 4% is effective in reducing pain associated with venepuncture, has an onset of 30 minutes (versus 60 minutes for EMLA®), and does not require an occlusive dressing (Eldeman et al. 2005).
- The use of liposomal lignocaine 4% is associated with higher cannulation success rates, less pain, and shorter procedure time when compared to placebo (Taddio et al. 2005).

BOX 10.9

Timing of pharmacological options

- Lignocaine/prilocaine (EMLA®): 45–60 minutes
- Amethocaine (tetracaine); liposomal lignocaine (lidocaine) (LMX®): 30–45 minutes
- Lignocaine (lidocaine) iontophoresis or heat-activated preparations: 15 minutes
- Needle-free 1% lignocaine (lidocaine) delivery (J-tip®); 1% buffered lignocaine (lidocaine) infiltration; ice/vibration (Buzzy®): 2 minutes
- Nitrous oxide: <1 minute
- Vapocoolant spray: 15 seconds

The timings for the various pharmacological options are outlined in Box 10.9.

Cryotherapy

Vapocoolant sprays (e.g. ethyl chloride or pentafluoropropane with tetrafluoroethane [Pain Ease®]) are available in some countries. These agents work by surface cooling the skin, act immediately and last up to 60 seconds (Soueid and Richard 2007; Page and Taylor 2010). Their effect is comparable to topical anaesthetics, with their greatest benefit seen in time-poor situations. Research has shown that vapocoolants:

- Significantly reduced pain and increased successful cannulation compared to placebo in children ($n = 80$), aged 6–12 years in the emergency department (Farion et al. 2008).
- Were associated with significantly greater cannulation success, took less time to administer and was more convenient for staff compared to 1% subcutaneous lignocaine in children ($n = 220$) undergoing IV cannulation (Page and Taylor 2010).

Other studies have found that:

- Oral morphine, in combination with topical local anaesthetic, did not provide any additional reduction in fear, distress or pain when compared to placebo in children for subcutaneous reservoir port access (Heden et al. 2011).
- At the current time there is insufficient evidence to recommend sweet-tasting solutions (sucrose) for needle-related pain in children aged 1–16 years (Harrison et al. 2011), or in children aged 1 month to 12 years (Kassab et al. 2012).

Practice point

Topical local anaesthetics and vapocoolant sprays:

- are widely available, safe, convenient to use and cost effective
- should be the mainstay of pharmacological interventions for needle-related pain

The choice of agent should be determined, at least in part, by the urgency of the procedure.

Psychological strategies

Distraction, hypnosis, breathing techniques and cognitive-behavioural therapies reduce pain and distress associated with needle-related pain (Uman et al. 2010). Psychological pain-relieving strategies are discussed in more depth in Chapter 5.

Physical strategies

The physical pain-relieving strategies that can be used to manage needle-related pain are discussed in more depth in Chapter 5. New devices that incorporate combinations of therapies (e.g. Buzzy®: www.buzzy4shots.com/) have been shown to be effective in managing needle pain (Baxter et al. 2011; Inal and Kelleci 2012).

Practice point

Children who have undergone previous medical procedures may have favourite strategies that have been successful. These strategies should be respected and used.

Pain related to burn wound care

Case study: Michael

Michael is a 15-year-old male admitted to the burns unit. He sustained full and partial thickness burns to his right forearm while putting petrol (gasoline) onto a campfire. He will require dressing changes and skin grafting.

- What pharmacological strategies would you use to reduce Michael's pain and anxiety related to his dressing changes?
- What physical strategies would you use to reduce Michael's pain and anxiety related to this procedure?
- What psychological strategies would you use to reduce Michael's pain and anxiety related to this procedure?

Burns are among the most intensely painful injuries experienced by children (Connor-Ballard 2009b; Gandhi et al. 2010). Children who have burn injuries require wound care to debride the wound, prevent infection and promote tissue healing. Burn wound care can be extremely painful and requires excellent pain management to minimise distress, suffering and psychological harm (Connor-Ballard 2009b; Gandhi et al. 2010).

Pharmacological management

Opioids are the mainstay for burn wound care:

- Opioids should be administered prior to commencement of procedures and can be given by oral, transmucosal, intranasal or IV routes according to patient preference, institutional guidelines and availability of suitable preparations (Gandhi et al. 2010; APA 2012).
- Children undergoing long-term wound care can develop tolerance to opioids and may require higher doses to manage the pain (Connor-Ballard 2009a). (See Chapter 4 regarding opioid tolerance.)
- Using multimodal analgesia can enhance pain management (e.g. combining opioids with ketamine) (Fabia and Groner 2009; Gandhi et al. 2010). (See Chapter 4 for a discussion about multimodal analgesia.)
- The use of sedation (e.g. nitrous oxide or intravenous agents) should also be considered, particularly for major burns (Gandhi et al. 2010; APA 2012).
- If there is a pain management service it should be involved to optimise pain management.

Psychological strategies

These are discussed in detail in Chapter 5 and include: breathing techniques, distraction and relaxation (Connor-Ballard 2009a). It is important to note that these techniques should not replace analgesic drugs for severely painful procedures (APA 2012).

Physical strategies

Physical strategies that have been shown to decrease pain and increase comfort during burn wound care include: warming the cleansing solutions, ensuring that the room temperature is comfortable (Kavanagh and de Jong 2004) and using non-adherent wound care products that minimise pain while promoting wound healing (Edwards 2011). Massage therapy involving healthy tissues prior to dressing changes was shown to significantly reduce pain, itch and anxiety in adolescents with burns (Parlak Gurol et al. 2010). See Chapter 5 for further information about these physical strategies.

Pain related to cancer investigations

Case study: Briannna

Brianna is a 6-year-old who has presented to the ED with fever, lethargy and leg pain. Her parents note that she's not been well since a cold a few weeks ago. Her blood count and differential has just returned from the laboratory – haemoglobin is 62, platelet count is 10 and white blood cell count is 27 with blast cells. A bone marrow aspiration and biopsy are required to determine if she has leukaemia.

- What pharmacological strategies would you use to reduce Brianna's pain and anxiety related to this procedure?
- What physical strategies would you use to reduce Brianna's pain and anxiety related to this procedure?
- What psychological strategies would you use to reduce Brianna's pain and anxiety related to this procedure?

Children undergoing investigations for a possible cancer diagnosis present a unique challenge to healthcare professionals. In addition to the pain and distress from the procedure itself is the further stress and anxiety related to the possible diagnosis. It is important that clinicians manage procedural pain optimally as it likely these children will undergo multiple painful procedures during their treatment, including bone marrow aspiration, lumbar puncture, venepuncture and IV cannulation. As already mentioned, children report these procedures to be more distressing than the cancer itself (Zernikow et al. 2006; Blount et al. 2006). Indeed, Weisman et al. (1998) found that, in children aged less than 8 years, inadequate analgesia for the first painful procedure diminished the effects of adequate analgesia for subsequent procedures.

Pharmacological management

Sedation in combination with analgesic drugs is the mainstay for the management of painful cancer procedures such as bone marrow aspiration (Mowery et al. 2008; NICE 2010). Typically, conscious sedation or brief (inhalational) general anaesthesia is used. Topical local anaesthetics and other local anaesthetics (see Chapter 4) can be administered as an adjunct (Hockenberry et al. 2011).

Sedation and analgesic drugs are both required for severely painful procedures such as bone marrow aspiration.

Psychological strategies

Landier and Tse (2010) carried out an integrative review of the physical and psychological interventions that can be used for managing procedure-related pain in children with cancer. They found that:

- hypnosis may be more effective than distraction, particularly for bone marrow aspiration and lumbar punctures;
- cognitive behavioural therapy (CBT) reduced fear and distress in some children.

Music has been shown to lower pain scores, anxiety scores, heart rate and respiratory rate during lumbar puncture in children with cancer aged 7–12 years (Nguyen et al. 2010). Further psychological interventions are discussed in Chapter 5.

Physical strategies

As pharmacological agents aimed at both sedation and analgesia are effective in managing pain, few physical interventions are required. However, it is recommended that children:

- should have personal comfort items to help them with relaxation and to feel as safe as possible (Young 2005; Hockenberry et al. 2011);
- are supported by their parents until sedation is achieved (Hockenberry et al. 2011).

Pain related to immunisations

Traditionally no pain-relieving interventions were used for childhood immunisations. This was partly due to a belief that using these techniques would be time consuming. However, concerns that using these techniques disrupts workflow have been shown to be untrue (Taddio et al. 2012). Two systematic reviews have examined the effectiveness of pain-relieving interventions for immunisations:

- Chambers et al. (2009) explored the effectiveness of psychological interventions for childhood immunisations. They found evidence to support the use of breathing exercises, child-directed and nurse-led distraction and CBT interventions to reduce the pain and distress associated with childhood immunisations.
- Harrington and colleagues (2012) looked at the use of physical interventions to manage the pain associated with infant immunisations and concluded that swaddling, side/stomach position, shushing, swinging and sucking (the 5 Ss) decreased pain scores and crying time for infants aged 2 and 4 months.

Best practice guidelines for managing pain associated with immunisations have been developed (Taddio et al. 2010). These recommendations are summarised in Box 10.10.

The best practice guidelines are available from: www.ncbi.nlm.nih.gov/pmc/articles/PMC3001531/pdf/182e843.pdf

More information about these guidelines, including posters for healthcare providers and information for parents, can be found at: www.cmaj.ca/content/182/18/E843/suppl/DC1

This YouTube video educates parents about managing the pain associated with immunisations: www.youtube.com/watch?v=jxnDc2PxGUc

> **BOX 10.10**
>
> ### Best practice guidelines for managing immunisation pain
>
> - Use topical local anaesthetics
> - Use distraction techniques, including deep breathing for older children
> - Encourage breastfeeding mothers to breastfeed during the vaccinations
> - Children up to 12 months of age who cannot be breastfed should be administered a sweet-tasting solution
> - *Do not* lie children down during the immunisation
> - *Do not* tell children 'it won't hurt'
> - Inject the least painful brand of vaccine available
> - Use rapid injection technique for intramuscular injections
> - When administering multiple injections on the same visit, inject the most painful vaccine last
>
> *Source:* Taddio et al. (2010)

Procedural pain management in neonates

Procedural pain in neonates is not managed as well as it could be. Neonates ($n = 582$) in Canadian neonatal intensive care units (NICUs) underwent a total of 3,508 skin-breaking procedures and 14,085 non-tissue-damaging procedures in one week (Johnston et al. 2011). Almost half these procedures were performed without analgesia. This is of concern, given the consequences of unrelieved pain discussed in Chapter 1. A better picture was seen in a study in one NICU in Australia. Neonates ($n = 55$), whose length of stay exceeded 28 days, underwent a total of 3,605 minor painful procedures with only 15% of these procedures performed without analgesia (Harrison et al. 2009).

Managing procedural pain in neonates is important.
Despite pharmacological, physical and psychological strategies being available, practices remain suboptimal.

Pharmacological management

Topical local anaesthetics are used to manage painful procedures in neonates. EMLA® is the most studied agent in this age group; however, concerns about the rare complication of methaemoglobinaemia limit its use (APA 2012). In many countries, amethocaine (tetracaine) is not recommended for use in infants under 1 month of age. Other research has found the following:

- EMLA® reduces pain during circumcision, venepuncture, arterial puncture, IV cannulation but not during heel-stick procedures (Taddio et al. 1998, 2009).
- Amethocaine (tetracaine) has been shown to be beneficial for venepuncture, immunisation and IV cannulation but is ineffective for heel-sticks and peripherally inserted central catheters (O'Brien et al. 2005).
- EMLA® with sucrose during venepuncture in preterm infants was more effective than placebo cream and sucrose (Biran et al. 2011).
- Sucrose was more effective than liposomal lignocaine (lidocaine) for reducing pain during venepuncture in term newborns ($n = 330$). The addition of liposomal lignocaine to sucrose did not confer any additional benefit compared with sucrose alone (Taddio et al. 2011).

Psychological strategies

Psychological strategies that can be used to manage procedural pain in neonates include:

- planning procedures so that sleep and feeding times are not interrupted (Lago et al. 2009);
- providing developmental care which involves reducing the stress of the NICU environment and supporting family-centred care (Fernandes et al. 2011).

Physical strategies

There are several physical strategies that can be used to manage procedural pain in neonates. These are discussed in Chapter 5 and include:

- breastfeeding (Leite et al. 2009);
- facilitated tucking (Fernandes et al. 2011);
- kangaroo care (skin-to-skin contact) (Campbell-Yeo et al. 2011);
- non-nutritive sucking (Fernandes et al. 2011);
- sucrose (Harrison et al. 2011; Stevens et al. 2010).

Summary

- Healthcare professionals need to be involved in implementing best practices to manage procedural pain in children of all ages.
- Pharmacological, physical and psychological therapies are effective and should be used in combination.
- Managing a child's procedure-related pain effectively will reduce the fear and anxiety associated with subsequent procedures.
- If procedure-related pain is not managed effectively this has long-term consequences for the child.
- All children are entitled to optimal comfort measures, and healthcare professionals have a responsibility to manage pain, distress and anxiety associated with procedures.

Additional information

Websites for children and families

Parent information sheets on burn care: www.chw.edu.au/prof/services/burns_unit/05_factsheets.htm

Parent information sheet on the use of Entonox®: www.gosh.nhs.uk/EasysiteWeb/getresource.axd?AssetID=106884&type=full&servicetype=Attachment

Parent information sheets about the use of sedation: www.rch.org.au/comfortkids/for_parents/#sedation

Helpful websites for healthcare professionals

Great Ormond Street Hospital Guidelines for the use of nitrous oxide: www.gosh.nhs.uk/health-professionals/clinical-guidelines/entonox-ward-administration-of/?locale=en

Immunisation Pain Guidelines (fact sheets translated into 13 languages): www.toronto.ca/health/immunization_children/howtoreducepain.htm

Royal Children's Hospital, Melbourne Clinical Guidelines Procedural Pain Guidelines: www.rch.org.au/rchcpg/index.cfm?doc_id=10245

Royal Children's Hospital, Melbourne Clinical Guidelines Sedation Guidelines: www.rch.org.au/rchcpg/hospital_clinical_guideline_index/Sedation_Procedural_Sedation_Guideline_Ward_and_Ambulatory_Areas/

Society for Pediatric Sedation: www.pedsedation.org

Acknowledgements
We would like to thank Mathew Martin, a photographer at Stollery Children's Hospital, Alberta, Canada, for taking the photo included in this chapter.

Key to Case Studies

See Boxes 10.11, 10.12 and 10.13.

BOX 10.11

Sophia

Introduce yourself and your role to both Sophia and her family.

Assess Sophia's fear and anxiety using a recognised tool.

Explain the procedure to Sophia at her developmental level. Use words such as 'magic cream'. Be truthful. Don't say 'It won't hurt', instead offer an explanation such as 'It may pinch for a few seconds and then this will go away.'

Play therapists (child life specialists) can provide preparation using medical play.

Create a calm and relaxing environment.

Give her developmentally appropriate choices whenever possible, such as 'Do you want to sit on Mum's lap or Dad's lap?'

Only give choices that are realistic. Asking 'are you ready?' may create further anxiety if Sophia says 'No'.

Apply topical local anaesthetic prior to procedure and allow time for it to be effective. Consider using a faster-acting agent if required.

Consider location of IV in non-dominant hand.

Be sure Sophia has her favourite comfort item.

Demonstrate comfort positioning to her parents. Allow her parents to remain with her and be active participants in the procedure.

Provide a distraction toy with lights and sounds.

Provide Sophia with a job to do, e.g. 'Your job is to press the buttons on the story book.'

Allow her to cry – 'It's OK to cry.'

Acknowledge her specific positive behaviours after the procedure – 'You held really still and pressed the button.'

BOX 10.12

Michael

Consider Michael's age, needs and fears in giving information and include him in the planning and preparation for the dressing change.

Assess Michael's pain prior to beginning the intervention. Ensure his pain is at an acceptable level for him.

Administer opioids, or encourage self-administration via PCA (if in use).

Utilise distraction techniques and involve Michael in choosing these.

Time the dressing change to peak effect of the opioid dose.

Have further analgesic doses available if the procedure is prolonged or Michael reports increased pain.

Consider sedation if necessary.

Consider the environment – ensure room temperature is comfortable and any wound cleansing supplies are warmed to a comfortable temperature.

Allow debriefing time for Michael after the procedure. Discuss possible changes to make for future burn wound care.

BOX 10.13

Brianna

Prior to the procedure: prepare Brianna and her family by explaining the procedure at her developmental level.

Play therapists (child life specialists) can provide preparation using medical play.

Prepare Brianna's parents for what to expect when sedation is provided.

Introduce relaxation techniques, breathing and guided imagery.

Consider use of a psychological strategy such as distraction with a movie or music in addition to sedation.

Consider use of topical local anaesthetic.

Assess pain and anxiety prior to starting the procedure.

The sedation (usually combined sedative and analgesic drugs) should be delivered by an appropriately trained clinician.

Where possible, allow a parent to stay with her until sedated.

After the procedure, assess her pain, and ensure her parents are able to be with her when she awakes.

Answer her parents' questions as to how she tolerated the procedure if they were not present.

References

American Academy of Pediatrics (2006) Committee on Hospital Care. Child Life Services. *Pediatrics* 18, 1757–1763.

American Academy of Pediatrics, American Academy of Pediatric Dentistry, Cote, C.J. and Wilson, S. (AAP et al.) (2006) Guidelines for monitoring and management of pediatric patients during and after sedation for diagnostic and therapeutic procedures: An update. *Pediatrics* 118(6) 2587–2602 (reaffirmed March 2011).

Association of Paediatric Anaesthetists of Great Britain and Ireland (APA) (2012) *Good Practice in Postoperative and Procedural Pain*, 2nd edition. Available from: http://onlinelibrary.wiley.com/doi/10.1111/pan.2012.22.issue-s1/issuetoc#group1 (accessed January 2013).

Babl, F., Oakley, E., Puspitadewi, A. and Sharwood, L. (2008a) Limited analgesic efficacy of nitrous oxide for painful procedures in children. *Emergency Medicine Journal* 25(11), 717–721.

Babl, F., Oakley, E., Seaman, C., Barnett, P., and Sharwood, L. (2008b) High-concentration nitrous oxide for procedural sedation in children: Adverse events and level of sedation. *Pediatrics* 121(3), e528–e532.

Babl, F.E., Crellin, D., Cheng, J., Sullivan, T.P. O'Sullivan, R. and Hutchinson, A. (2012) The use of the Faces, Legs, Activity, Cry and Consolability Scale to assess procedural pain and distress in young children. *Pediatric Emergency Care* 28(12), 1281–1296.

Bandstra, N.F., Skinner, L., LeBlanc, C. et al. (2008) The role of child life specialist in pediatric pain management: A survey of child life specialists. *Journal of Pain* 9(4), 320–329.

Baum, V., Willschke, H., and Marciniak, B. (2012). Is nitrous oxide necessary in the future? *Pediatric Anaesthesia* 22, 981–987

Baxter, A., Cohen, L., McElvery, H. Lawson, M. and von Baeyer, C. (2011) An integration of vibration and cold relieves venipuncture pain in a pediatric emergency department. *Pediatric Emergency Care* 27(12), 1151–1156.

Bearden, D.J., Feinstein, A. and Cohen, L.L. (2012) The influence of parent preprocedural anxiety on child procedural pain: Mediation by child procedural anxiety. *Journal of Pediatric Psychology* 37(6), 680–686.

Biran, V., Gourrier, E., Cimerman, P., Walter-Nicolet, E., Mitanchez, D. and Carbajal, R. (2011) Analgesic effects of EMLA cream and oral sucrose during venipuncture in preterm infants. *Pediatrics* 128(1), e63–70.

Blount, R.L., Piira, T., Cohen, L.L., and Cheng, P.S. (2006) Pediatric procedural pain. *Behavior Modification* 30, 24–49.

Bruce, E., Franck, L. and Howard, R.F. (2006) The efficacy of morphine and Entonox analgesia during chest drain removal in children. *Pediatric Anesthesia* **16**, 203–208.

Campbell-Yeo, M., Fernandes, A. and Johnston, C.C. (2011) Procedural pain management for neonates using non-pharmacological strategies. Part 2: Mother-driven interventions. *Advances in Neonatal Care* **11**(5), 312–318.

Chambers, C.T., Taddio, A., Uman, L.S., McMurtry, C.M. and HELPinKIDS team (2009) Psychological interventions for reducing pain and distress during routine childhood immunizations: A systematic review. *Clinical Therapeutics* **31**(S2), S77–S103.

Cohen, L. (2008) Behavioural approaches to anxiety and pain management for pediatric venous access. *Pediatrics* **122**(S3), S134–S139.

Connor-Ballard, P. (2009a) Understanding and managing burn pain: Part 2. *American Journal of Nursing* **109**(5), 54–62.

Connor-Ballard, P. (2009b) Understanding and managing burn pain: Part 1. *American Journal of Nursing* **109**(4), 48–54.

Crowley, M.A., Storer, A., Heaton K. et al.; 2010 ENA Emergency Nurses Resources Development Committee (2011) Emergency nursing resource: Needle-related procedural pain in pediatric patients in the emergency department. *Journal of Emergency Nursing* **37**(3), 246–251.

Curtis, S., Wingert, A. and Ali, S. (2012) The Cochrane Library and procedural pain in children: An overview of the reviews, *Evidence-Based Child Health* **7**, 1363–1399.

Czarnecki, M., Turner, H., Collins, P., Doellman, D., Wrona, S. and Reynolds, J. (2011) Procedural pain managment: A position statement with clinical practice guidelines. *Pain Management Nursing* **12**(2), 95–111.

Edwards, J. (2011) Managing wound pain in patients with burns using soft silicone dressings. *Wounds UK* **7**(4), 122–126.

Ekbom, K., Kalman, S., Jakobsson, J. and Marcus, C. (2011) Efficient intravenous access without distress: A double-blind randomized study of midazolam and nitrous oxide in children and adolescents. *Archives of Pediatric and Adolescent Medicine* **165**(9), 785–791.

Ellis, J., Villeneuve, K., Newhook, K. and Ulrichsen, J. (2007) Pain management practices for lumbar punctures: Are we consistent? *Journal of Pediatric Nursing* **22**(6), 479–487.

Eldeman, A., Weiss, J., Lau, J. and Carr, D. (2005) Topical anaesthetics for dermal instrumentation: A systematic review of randomized controlled trials. *Annals of Emergency Medicine* **46**(4), 343–351.

Emmanouil, D.E. and Quock, R.M. (2007) Advances in understanding the actions of nitrous oxide. *Anesthesia Progress* **54**(1), 9–18.

Esteve, R. and Marquina-Aponte, V. (2012) Children's pain perspectives. *Child: Care, Health and Development* **3**, 441–452

Fabia, R. and Groner, J. (2009) Advances in the care of children with burns. *Advances in Pediatrics* **56**. 219–248.

Farion, K., Splinter, K., Newhook, K. and Gaboury, I.A.S.W. (2008) The effect of vapocoolant spray on pain due to intravenous cannulation in children: A randomized controlled trial. *Canadian Medical Association Journal* **179**(1), 31–36.

Fein, D., Avner, J. and Khine, H. (2010) Pattern of pain management during lumbar puncture in children. *Pediatric Emergency Care* **26**(5), 357–360.

Fein, J.A., Zempsky, W.T., Cravero, J.P. and the Committee on Pediatric Emergency Medicine and Section on Anesthesiology and Pain Medicine (2012) Relief of pain and anxiety in pediatric patients in emergency medical systems. *Pediatrics* **130**(5), e1391–e1405.

Fernandes, A., Campbell-Yeo, M. and Johnston, C.C. (2011) Procedural pain management for neonates using non-pharmacological strategies. Part 1: Sensorial interventions. *Advances in Neonatal Care* **11**(4), 235–241.

Gandhi, M., Thomson, C., Lord, D. and Enoch, S. (2010) Management of pain in children with burns. *International Journal of Pediatrics*. doi:10.1155/2010/825657.

Gorchynski, J. and McLaughlin, T. (2011) The routine utilization of procedural pain management for pediatric lumbar puncture: Are we there yet? *Journal of Clinical Medical Research* **3**(4), 164–167.

Grunau, R.V.E., Whitfield, M.F., Petrie, J. et al. (2009) Neonatal pain, parenting stress and interaction, in relation to cognitive and motor development at 8 and 18 months in preterm infants. *Pain* **143**(1–2), 138–146.

Gursky, B., Kestle, L. and Lewis, M. (2010) Psychological intervention on procedure-related distress in children. *Journal of Developmental and Behavioral Pediatrics* **31**(3), 217–222.

Harrington, J.W., Logan, S., Harwell, C. et al. (2012) Effective analgesia using physical interventions for infant immunizations. *Pediatrics* **129**, 815–822.

Harrison, D., Loughnan, P., Manias, E. and Johnston, L. (2009) Analgesics administered during minor painful procedures in a cohort of hospitalized infants: A prospective clinical audit. *Journal of Pain* **10**(7), 715–722.

Harrison, D., Yamada, J., Adams-Webber, T., Ohlsson, A., Beyene, J. and Stevens, B. (2011) Sweet tasting solutions for reduction of needle-related procedural pain in children aged one to 16 years (Review). *Cochrane Database of Systematic Reviews* issue 10.

Harvey, A.J. and Morton, N.S. (2007) Management of procedural pain in children. *Archives of Disease in Childhood* **92**, ep20–ep26.

Heden, L., von Essen, L. and Ljungman, G. (2011) Effect of morphine in needle procedures in children with cancer. *European Journal of Pain* **15**(10), 1056–1060.

Hockenberry, M.J., McCarthy, K., Taylor, O. et al. (2011) Managing painful procedures in children with cancer. *Journal of Pediatric Hematology and Oncology* **33**(2), 119–127.

Hoyle, J., Rogers, A., Reischman, D. et al. (2011) Pain intervention for infant lumbar puncture in the emergency department: Physician practice and beliefs. *Academic Emergency Medicine* **18**(2), 140–144.

Inal, S. and Kelleci, M. (2012) Relief of pain during blood specimen collection in pediatric patients. *American Journal of Maternal and Child Nursing* **37**(5), 339–345.

Jaaniste, T., Hayes, B. and von Baeyer, C.L. (2007a) Providing children with information about forthcoming medical procedures: A review and synthesis. *Clinical Psychology: Science and Practice* **14**, 124–143.

Jaaniste, T., Hayes, B. and von Baeyer, C.L. (2007b) Effects of preparatory information and distraction on children's cold-pressor pain outcomes: A randomized controlled trial. *Behaviour Research and Therapy* **45**, 2789–2799.

Johnston, C., Barrington, K., Taddio, A., Carbajal, R. and Fillion, F. (2011) Pain in Canadian NICUs: Have we improved over the past 12 years? *Clinical Journal of Pain* **27**(3), 225–232.

Kassab, M., Foster, J.P., Foureur, M. and Fowler, C. (2012) Sweet-tasting solutions for needle-related procedural pain in infants one month to one year of age. *Cochrane Database of Systematic Reviews* **issue 12**.

Kavanagh, S. and de Jong, A. (2004) Care of burn patients in the hospital. *Burns* **30**(8), A2–A6.

Kortesluoma, R. and Nikkonen, M. (2004) 'I had this horrible pain': The sources and causes of pain experiences in 4–11 year old hospitalized children. *Journal of Child Health Care* **8**(3), 210–231.

Kristjansdottir, O., Unruh, A.M., McAlpine, L. and McGrath, P.J. (2012) A systematic review of cross-cultural comparison studies of child, parent, and health professional outcomes associated with pediatric medical procedures. *Journal of Pain* **12**(3), 207–219.

Kuttner, L. (2010) *A Child in Pain: What health professionals can do to help*. Crown House Publishing, Bethel, CT.

Lambrenos, K. and McArthur, K. (2003) Introducing a clinical holding policy. *Paediatric Nursing* **15**(4), 30–33.

Lago, P., Garetti, E., Merazzi, D. et al. (2009) Guidelines for procedural pain in the newborn. *Acta Pediatrica* **98**(6), 932–939.

Landier, W. and Tse, A. (2010) Use of complementary and alternative medical interventions for the management of procedure-related pain, anxiety and distress in pediatric oncology: An integrative review. *Journal of Pediatric Nursing* **25**(6), 566–579.

Lee, J.H., Kim, K., Kim, T.Y. et al. (2012) A randomized comparison of nitrous oxide versus intravenous ketamine for laceration repair in children. *Pediatric Emergency Care* **28**(12), 1297–301.

Leite, A., Linhares, M., Lander, J., Castral, T., dos Santos, C. and Silvan Scochi, C. (2009) Effects of breastfeeding on pain relief in full-term newborns. *Clinical Journal of Pain* **25**(9), 827–832.

Lightdale, J., Mahoney, L., Fredette, M., Valim, C., Wong, S. and DiNardo, J. (2009) Nurse reports of adverse events during sedation procedures at a pediatric hospital. *Journal of PeriAnesthesia Nurisng* **24**(5), 300–306.

Maclaren, J. and Cohen, L.L. (2007) Interventions in paediatric procedure-related pain in primary care, *Paediatrics and Child Health* **12**(2), 111–116.

March, J.S., Parker, J.D.A., Sullivan, K., Stallings, P. and Conners, C.K. (1997) The Multidimensional Anxiety Scale for Children (MASC): Factor structure, reliability and validity. *Journal of American Academy of Child and Adolescent Psychiatry* **36**(4), 554–565.

Marteau, T.M. and Bekker, H. (1992) The development of a six-item short-form of the state scale of Speilberger-State-Trait Anxiety Inventory (STAI). *British Journal of Clinical Psychology* **31**(3), 301–306.

McCarthy, A., Kleiber, C., Hanrahan, K., Zimmerman, M. B., Westhus, N. and Allen, S. (2010) Factors explaining children's responses to intravenous needle insertions. *Nursing Research* **59**(6), 407–416.

McGrath, P.A., Selfert, C.E., Speechley, K.N., Booth, J.C., Stitt, L. and Gibson, M.C. (1996) A new analogue scale for assessing children's pain. *Pain* **64**(3), 435–443.

McMurtry, C.M., Chambers, C.T., McGrath, P.J. and Asp, E. (2010) When 'don't worry' communicates fear: Children's perceptions of parental reassurance and distraction during a painful medical procedure. *Pain* **150**(1), 52–58.

McMurtry, C.M., Noel, M., Chambers, C.T. and McGrath, P.J. (2011) Children's fear during procedural pain: Preliminary investigation of the Children's Fear Scale. *Health Psychology* **30**(6), 780–788.

Mowery, B., Suddaby, E., Kang, K. and Cooper, L. (2008) The art of procedural sedation and analgesia. *Pediatric Nursing* **34**(6), 490–492.

Nguyen, T., Nilsson, S., Hellstrom, A. and Bengtson, A. (2010) Music therapy to reduce pain and anxiety in children with cancer undergoing lumbar puncture: A randomized clinical trial. *Journal of Pediatric Oncology Nursing* **27**(3), 146–155.

National Institute for Health and Care Excellence (NICE) (2010) Sedation in children and young people. Available from: www.nice.org.uk/nicemedia/live/13296/52130/52130.pdf (accessed November 2012).

Nilsson, S., Finnstrom, B. and Kokinsky, E. (2008) The FLACC behavioral scale for procedural pain assessment in children. *Paediatric Anaesthesia* **18**(8), 767–774.

Nilsson, S. and Renning, A-C. (2012) Pain management during wound dressing in children. *Nursing Standard* **26**(32), 50–55.

Noel, M., Chambers, C. McGrath, P.J., Klein. R. and Stewart, S. (2012) The influence of children's pain memories on subsequent pain experience. *Pain* **153**(8), 1563–1572.

Oakes, L. (2011) *Infant and Child Pain Management: An Evidence-Based Approach for Nurses.* Springer Publishing Company, New York.

O'Brien, L., Taddio, A., Lyszkiewicz, D.A. and Koren, G. (2005) A critical review of the topical local anesthetic amethocaine (Ametop) for pediatric pain. *Paediatric Drugs* **7**(1), 41–54.

Ozil, C., Vialle, R., Thevenin-Lemoine, C., Conit, E. and Annequin, D. (2010) Use of a combined oxygen/nitrous oxide/morphine chlorydrate protocol for analgesia in burned children requiring painful local care. *Pediatric Surgery International* **26**(3), 263–267.

Page, D.E. and Taylor, D.McD. (2010) Vapocoolant spray vs subcutaneous lidnocaine injection for reducing the pain of intravenous cannulation: A randomized controlled clinical trial. *British Journal of Anaesthesia* **105**(4), 519–525.

Page, M.G., Fuss, S., Martin, A.L., Escobar, E.M. and Katz, J. (2010) Development and preliminary evaluation of the Child Pain Anxiety Symptoms Scale in a community sample. *Journal of Pediatric Psychology* **35**(10), 1071–1082.

Parlak Gurol, A., Polat, S. and Nurna Akcay, M. (2010) Itching, pain and anxiety levels are reduced with massage therapy in burned adolescents. *Journal of Burn Care and Research* **31**(3), 429–432.

Pershad, J., Steinberg, S. and Water, T. (2008) Cost-effectiveness analysis of anesthetic agents during peripheral intravenous cannulation in the pediatric emergency department. *Archives of Pediatric and Adolescent Medicine* **162**(10), 952–961.

Polkki, T., Pietila, A-M. and Vehvilamen-Julkunen, K. (2003) Hospitalized children's descriptions of their experiences with postsurgical pain relieving methods. *International Journal of Nursing Studies* **40**, 33–44.

Reinoso-Barbero, F., Pascual-Pascual, S., de Lucas, R. et al. (2011) Equimolar nitrous oxide/oxygen vs placebo for procedural pain in children: a randomized trial. *Pediatrics* **127**(6) e1464–e1470.

Rocha, E., Marche, T. and von Baeyer, C. (2009) Anxiety influences children's memory for procedural pain. *Pain Research and Management* **14**(3), 233–237.

Royal Australasian College of Physicians Paediatrics and Child Health Division (RACP) (2006) Guideline Statement: Management of Procedure-related Pain in Children and Adolescents. *Journal of Paediatrics and Child Health* **12**(1), S2–S29.

Royal Children's Hospital, Melbourne (2011) *Procedural Pain Management.* Available at: www.rch.org .au/rchcpg/hospital_clinical_guideline_index/Procedural_Pain_Management/. (accessed January 2013).

Royal College of Nursing (RCN) (2010) *Restrictive Physical Intervention and Therapeutic Holding for Children and Young People*. RCN Publishing, London.

Seith, R.W., Theophilos, T. and Babl, F.E. (2012) Intranasal fentanyl and high-concentration inhaled nitrous oxide for procedural sedation: A prospective observational pilot study of adverse events and depth of sedation. *Academy of Emergency Medicine* 19(1), 31–36.

Soueid, A. and Richard, B. (2007) Ethyl chloride as a cryoanalgesic in pediatrics for venipuncture. *Pediatric Emergency Care* 23, 380–383.

Stevens, B., Abbott L, Yamada, J. et al. (2011) Epidemiology and management of painful procedures in children in Canadian hospitals. *Canadian Medical Association Journal* 183(7), 1–8.

Stevens, B., Yamada, J. and Ohlsson, A. (2010) *Sucrose for analgesia in newborn infants undergoing painful procedures*. *Cochrane Database of Systematic Reviews* issue 13.

Stinson, J., Yamada, J., Dickson, A., Lamba, J. and Stevens, B. (2008) Review of systematic reviews on acute procedural pain in children in the hospital setting. *Pain Research and Management* 13(1), 51–57.

Summer, G.J., Puntillo, K.A., Miakowski, C., Green, P.G. and Levine, J.D. (2007) Burn injury pain: The continuing challenge. *Journal of Pain* 8(7), 533–548

Taddio, A., Katz, J., Ilersich, A. and Koren, G. (1997) Effect of neonatal circumcision on pain response during subsequent routine vaccination. *Lancet* 349(9052), 599–603.

Taddio, A., Ohlsson, A., Einarson, T.R., Stevens, B. and Koren, G. (1998) A systematic review of lidocaine-prilocaine cream (EMLA) in the treatment of acute pain in neonates. *Pediatrics* 101(2), E1.

Taddio, A. Soin, H.K., Schuh, S., Koren, G. and Scolnik, D. (2005) Liposomal lidocaine to improve procedural success rates and reduce procedural pain among children: A randomized controlled trial. *Canadian Medical Association Journal* 172(13), 1691–1695.

Taddio, A., Ohlsson, A. and Ohlsson, K. (2009) Lidocaine-prilocaine cream for analgesia during circumcision in newborn boys. *Cochrane Database Systematic Review* issue 1.

Taddio, A., Appleton, M., Bortolussi, R. et al. (2010) Reducing the pain of childhood vaccination: An evidence-based clinical practice guideline. *Canadian Medical Association Journal* 182(18), E843–E855.

Taddio, A., Shah, V., Stephens, D. et al. (2011) Effect of liposomal lidocaine and sucrose alone and in combination for venipuncture pain in newborns. *Pediatrics* 127(4):e940–947.

Taddio, A., Hogan, M., Gerges, S., et al. (2012) Addressing parental concerns about pain during childhood vaccination. *Clinical Journal of Pain* 28(3), 238–242.

Uman, L.S., Chambers, C.T., McGrath, P.J. and Kisely, S. (2010) Psychological interventions for needle-related procedural pain and distress in children and adolescents. *Cochrane Database of Systematic Reviews* issue 10.

van Staa, A., Jedeloo, S. and van der Stege, H. (2011) 'What we want': Chronically ill adolescents' preferences and priorities for improving health care. *Patient Preference and Adherence* 5, 291–305.

von Baeyer, C.L., Marcher, T.A., Rocha, E.M. and Salomon, K. (2004) Children's memory for pain: Overview and implications for practice. *Journal of Pain* 5(5), 241–249.

Weisman, S., Bernstein, B. and Schechter, N. (1998) Consequences of inadequate analgesia during painful procedures in children. *Archives of Pediatric Adolescent Medicine* 152(2), 147–149.

Wilson-Smith, E. (2011) Procedural pain management in neonates, infants and children. *Reviews in Pain* 5(3), 4–12.

World Health Organization (2011) Immunization surveillance, assessment and monitoring. Available from: www.who.int/immunization_monitoring/en/ (accessed February 2013).

Young, K.D. (2005) Pediatric procedural pain. *Annals of Emergency Medicine* 45, 160–171.

Zier, J. and Liu, M. (2011) Safety of high-concentration nitrous oxide by nasal mask for pediatric procedural sedation: Experience with 7802 cases. *Pediatric Emergency Care* 27(12), 1107–1112.

Zempsky, W.T. (2008a) Optimizing the management of peripheral venous access pain in children: Evidence, impact and implementation. *Pediatrics* 122(Suppl 3) S121–124.

Zempsky, W.T. (2008b) Pharmacological approaches for reducing venous access pain in children. *Pediatrics* 122(S3), S140–S153.

Zernikow, B., Smale, H., Michel, E., Hasan, C., Jorch, N., and Andler, W. (2006) Paediatric cancer pain management using the WHO analgesic ladder: Results of a prospective analysis from 2265 treatment days during a quality improvement study. *European Journal of Pain* 10, 587–595.

CHAPTER 11

Where To From Here?

Alison Twycross

Department for Children's Nursing and Children's Pain Management,
London South Bank University, United Kingdom

Jennifer Stinson

Chronic Pain Programme, The Hospital for Sick Children;
Lawrence S. Bloomberg Faculty of Nursing, University of Toronto, Canada

Introduction

In this chapter the factors contributing to suboptimal pain management practices will be discussed, demonstrating that a multifactorial approach is needed to improve the management of pain in children. The use of a knowledge translation model to help nurses improve practice is discussed. Areas where research is still needed to guide clinical practice are identified and the ethical issues relating to carrying out research with children are outlined.

Reasons for Suboptimal Practices

The evidence to guide pain management practices is readily available, in the form of clinical guidelines (see Chapter 1). However, practices continue to fall short of the ideal (Shrestha-Ranjit and Manias 2010; Twycross and Collis 2012) with children experiencing moderate to severe unrelieved pain while in hospital (Shrestha-Ranjit and Manias 2010; Kozlowski et al. 2012; Twycross and Collis 2012). Several factors have been suggested as reasons why children's pain is still not managed effectively. These include:

- knowledge deficits;
- incorrect or outdated beliefs about pain and pain management;
- the decision-making strategies used;
- organisational culture.

Managing Pain in Children: A Clinical Guide for Nurses and Healthcare Professionals, Second Edition.
Edited by Alison Twycross, Stephanie Dowden, and Jennifer Stinson.
© 2014 John Wiley & Sons, Ltd. Published 2014 by John Wiley & Sons, Ltd.

Knowledge deficits

Limited theoretical knowledge about managing pain in children has been suggested as one reason paediatric nurses do not manage pain effectively. Several studies have examined nurses' theoretical knowledge about pain in children (Table 11.1). The results of these studies suggest that knowledge gaps remain, particularly with pain assessment, analgesic drugs and the use of psychological and physical methods.

> Gaps remain in nurses' knowledge about pain in children, and in particular in relation to pain assessment, analgesic drugs and physical and psychological methods.

Other studies have examined the influence of nurses' theoretical knowledge on the quality of pain management practices:

Table 11.1 Summary of studies examining nurses' knowledge

Author	Sample and questionnaire	Gaps in knowledge and mean score
Salantera et al. (1999)	Paediatric nurses (*n* = 265) in Finland Completed a knowledge and attitudes questionnaire.	• Analgesic drugs • Non-pharmacological methods *Mean knowledge score: 63%*
Twycross (2004)	Paediatric nurses (*n* = 12) Used a modified version of Salantera's questionnaire	• Analgesic drugs • Non-pharmacological methods • Physiology of pain • Psychology and sociology of pain *Mean knowledge score: 78%*
Manworren (2000)	Paediatric nurses (*n* = 274) *Pediatric Nurses' Knowledge and Attitudes Regarding Pain Survey (PNKARPS)*	• Pain assessment • Pharmacology of analgesic drugs • Use of analgesic drugs • Non-pharmacological methods *Mean knowledge score: 66%*
Vincent (2005)	Paediatric nurses (*n* = 67) Adapted version of the *Nurses' Knowledge and Attitudes Regarding Pain Survey*	• Non-pharmacological methods • Analgesic drugs • Incidence of respiratory depression *Mean knowledge score: 76%*
Rieman et al. (2007)	Paediatric nurses (*n* = 295) working in Shriner's Hospitals in the USA Revised version of *PNKARPS*	• Pharmacology • Incidence of respiratory depression *Mean knowledge score: 74%*
Tiernan (2009)	Paediatric nurses (*n* = 292) in Ireland *PNKARPS*	• Pharmacology (particularly opioids) • Pharmacokinetics • Non-pharmacological methods *Mean knowledge score: 62%*
Ekim and Ocakci (2012)	Paediatric nurses (*n* = 224) from five paediatric hospitals in Turkey *PNKARPS*	• Pharmacology and the use of opioid analgesia • Addiction • Accuracy of child's self-report of pain *Mean knowledge score: 38%*

- Vincent and Denyes (2004) observed the care of children ($n = 132$), aged 3½ to 17 years, by nurses ($n = 67$) and found that a better theoretical knowledge about pain did not make it more likely they would administer analgesia.
- No positive relationship between paediatric nurses' level of knowledge and how well they actually managed pain was found by Twycross (2007). Even when nurses ($n = 12$) had a good level of theoretical knowledge, this was not reflected in their pain management practices.
- No relationship was found between adult nurses' ($n = 80$) knowledge and patients' ratings of pain and the amount of analgesia administered, although the nurses had moderately good levels of knowledge about pain management (Watt-Watson et al. 2001).

> Gaps in nurses' theoretical knowledge levels do not appear to provide the sole explanation for deficits in pain management practices.

Recent reviews of curricula content in the UK and Canada suggest that prequalification curricula contain limited input about pain (Watt-Watson et al. 2009; Briggs et al. 2011; Twycross and Roderique 2011). This may explain the apparent gaps in knowledge and is of concern as the lack of pain content may impact on nursing care provided to children.

> Limited pain conent in prequalification curricula may explain, at least in part, the gaps in knowledge.

Beliefs about pain in children

Nurses' beliefs about pain and, particularly, the priority they attribute to pain management have also been suggested as reasons for suboptimal pain management practices in children. Nurses' beliefs about pain management have been examined in several studies:

- Nurses ($n = 13$) were observed to negate (ignore) children's ($n = 16$) pain in Byrne et al.'s (2001) observational study.
- Vincent and Denyes (2004) found nurses believed that 20% or more of children over-reported their pain.
- Nurses may believe that pain management is synonymous with administering analgesic drugs alone and not see the need to evaluate the effectiveness of interventions or to use other pain-relieving strategies (Twycross 2004; Twycross et al. 2013).

Two studies have examined the priority nurses' attribute to managing children's pain:

- Nurses ($n = 22$) completing a training needs questionnaire about several aspects of nursing attributed a significantly lower priority to pain management than to other aspects of their role (Twycross 1999).
- Twycross (2008) compared data regarding the perceived importance of pain management tasks with observational data relating to individual nurses' ($n = 12$) practices. The importance nurses attributed to the pain management task did not reflect the likelihood of the task being undertaken in practice.

Many factors impact on pain management practices including outdated and incorrect beliefs about pain management, and not making pain a priority. Changing practices is complex and requires a multifaceted approach.

Parents' beliefs about pain and pain management

Parents' beliefs about pain and pain management also affect children's pain care. Studies exploring parents' management of children's pain at home found that even when they recognise that their child is in pain, they often give inadequate doses of pain medication (Finley et al. 1996; Fortier et al. 2009). Other studies have found that parents:

- fear the side-effects of analgesic drugs (Zisk-Rony et al. 2010; Vincent et al. 2012);
- think pain medications are addictive (Zisk et al. 2007; Zisk-Rony et al. 2010);
- believe children should receive as little pain medication as possible (Zisk et al. 2007, Zisk-Rony et al. 2010, Lim et al. 2011).

Other studies in the UK and Canada have found that parents are satisfied with their child's pain care even if they experience moderate to severe pain while in hospital (Twycross and Collis 2012; Twycross and Finley 2013). Parents may assume that pain is to be expected during a hospital stay.

Parents' views about pain and pain management impact on their child's pain management. Adolescents also have similar views, which can affect their care (Stinson et al. 2013).

Decision-making strategies

Several factors have been identified as affecting paediatric nurses' decision-making about pain. These are discussed in Chapter 1. However, little is known about how nurses make decisions. Twycross and Powls (2006) examined paediatric nurses' decision-making in relation to both managing pain and care for children with acute medical conditions and found that:

- nurses ($n = 12$) appeared to use an analytical model of decision-making;
- all the nurses used backward reasoning strategies and collected similar types and amounts of information before making a decision about appropriate nursing care. This is indicative of non-expert decision-making;
- no differences were noted between nurses with 5 or more years' experience in paediatric surgery and less experienced nurses;
- no differences were apparent between graduate and non-graduate nurses.

An *analytical model* of decision-making is a step-by-step process. For example:

- gathering information;
- generating hypothesis;
- using the data gathered data to rule the hypothesis in or out;
- deciding on a plan of action from the data gathered/hypothesis generated.

Adapted from Elstein et al. (1978)

In *forward reasoning* an individual works forward from a hypothesis to find a problem solution, while in *backward reasoning* an individual works backwards from a hypothesis to evaluate different options or find a solution. Experts are thought to use more forward reasoning while novices tend to use backward reasoning strategies (Lamond et al. 1996).

Suboptimal decision-making strategies might explain, at least in part, why children continue to experience unrelieved pain. Further research is needed about the factors affecting paediatric nurses' decision-making.

Organisational culture

Organisational (or unit) culture may also be an important factor in relation to pain management practices. Organisational culture has been defined as:

'Characteristic ideologies, language, dress codes, behaviour patterns, signs of status and authority, modes of deference and misbehaviour, rituals, myths and stories, prevailing beliefs, values, unspoken assumptions, etc.' (Scott et al. 2003, p. 1).

Organisational culture (context) was found to influence the care provided in paediatric acute settings in eight hospitals in Canada, with contextual factors explaining many of the variations noted in practice (Estabrooks et al. 2011). More detail about the specific contextual factors can be seen in Table 11.2. Cummings et al. (2010) found that a more positive organisational culture was associated with higher reports of research use in paediatric nursing practice. Similar findings have been found in other healthcare settings (Wallin et al. 2006; Cummings et al. 2007).

Table 11.2 Contextual factors

Factor	Definition
Leadership	The actions of formal leaders in an organisation to influence change and excellence in practice
Culture	The way 'we do things' in our organisations and work units
Evaluation	The process of using data to assess group or /team performance and to achieve outcomes in organisations
Social capital	The 'stock of active connections' among people (bonding, bridging and linking)
Formal interactions	Formal exchanges that occur between individuals working within an organisation to promote transfer of knowledge
Informal interactions	Informal exchanges that occur between individuals working within an organisation to promote transfer of knowledge
Structural/electronic resources	The structural and electronic elements of an organisation that facilitate the ability to use knowledge
Organisational slack	The cushion of actual or potential resources, which allows an organisation to adapt successfully to internal or external pressures for changes

Source: Estabrooks et al. (2009). © 2013 BioMed Central Ltd.

Over the past decade there has been a growing awareness that a unit (ward) has a set of *informal rules* that determine how pain is managed. This was demonstrated by the results of Lauzon Clabo's (2008) ethnographic study on two (adult) units in one hospital in the USA. Participants described a clear but different pattern of pain assessment on each ward. The social context of the ward appeared to influence practices. Further, in one Canadian study, paediatric nurses described the unit's pain management culture as *giving pain medications regularly even if they are prescribed prn;* this appeared to be the factor that impacted most on practice (Twycross et al. 2013). Another study exploring neonatal pain management also found that organisational context affected practices (Stevens et al. 2011).

Organisational (unit) culture appears to have an impact on pain management practices.

A key organisational factor that influences pain management practices is the relationship between medical and nursing staff. This was clearly described in Van Niekerk and Martin's (2003) study where (adult) nurses who did not feel adequately consulted by medical staff were significantly more likely to report encountering barriers such as insufficient cooperation and inadequate prescription of analgesic medications. Similar findings about a lack of cooperation between nurses and medical staff have been found in paediatric settings (Vincent 2005; Gimbler-Berglund et al. 2008; Czarnecki et al. 2011).

Interactions between medical and nursing staff about pain in children may affect pain management practices.

The Way Forward: Using a Knowledge Translation Model as a Framework for Improving Practice

Clearly there is no easy answer to improving the management of pain in children. However, if the factors identified in this chapter are addressed, practices may improve. Figure 11.1 provides a pictorial representation of the factors that impact on pain management practices. Knowledge translation (KT) strategies have been used to improve pain management practices in one Canadian children's hospital (Zhu et al. 2012) and have also been shown to have some effect on the management of cancer pain in adults (Cummings et al. 2011).

Knowledge translation is the process by which specific research-based knowledge (science) is implemented in practice (Estabrooks et al. 2003).

The Promoting Action on Research Implementation in Health Services (PARIHS) model was developed as a way of understanding the complexity of implementing evidence (and knowledge) in practice (Rycroft-Malone 2010). The model provides a structure to support behaviour change and consists of three elements (Table 11.3),

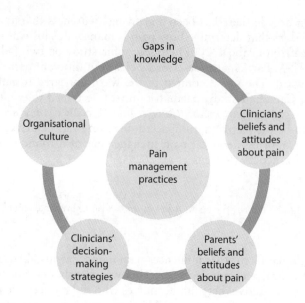

Figure 11.1   Factors that impact on pain management practices.

Table 11.3 Elements of the PARIHS model

Element	Sub-element
Evidence	Research
	Clinical experience
	Patient experience
	Local data/information
Context	Culture
	Leadership
	Evaluation
Facilitation	Low inappropriate facilitation
	High appropriate facilitation

Source: Rycroft-Malone (2010)

focusing on the interaction of the quality of the evidence with the context, and methods of facilitating knowledge translation. All three elements impact on healthcare professionals' readiness to change their pain practices and provide a framework to identify strategies to support change in practice. The PARIHS model can be used to help clinicians improve pain management practices.

A pictorial representation of how the PARIHS model and associated KT strategies can be used to improve pain management practices can be seen in Figure 11.2.

Evidence

Gaps in knowledge about the pharmacology of analgesic drugs and the anatomy and physiology of pain may mean that the rationale for implementing pain-relieving interventions is not understood. If healthcare professionals lack knowledge about pain

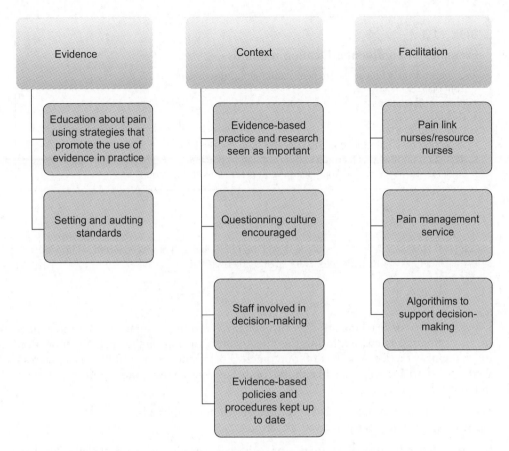

Figure 11.2   Using the PARIHS model to improve pain management practices.

assessment they may be unable to assess children's pain. Similarly, if knowledge deficits exist in relation to other methods of pain relief, healthcare professionals may not feel confident using these strategies.

Educational strategies

To support healthcare professionals to use their knowledge in practice, different educational strategies need consideration. A review of this literature by Twycross (2002) found that:

- nurse education does not prepare nurses to manage pain in practice;
- nurses continue to have educational deficits about pain management;
- not all educational interventions result in improvements in pain management practices.

Successful programmes used a variety of teaching methods (interactive and didactic) and encouraged students to reflect on practice. Francke et al. (1995) had some success using *confluent education methods* that emphasise the importance of integrating left-brain knowledge with right-brain creativity. Examples of teaching methods used in confluent education can be seen in Box 11.1.

BOX 11.1

Examples of confluent education methods

- Using students' clinical experiences within group discussions
- Role-play
- Clinical simulations
- Gaming
- Case studies
- Reflection on what individuals have learnt from the sessions
- Reflection on how this learning will be applied in practice
- Students sharing how will apply learning in practice (with the group)

Confluent education helps to ensure the integration of theory and practice, and to acknowledge learner's feelings and experiences (Francke and Erkens 1994).

Using a variety of teaching strategies to enhance learning is supported by the results of a systematic review, exploring the effectiveness of continuing medical education in changing practice and health outcomes (Forsetlund et al. 2009). Two factors were found to increase the likelihood of behaviour change and improved patient outcomes:

- using a mixture of interactive and didactic teaching methods;
- focusing on outcomes perceived as serious.

Several other educational strategies have been suggested as particularly helpful in promoting the use of knowledge in practice (Table 11.4).

Details of two web-based courses about paediatric pain are provided In Box 11.2.

BOX 11.2

Web-based courses about paediatric pain

Course 1

An interprofessional pain curriculum designed for novice healthcare practitioners and trainees based on the IASP's (2005) *Core Curriculum for Professional Education in Pain*. The online programme will be launched in 2013 and will be available via: www.sickkids.ca/Centres/pain-centre/index.html.

Course 2

Developed and run by the International Children's Palliative Care Network (ICPCN) and covers pain assessment and management for children linked to the WHO (2012) guidelines on the pharmacological treatment of persisting pain in children with medical illnesses. Further information can be found at: www.icpcn.org.uk/page.asp?section=000100010043&sectionTitle=ICPCN%27s+new+elearning+programme

Table 11.4 Other educational strategies that promote the use of knowledge in practice

Educational strategy	Evidence

Interprofessional education	**Hunter et al. (2012)**
	• A 2-hours per week interprofessional paediatric pain clinical placement intervention was pilot tested over a 5-week period with an average of 6 undergraduate students per cycle ($n = 21$) in Canada
	• After the programme, trainees were more:
	  ○ knowledgeable about paediatric pain
	  ○ positive towards interprofessional pain training
	  ○ competent about interprofessional pain care
	• It is essential that medical students are involved in this clinical training

Educational outreach visits	**Schechter et al. (2010)**
	• A 1-hour teaching session on pain reduction strategies during childhood immunisations was provided to staff in 13 GP practices in one state in the USA
	• One month later parents were:
	  ○ more likely to report receiving information
	  ○ using strategies to reduce pain
	  ○ learning something new
	  ○ using Shotblocker®
	  ○ reported higher levels of satisfaction
	• Rates remained higher at 6 months except for satisfaction
	• Clinician surveys at 6 months revealed significant increases in the use of:
	  ○ longer needles
	  ○ sucrose
	  ○ pinwheels
	  ○ focused breathing
	  ○ Shotblocker®

Individual feedback	**Duncan and Pozehl (2001)** • Coaching was used with nurses ($n = 30$) caring for (adult) patients undergoing arthroscopy • Nurses received individual feedback on their past performance on three recommended pain management practices (4-hourly pain assessment; reassessment following pain medications; follow-up for unacceptable levels of pain) • Nurses' performance in the three areas improved significantly over the 15 weeks after the intervention **Johnston et al. (2007)** • Coaching with individual audit feedback from a chart review was provided to nurses every 2 weeks, for 6 months in six Canadian paediatric hospitals • Some changes were found between the experimental and control groups such as an increase in documented pain assessments and the use of psychological and physical methods • However, there were inconsistencies across sites

Continued

Table 11.4 Continued

Educational strategy	Evidence
Web-based learning	**Dy et al. (2008)** • Explored the effect of a web-based palliative care module for medical residents (*n* = 612) • Knowledge about palliative care did not increase simply by completing the 4-year residency programme but undertaking the web-based course resulted in a larger increase in knowledge **Sullivan et al. (2010)** • Evaluated the effectiveness of internal medicine residents (*n* = 213) having web-based training about the use of opioid therapy for chronic pain compared with being given a copy of current clinical guidelines • The web-based group had a greater increase in knowledge (*p* < 0.00001) and higher self-ratings of their competence in overall management (*p* = 0.02) and in prescribing opioids (*p* = 0.02). However, the web-based training also covered shared decision-making (patient and doctor) and communication skills; it may have been this difference rather than the content relating to the use of opioids that was effective **Vincent et al. (2011)** • Nurses (*n* = 24) undertook a web-based teaching package with a variety of educational strategies • Nurses completed a questionnaire before and after using the teaching package • After completing the package nurses administered more ibuprofen and ketorolac, and children's pain intensity scores decreased

A variety of educational strategies (interactive and didactic) should be used that facilitate the use of knowledge in practice.

Web-based courses need evaluating to ascertain their effectiveness in increasing knowledge and changing practice, as well as comparison with courses taught face-to-face.

Some of the methods advocated are resource intensive (e.g. individual feedback) and an economic evaluation needs to be undertaken before implementing these more widely.

Local data

Setting and auditing pain standards is a way of providing local data about areas where practice may need improving. A recent systematic review found that audit and feedback leads to small but potentially important improvements in professional practice (Ivers et al. 2012). There are a several national pain standards and guidelines (see Chapter 1). These pain management standards should be audited on a regular basis (at least every 6 months). Following completion of the audit an action plan should be drawn up. Staff need to be actively involved in this process to determine realistic and achievable priorities. Once sufficient time has been given for changes to be implemented, practice should be re-audited. Figure 11.3 outlines the process of auditing pain management practices.

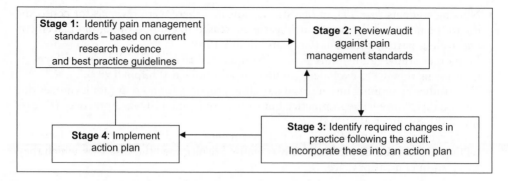

Figure 11.3   Auditing pain management practices.

> Pain management standards should be audited on a regular basis and an action plan agreed with unit staff to address areas where improvements are needed.

Context

As discussed earlier in the chapter, organisational culture (context) has a place in ensuring that knowledge is used in practice. Indeed, it has been postulated that pain management practices remain poor because contextual factors are not taken into account (Craig 2009). The importance of context becomes clear when evidence that nurses learn by role-modelling on senior staff is considered:

- Novice (adult) nurses ($n = 15$) in Taylor's (1997) study commented: 'they just followed the [more experienced] nurse's lead'.
- Nursing students ($n = 99$), interviewed by Fitzpatrick et al. (1996), discussed modelling their practices on those of more experienced nurses.
- In Twycross' (2004) study two participants indicated they had learnt about paediatric pain management by observing and working with more senior staff, and another participant reported that she had had no formal education in pain management 'except what I picked up as I've gone along'.

If nurses learn by mirroring the behaviours of role models, the quality of their practice will depend on the practices of the role model. If role models have, for example, poor pain assessment skills or use limited physical and psychological methods of pain relief and merely administer analgesic drugs when a child complains of pain, the novice nurse is likely to develop a similar approach. Thus, even if a nurse has a good level of knowledge, it is unlikely to be applied in practice.

> Junior staff modelling their pain management practices on those of more senior staff who have suboptimal practices offers another explanation of why pain management practices remain poor.

Professional socialisation also plays a part in perpetuating non-evidenced-based practice and is inextricably linked to organisational culture. When starting a new placement or job, all clinicians undergo a period of socialisation, during which they learn the rules (formal and informal) that guide behaviour:

- Nursing students (*n* = 17), in one study, indicated there were rewards for conforming to the norms of the ward, such as the increased likelihood of a good placement and feeling part of the team (Gray and Smith 1999).
- In another study, (adult) nurses (*n* = 18) indicated that if they did not conform to unit norms they were excluded, shouted at and bullied (Philpin 1999).
- Two studies examining moving and handling practices found that (adult) nurses did not use their knowledge in practice but rather conformed to ward practices (Kneafsey 2000; Swain et al. 2003).
- More recently, Mooney (2007) found that newly qualified (adult) nurses' (*n* = 12) willingness to become professionally socialised determined the ease with which they survived in clinical practice.

A nurse's need to *fit in* may mean that they adopt the ward's (poor) pain management practices, despite having (at least some) knowledge about how children's pain should be managed and believing that pain management is important. If nurses acting differently to the ward culture are *picked on* this is likely to discourage them from using their own discretion, or from questioning practice.

> Professional socialisation may allow non-evidence-based practices to be perpetuated. Strategies to promote change in organisational culture may help to address this. Further research is needed in this area.

Leadership

If the tendency for nurses to follow a role model is considered alongside the impact of professional socialisation, leadership can be seen to be particularly important. Leadership has been identified as key to ensuring evidence is used in practice (Gifford et al. 2007; Sandstrom et al. 2011). Indeed, resistant leadership and a lack of support from leaders may negatively impact on the use of evidence in practice (Hutchinson and Johnston 2006; Newhouse et al. 2007). However, research regarding leadership activities that support the use of evidence in practice remains inconclusive (Sandstrom et al. 2011). Leadership attributes and qualities that appear to help change organisational culture and support the use of KT are outlined in Box 11.3.

BOX 11.3

Leadership attributes and qualities that support the use of evidence in practice

- Valuing research e.g. research incorporated into annual appraisal
- Knowledgeable about research
- Role-modelling evidence-based care
- Effective communicator
- Encouraging staff to question practice
- Staff involved in decision-making
- Supportive of changes in practice
- Providing feedback to staff
- Ensuring policy and procedures are evidence-based and kept up to date

Adapted from Sandstrom et al. (2011)

Facilitating change

Use of local opinion leaders

Human sources of information have been shown to be important in changing practices and in the dissemination of research evidence into practice (Spenceley et al. 2008). The PARIHS model describes *facilitators* as having a key role in changing practice (Harvey et al. 2002). Indeed, a systematic review concluded that the use of local opinion leaders was an effective way of promoting evidence-based practice (Flodgren et al. 2011). The use of opinion leaders (link nurses/resource nurses) has been suggested as a way of increasing the application of research in practice in relation to pain management (McCleary et al. 2004; Ladak et al. 2011), but such roles need to be resourced adequately.

The use of pain link nurses (or pain resource nurses) as a way of improving patient outcomes has been evaluated in two Australian hospitals (Williams et al. 2012). Eleven months after their introduction:

- more patients had a pain score recorded on the daily observational chart and in the nursing care plan;
- there was an increase in the number of patients with a pain score documented each nursing shift;
- no differences were noted in other areas.

These results suggest that pain link nurses may be a useful strategy for improving documentation practices. Further evaluation is needed to explore the impact on patient outcomes.

> Pain link nurses/resource nurses appear to be an effective strategy for improving practice.

Pain management services

Facilitation can also be provided by pain management services. The Royal College of Anaesthetists (2010) in the UK recommend that a member of the acute pain service should visit all children's surgical wards every day and see all children having major surgery. A nurse from the pain management service visiting the wards each day can provide support to the nurses caring for children in pain. This could reduce the stress associated with decision-making and caring for children in pain and may increase nurses' confidence regarding pain management. The implementation of an acute pain service has been found to improve the postoperative pain care of children (Frigon et al. 2009). Similar findings have been found in relation to adult patients' pain (Bardiau et al. 2003; McDonnell et al. 2005).

> Pain management services appear to facilitate the use of evidence in practice.

Supporting decision-making

A review of the decision-making literature provides no definitive answers about ways to improve nurses' decision-making strategies or how to ensure that current best practice guidelines are used when making clinical decisions. One possible method would be the use of a decision-making algorithm. The effectiveness of an algorithm in conjunction with the administration of regular multimodal analgesia has been tested (Falanga et al. 2006). When the algorithm was used, children received more analgesia and had lower pain intensity scores. (Algorithms to support clinical decision-making can be found in Chapters 6, 7, 8 and 10.)

> Developing and using algorithms from best practice guidelines decreases the stress of decision-making and guides nurses in a step-by-step manner. This might help ensure that best practice guidelines are adhered to and thus improve pain management practices.

Researching Children's Pain

There is limited research regarding children's views about the quality of pain management practices (see Chapter 1). This is perhaps attributable to the ethical issues that need to be considered when involving children in research, such as:

- obtaining informed consent from the child;
- determining whether parental consent is required;
- limiting the guarantees of confidentiality if child protection issue arise;
- deciding whether payments should be made to children who take part in research;
- protecting children who are research participants;
- monitoring researchers' adherence to ethical codes.

Several organisations have ethical guidelines relating to research with children and young people (Box 11.4).

> Further information about the ethical issues relating to undertaking research with children can be found in:
> Gibson, F. and Twycross, A. (2007) Children's participation in research: A position statement on behalf of the Royal College of Nursing's Research in Child Health (RiCH) Group and Children's and Young People's Rights and Ethics Group. *Paediatric Nursing* **19**(4), 14–17.
> Noel, M. and Birnie, K. (2010) Ethical challenges in pediatric pain research. *Pediatric Pain Letter* **12**(2), 18–22. Available from: http://childpain.org/ppl/issues/v12n2_2010/v12n2.shtml
> Soloduik, J. and Berde, C. (2012) Balancing ethics and science in pediatric pain intervention trials. *Pain* **153**, 939–940.
> Twycross, A. (2008) An inter-professional approach to the ethics of undertaking research with children in the United Kingdom. *Nurse Researcher* **16**(3), 7–20.

BOX 11.4

Ethical guidelines relating to undertaking research with children

- Canadian Paediatric Society (2008) position statement on ethical issues in health research in children. Available at: www.cps.ca/en/documents/position/ethical-issues-in-health-research -in-children
- Medical Research Council (2004) *Medical Research Involving Children*. Available from: www .mrc.ac.uk/Utilities/Documentrecord/index.htm?d=MRC002430
- National Children's Bureau (2011) *Guidelines for Research with Children and Young People*. Available from: www.ncb.org.uk/media/434791/guidelines_for_research_with_cyp.pdf
- Royal College of Nursing (2012) *Planning a new qualitative study with children, young people and families*. Available from: www.rcn.org.uk/__data/assets/pdf_file/0012/451101/Planning_a _New_Qual_Study_with_CYP_and_Families_12May.pdf

Areas for Future Research

Despite the growth in paediatric pain research over the past two decades, more research is needed in the following areas:

- Cross-cultural views on children's pain management.
- Evaluating the impact of paediatric pain protocols, clinical practice guidelines and knowledge translation activities on both process and clinical outcomes.
- Impact of early pain experience on pain behaviour and sensitivity later in life, especially related to the risk of not treating pain compared to the risks with administration of opioids in this population.
- Influence of age, gender and genetics on pain responses.
- Development and validation of tools to assess pain in children with cognitive impairment, medical complexity and those ventilated/paralysed in intensive care units.
- Understanding the factors that influence acute and persistent pain in children using real-time data capture approaches such as electronic pain diaries.
- Management of acute postoperative pain in the home setting.
- Effectiveness of face-to-face, Internet and smartphone-based pain self-help programmes.
- Long-term outcomes of children with chronic pain who do and do not receive treatment.
- Appropriate timeframes for preparing children of different developmental stages for painful procedures.
- How needle pain, specifically immunisation needle pain, affects immunisation rates in developed and developing countries.
- Efficacy of the WHO two-step strategy for pain management.
- Long-term safety data and dosing of non-opioids and opioids for different age groups of children.
- Clinical studies of paracetamol (acetaminophen), NSAIDs, opioids and adjuvants in children for acute and chronic pain.
- Clinical studies/RCTs on opioid dose conversion, opioid switching and dose equivalence for different age groups.
- Studies evaluating effectiveness of physical pain-relieving strategies (exercise, massage, TENS, mirror therapy, desensitisation).
- Multidimensional symptom assessment tools for different patient groups in palliative care.
- Symptom profiles of children with non-oncology conditions at end of life.
- Best practice in pain management during end-of-life care.

Summary

- Factors that contribute to continuing poor pain management practices include:
  - knowledge deficits among clinicians;
  - incorrect or outdated beliefs about pain and pain management (by clinicians, children and parents);
  - the decision-making strategies used by clinicians;
  - organisational culture.
- When several knowledge translation strategies are used simultaneously this appears to facilitate improvements in pain management.

- Further research needs to be carried out to explore the most effective strategies for ensuring that evidence is used in practice.
- When undertaking research with children, ethical principles need to be upheld.

References

Bardiau, F.M., Taviaux, N.F., Albert, A., Boogaerts, J.G. and Stadler, M. (2003) An intervention study to enhance postoperative pain management. *Anesthesia and Analgesia* 96(1), 179–185.

Briggs, E., Carr, E.C.J. and Whittaker, M. (2011) Survey of undergraduate pain curricula for health-care professionals in the United Kingdom. *European Journal of Pain* 15, 789–795.

Byrne, A., Morton, J. and Salmon, P. (2001) Defending against patients' pain: A qualitative analysis of nurses' responses to children's postoperative pain. *Journal of Psychosomatic Research* 50, 69–76.

Craig, K.D. (2009) The social communication model of pain. *Canadian Psychology* 20(1), 22–32.

Cummings, G.G., Estabrooks, C.A., Midozi, W.K., Wallin, L. and Hayduk, L. (2007) Influence of organizational characteristics and context on research utilization. *Nursing Research* 56(45), S24–S39.

Cummings, G.G., Hutchinson, A.M., Scott, S.D., Norton, P.G. and Estabrooks, C.A. (2010) The relationship between characteristics of context and research utilization in a pediatric setting. *BMC Health Services Research* 10(168), 1–10.

Cummings, G.G., Armijo Olivo, S., Biondo, P.D et al. (2011) Effectiveness of knowledge translation interventions to improve cancer pain management. *Journal of Pain and Symptom Management* 41(5), 915–939.

Czarnecki, M.L., Simon, K., Thompson, J.J. et al (2011) Barriers to pediatric pain management: A nursing perspective. *Pain Management Nursing* 12, 154–162.

Duncan, K. and Pozehl, B. (2001) Effects of individual performance feedback on nurses' adherence to pain management clinical guidelines. *Outcomes Management for Nursing Practice* 5, 57–62.

Dy, S.M., Hughes, M., Weiss, C. and Sisson, S. (2008) Evaluation of a web-based palliative care pain management programme for house staff. *Journal of Pain and Symptom Management* 36(6), 596–603.

Ekim, A. and Ocakci, A.F. (2012) Knowledge and attitudes regarding pain management of pediatric nurses in Turkey. *Pain Management Nursing*, online early.

Elstein, A.S., Schulman, L.S. and Sprafka, S.A. (1978) *Medical Problem Solving: An Analysis of Clinical Reasoning*. Harvard University Press, Cambridge, MA.

Estabrooks, C.A., Floyd, J.A., Scott-Findlay, S., O'Leary, K.A. and Gushta, M. (2003) Individual determinants of research utilization: A systematic review. *Journal of Advanced Nursing* 43, 506–520.

Estabrooks, C.A., Squires, J.E., Cummings, G.G., Birdsell, J.M. and Norton, P.G. (2009) Development and assessment of the Alberta context tool. *BMC Health Services Research* 9, 234, 1–12.

Estabrooks, C.A., Squires, J.E., Hutchinson, A.M. et al. (2011) Assessment of variation in the Alberta context tool: The contribution of unit level contextual factors and speciality in Canadian pediatric acute care settings. *BMC Health Services Research* 11(251), 1–17.

Falanga, I.J., Lafrenaye, S., Mayer, S.K. and Tetrault, J-P. (2006) Management of acute pain in children: Safety and efficacy of a nurse-controlled algorithm for pain relief. *Acute Pain* 8(2), 45–54.

Finley, G.A., McGrath, P.J., Forward, P.S., McNeill, G. and Fitzgerald, P. (1996) Parents' management of children's pain following 'minor' surgery. *Pain* 64, 83–87.

Fitzpatrick, J.M., While, A.E. and Roberts, J.D. (1996) Key influences on the professional socialisation and practice of students undertaking different pre-registration nurse education programmes in the United Kingdom. *International Journal of Nursing Studies* 33(5), 506–518.

Flodgren, G., Parmelli, E., Doumit, G. et al. (2011) Local opinion leaders: Effects on professional practice and health care outcomes. *Cochrane Database of Systematic Reviews*, issue 8.

Forsetlund, L., Bjørndal, B.A., Rashidian, A. et al. (2009). Continuing education meetings and workshops: Effects of professional practice and health care outcomes. *Cochrane Database of Systematic Reviews*, issue 2.

Fortier, M.A., MacLaren, J.E., Perrett-Karimi, D. and Kain, Z.N. (2009). Pediatric pain after ambulatory surgery: Where's the medication? *Pediatrics* 134(4), e588–e595.

Francke, A.L. and Erkens, T. (1994) Confluent education: An integrative method for nursing (continuing education). *Journal of Advanced Nursing* 19, 3564–3361.

Francke, A.L., Garssen, B. and Abu-Saad, H.H. (1995) Determinants of changes in nurses' behaviour after continuing education: A literature review. *Journal of Advanced Nursing* 21, 371–377.

Frigon, C., Loetwiriyakul, W., Ranger, M. and Otis, A. (2009) An acute pain service improves postoperative pain management for children undergoing selective dorsal rhizotomy. *Pediatric Anesthesia* 19, 1213–1219.

Gifford, W., Davies, B., Edwards, N., Griffin, P. and Lybanon, V. (2007) Managerial leadership for nurses' use of research evidence: An integrative review of the literature. *Worldviews on Evidence-Based Nursing* Q3, 126–145.

Gimbler-Berglund, I., Ljusegren, G. and Ensker, K. (2008) Factors influencing pain management in children. *Paediatric Nursing* 20, 21–24.

Gray, M. and Smith, L.N. (1999) The professional socialization of diploma of higher education in nursing students (Project 2000): A longitudinal study. *Journal of Advanced Nursing* 29(3), 639–647.

Harvey, G., Loftus-Hills, A., Rycroft-Malone, J. et al. (2002) Getting evidence into practice: The role and function of facilitation. *Journal of Advanced Nursing* 37(6), 577–588.

Hunter, J.P., Stinson, J., Campbell, F. et al. (2012). A unique interprofessional clinical experience for health care trainees in pediatric pain: Impact on knowledge and interprofessional competencies. Poster presented at the IASP 14th World Congress on Pain, 29 August 2012, Milan, Italy.

Hutchinson, A.M and Johnston, L. (2006) Beyond the barriers scale: Commonly reported barriers to research use. *Journal of Nursing Administration* 36(4), 189–199.

Ivers, N., Jamtvedt, G., Odgaard-Jensen, J. et al. (2012) Audit and feedback: effects on professional practice and healthcare outcomes. *Cochrane Database of Systematic Reviews* issue 7.

Johnston, C. C., Gagnon, A. J., Rennick, J. et al. (2007) One-on-one coaching to improve pain assessment and management practices of pediatric nurses. *Journal of Pediatric Nursing* 22(6), 467–478.

Kneafsey, R. (2000) The effect of occupational socialization in nurses' patient handling practices. *Journal of Clinical Nursing* 9(4), 585–593.

Kozlowski, L.J., Kost-Byerly, S., Colantuoni, E. et al. (2012) Pain prevalence, intensity, assessment and management in a hospitalized pediatric population. *Pain Management Nursing*, online early.

Ladak, S.S.J., McPhee, C., Muscat, M. et al. (2011) The journey of the pain resource nurse in improving pain management practices: Understanding role implementation. *Pain Management Nursing*, online early.

Lamond, D., Crow, R.A. and Chase, J. (1996) Judgements and processes in care decision in acute medical and surgical wards. *Journal of Evaluation in Clinical Practice* 2(3), 211–216.

Lauzon Clabo, L.M. (2008). An ethnography of pain assessment and the role of social context on two postoperative units. *Journal of Advanced Nursing* 61(5), 531–539.

Lim, S.H., Mackey, S., Liam, J.L.W. and He, H.-G. (2011) An exploration of Singaporean parental experiences in managing school-aged children's post-operative pain: A descriptive qualitative approach. *Journal of Clinical Nursing*, 21, 860–869.

Manworren, R.C.B. (2000) Pediatric nurses' knowledge and attitudes survey regarding pain. *Pediatric Nursing* 26(6), 610–614.

McCleary, L., Ellis, J.A. and Rowley, B. (2004) Evaluation of the pain resource nurse role: A resource for improving pediatric pain management. *Pain Management Nursing* 5(1), 29–36.

McDonnell, A., Nicholl, J. and Read, S. (2005) Focus. Exploring the impact of Acute Pain Teams (APTs) on patient outcomes using routine data: can it be done? *Journal of Research in Nursing* 10(4), 383–402.

Mooney, M. (2007) Professional socialisation: The key to survival as newly qualified nurses. *International Journal of Nursing Practice* 13(2), 75–80.

Newhouse, R.P., Dearholt, S., Poe, S., Pugh, L.C. and White, M.K. (2007) Organizational change strategies for evidence-based nursing practice. *Journal of Nursing Administration* 37(12), 552–557.

Philpin, S.M. (1999) The impact of 'Project 2000' educational reforms on the occupational socialization of nurses: An exploratory study. *Journal of Advanced Nursing* 29(6), 1326–1331.

Rieman, M.T., Gordon, M. and Marvin, J.M. (2007) Pediatric nurses' knowledge and attitudes survey regarding pain: A competency tool modification. *Pediatric Nursing* 33(4), 303–313.

Royal College of Anaesthetists (2010) *Guidance on the Provision of Paediatric Anaesthetic Services*, 2nd edition. Royal College of Anaesthetists, London.

Rycroft-Malone, J. (2010) Promoting Action of Research Implementation in Health Services (PARIHS). In *Models and Frameworks for Implementing Evidence-Based Practice: Linking Evidence to Action* (eds J. Rycroft-Malone and T. Bucknall), pp. 109–136. Wiley-Blackwell, Oxford.

Salantera, S., Lauri, S., Salmi, T.T. and Helenius, H. (1999) Nurses' knowledge about pharmacological and non-pharmacological pain management in children. *Journal of Pain and Symptom Management* 18(4): 289–299.

Sandstrom, B., Borglin, G., Nilsson, R. and Willman, A. (2011) Promoting the implementation of evidence-based practice: A literature review focusing on the role of nursing leadership. *Worldviews on Evidence-Based Nursing* Q4, 212–223.

Schechter, N.L., Bernstein, B.A., Zempsky, W., Bright, N.S. and Willard, A.K. (2010) Educational outreach to reduce immunization pain in office settings. *Pediatrics* 126(6), e1514–e1521.

Scott, T., Mannion, R., Davies, H. and Marshall, M. (2003) *Healthcare performance and organisational culture*. Radcliffe Medical Press Ltd, Oxford.

Shrestha-Ranjit, J.M. and Manias, E. (2010) Pain assessment and management practices in children following surgery of the lower limb. *Journal of Clinical Nursing* 19, 118–128.

Spenceley, S.M., O'Leary, K.A., Chizawsky, L.L.K., Ross, A.J. and Estabrooks, C.A. (2008) Sources of information used by nurses to inform practice: An integrative review. *International Journal of Nursing Studies* 45, 954–970.

Stevens, B., Riahi, S., Cardoso, R. et al. (2011) The influence of context on pain practices in NICU: Perceptions of health care professionals. *Qualitative Health Research* 21(6), 757–770.

Stinson, J., Lalloo, C., Harris, L. et al. (2013) Understanding the self-management needs of adolescents with chronic pain: Perspectives of adolescents and their healthcare providers. *European Journal of Pain*, in preparation.

Sullivan, M.D., Gaster, B., Russo, J. et al . (2010) Randomized trial of web-based training about opioid therapy for chronic pain. *Clinical Journal of Pain* 26(6), 512–517.

Swain, J., Pufahl, E. and Williamson, G.R. (2003) Do they practise what we teach? A survey of manual handling practice. *Journal of Clinical Nursing* 12(2), 297–306.

Taylor, C. (1997) Problem solving in clinical nursing practice, *Journal of Advanced Nursing* 26(2), 329–336.

Tiernan, E.P. (2009) A survey of registered nurses' knowledge and attitudes regarding paediatric pain assessment and management: An Irish perspective. *Archives of Disease in Childhood* 93(1002) n18.

Twycross, A. (1999) Pain management: A nursing priority? *Journal of Child Health Care* 3(3), 19–25.

Twycross, A. (2002) Educating nurses about pain management: The way forward. *Journal of Clinical Nursing* 11, 705–714.

Twycross, A. (2004) *Children's Nurses' Pain Management Practices: Theoretical Knowledge, Perceived Importance and Decision-Making*. Unpublished PhD Thesis, University of Central Lancashire.

Twycross, A. (2007) What is the impact of theoretical knowledge on children's nurses' postoperative pain management practices? An exploratory study. *Nurse Education Today* 27(7), 697–707.

Twycross, A. (2008) Does the perceived importance of a pain management task affect the quality of children's nurses' post-operative pain management practices? *Journal of Clinical Nursing* 17(23), 3205–3216.

Twycross, A. and Collis, S. (2012) How well is acute pain in children managed? A snapshot in one English hospital. *Pain Management Nursing*, online early.

Twycross, A. and Finley, G.A. (2013) Parents' and children's views about pain management, *Journal of Clinical Nursing*, online early.

Twycross, A. and Powls, L. (2006) How do children's nurses make clinical decisions? Two preliminary studies. *Journal of Clinical Nursing* 15, 1324–1335.

Twycross, A. and Roderique, L (2011) Review of pain content in three-year preregistration pediatric nursing courses in the United Kingdom. *Pain Management Nursing*, online early.

Twycross, A., Finley, G.A. and Latimer, M. (2013) Pediatric nurses' postoperative pain management practices: An observational study. *Journal for Specialists in Pediatric Nursing* 18(3), 189–201.

Van Niekerk, L.M. and Martin, F. (2003) The impact of the nurse–physician relationship on barriers encountered by nurses during pain management. *Pain Management Nursing* 4(1), 3–10.

Vincent, C.V.H. (2005) Nurses' knowledge, attitudes, and practices regarding children's pain. *American Journal of Maternal Child Nursing* 30(3), 177–183.

Vincent, C.V.H. and Denyes, M.J. (2004) Relieving children's pain: Nurses' abilities and analgesic administration practices. *Journal of Pediatric Nursing* 19(1), 40–50.

Vincent, C.V.H., Wilkie, D.J. and Wang, E. (2011) Pediatric nurses' beliefs and pain management practices: An intervention pilot. *Western Journal of Nursing Research* 33(6), 825–845.

Vincent, C., Chiappetta, M., Beach, A. et al. (2012) Parents' management of children's pain at home after surgery. *Journal for Specialists in Pediatric Nursing* 17, 108–120.

Wallin, L., Ewald, U., Wikblad, K., Scott-Findlay, S. and Arnetz, B.B. (2006) Understanding work contextual factors: A short-cut to evidence-based practice? *Worldviews on Evidence-Based Nursing* Q4, 153–164.

Watt-Watson, J, McGillon, M, Hunter, J. et al. (2009). A survey of prelicensure pain curricula in health science faculties in Canadian universities. *Pain Research and Management* 14(4), 439–444.

Watt-Watson, J., Stevens, B., Garfinkel, P., Streiner, D. and Gallop, R. (2001) Relationship between nurses' pain knowledge and pain management outcomes for their postoperative cardiac patients. *Journal of Advanced Nursing* 36(4), 535–545.

Williams, A.M., Toye, C., Deas, K., Fairclough, D., Curro, K. and Oldham, L. (2012) Evaluating the feasibilty and effect of using a hospital-wide coordinated approach to evidence-based changes for pain management. *Pain Management Nursing* 13(4), 202–214.

Zhu, L.M., Stinson, J., Palozzi, L. et al. (2012) Improvements in pain outcomes in a Canadian pediatric teaching hospital following implementation of a multifaceted, knowledge translation initiative. *Pain Research and Management* 17(3), 173–179.

Zisk, R.Y., Grey, M., Medoff-Cooper, B. and Kain, Z.N. (2007) Accuracy of parental-global-impression of children's acute pain. *Pain Management Nursing* 8(2), 72–76.

Zisk-Rony, R.Y., Fortier, M.A., MacLaren-Chorney, J., Perrett, D. and Zain, Z.N. (2010) Parental postoperative pain management: Attitudes, assessment and management. *Pediatrics* 125(8), 1372–1378.

Index

Notes Page numbers in *italics* denote figures and those in **bold** denote tables

Managing Pain in Children: A Clinical Guide for Nurses and Healthcare Professionals, Second Edition.
Edited by Alison Twycross, Stephanie Dowden, and Jennifer Stinson.
© 2014 John Wiley & Sons, Ltd. Published 2014 by John Wiley & Sons, Ltd.